CRASH COURSE

Third Edition

Anatomy

First and second edition authors:

Michael Dykes

Phillip Ameerally

CRASH COURSE

Third Edition

Anatomy

Series editor

Daniel Horton-Szar
BSc (Hons), MBBS (Hons), MRCGP

Northgate Medical Practice
Canterbury
Kent, UK

Faculty advisor

Susan Whiten
MD

Foundations of Medicine Module
Organiser
Bute Medical School
University of St Andrews
St Andrews, UK

Michael Dykes
BSc (Hons), MBChB (Hons)

Pre-registration House Officer
Northern General Hospital
Sheffield, UK

Will Watson

Undergraduate medical student
St Andrews University Medical School
St Andrews, UK

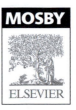

MOSBY

ELSEVIER

Edinburgh • London • New York • Oxford • Philadelphia • St Louis • Sydney • Toronto 2007

MOSBY
ELSEVIER

An imprint of Elsevier Limited

Commissioning Editor	**Fiona Conn**
Development Editor	**Helen Leng**
Project Manager	**Andrew Palfreyman**
Design Text	**Sarah Russell**
Icon Illustrations	**Geo Parkin**
Cover Design	**Stewart Larking**
Illustrations Buyer	**Gillian Richards**
Illustrator	**Jennifer Rose**

First edition 1998
Second edition 2002
Third edition 2007

ISBN: 9780723434177

British Library Cataloguing in Publication Data
A catalogue record for this book is available from the British Library

Library of Congress Cataloging in Publication Data
A catalog record for this book is available from the Library of Congress

Note
Neither the publisher nor the authors assume any responsibility for any loss or injury and/or damage to
persons or property arising out of or related to any use of the material contained in this book. It is the
responsibility of the treating practitioner, relying on independent expertise and knowledge of the patient, to
determine the best treatment and method of application for the patient.

ELSEVIER your source for books,
journals and multimedia
in the health sciences

www.elsevierhealth.com

Working together to grow
libraries in developing countries

www.elsevier.com | www.bookaid.org | www.sabre.org

ELSEVIER   BOOK AID International   Sabre Foundation

The
Publisher's
policy is to use
**paper manufactured
from sustainable forests**

Printed in China

Preface

Anatomy, medical students either love it or loathe it but we all need a good understanding of it (particularly at exam time!). It can often be a daunting task trying to commit this new vocabulary to memory, especially to those of us who have never studied it before. However, this book has been written to help remove this burden.

This Third Edition builds upon the Second to provide you with an ever-concise presentation of this subject but with better aids to help you learn. These include mnemonics, new hints and tips, clinical boxes to illustrate why anatomy is important, and new figures, including a radiological anatomy section for each chapter to introduce you to normal X-rays.

The final section content has 100 multiple-choice questions with explanations, 20 short-answer questions with model answers and 10 extended matching questions for you to attempt. I hope that you find this book useful throughout your study of this fascinating subject and good luck in your exams.

Michael Dykes

More than a decade has now passed since work began on the first editions of the Crash Course series, and over four years since the publication of the second editions. Medicine never stands still, and the work of keeping this series relevant for today's students is an ongoing process. These third editions build upon the success of the preceding books and incorporate a great deal of new and revised material, keeping the series up to date with the latest medical research and developments in pharmacology and current best practice.

As always, we listen to feedback from the thousands of students who use Crash Course and have made further improvements to the layout and structure of the books. Each chapter now starts with a set of learning objectives, and the self-assessment sections have been enhanced and brought up to date with modern exam formats. We have also worked to integrate points of clinical relevance into the basic medical science material, which will not only add to the interest of the text but will reinforce the principles being described.

Despite fully revising the books, we hold fast to the principles on which we first developed the series: Crash Course will always bring you all the information you need to revise in compact, manageable volumes that integrate basic medical science and clinical practice. The books still maintain the balance between clarity and conciseness, and providing sufficient depth for those aiming at distinction. The authors are medical students and junior doctors who have recent experience of the exams you are now facing, and the accuracy of the material is checked by senior faculty members from across the UK.

I wish you all the best for your future careers!

Dr Dan Horton-Szar
Series Editor

Acknowledgements

I would like to thank everyone who has helped in the production of this book, especially Susan Whiten and Dan Horton-Szar for reading my work and their suggestions. Will Watson for writing his chapters and Helen Leng for her help in making the whole process run smoothly and answering all my questions. It was a pleasure to work with all.

All radiological images were reproduced with permission from J Weir and P H Abrahams, *Imaging Atlas of Human Anatomy*, 2nd edition, Mosby 1997.

Michael Dykes

To Mum, Dad, Philip, Gran, Marilyn and Marisa. For your unconditional love and support.

Michael Dykes

Contents

Glossary

A- Absence of; lacking, e.g. avascular – an absence of a blood supply.

Abscess A localized collection of pus.

Adrenal Endocrine gland located near the kidney (literally meaning towards the kidney). It is also called suprarenal gland (i.e. above the kidney).

Afferent Carrying towards a given point. Afferent nerve impulses (i.e. sensory) are carried towards the brain and spinal cord.

Agonist A muscle that, when it contracts, causes a specific movement (prime mover), e.g. biceps brachii causes flexion of the elbow. Contraction of the agonist usually requires the relaxation of the antagonist. See antagonist.

Anaesthesia An absence of feeling caused by damage to a nerve through disease or trauma.

Anastomosis Network of communicating arteries, veins or nerves (plural anastomoses).

ANS Autonomic nervous system is part of the nervous system regulating bodily functions not under conscious control. It is divided into sympathetic and parasympathetic divisions.

Antagonist A muscle that has the opposite action of a given movement. Triceps is the antagonist to flexion of the elbow.

Antigen-presenting cell A macrophage cell that processes foreign material, e.g. bacteria for presentation to immune cells (lymphocytes).

Aneurysm A spherical swelling of an arterial wall.

Apex Pointed end of a cone-shaped structure, e.g. apex of the axilla (adjective apical).

Aponeurosis Strong, flattened tendon with a wide area of attachment, e.g. external oblique aponeurosis.

Appendicular Relating to the appendages, i.e. the limbs, as in appendicular skeleton.

Arachnoid Middle layer of the meninges.

Arteriogram Photographic film or digital image produced by arteriography.

Arteriography X-ray examination of an artery using a radio-opaque contrast medium.

Arthro- Relates to joints, e.g. articular, arthritis, arthroscope.

Atherosclerosis A degenerative disease affecting the inner and middle layers of arteries.

Atrium The two smaller chambers of the heart (plural atria, adjective atrial).

Atrophy Wasting of a tissue or organ due to cell loss.

Axial Relating to the axis of the body as in axial skeleton, which consists of the skull, vertebral column and thoracic cage.

Axilla Region where the upper limb joins the trunk, also armpit, e.g. axillary artery, axillary lymph nodes.

Axon A neuron(e) consists of a nerve cell body and fibre known as the axon. It conducts impulses away from the cell body.

Barium A water-insoluble salt which is used as a contrast medium for radiography of the gastrointestinal tract.

Bifurcate The point at which an anatomical structure, e.g. trachea, divides into two parts, i.e. primary bronchi.

Brachial Relates to the arm (between the shoulder and elbow) – hence brachial artery.

Branchial At the cranial end of the embryonic digestive system there are a series of branchial arches (primitive gill arches) that give rise to specific structures of the head and neck.

Bronchiole Microscopic branches of the bronchi.

Bronchus First branches of the trachea (plural bronchi, adjective, bronchial).

Buccal Relates to the mouth.

Bursa Small sac lined by synovial membrane that ensures free movement of tendons close to joints, e.g. infrapatellar bursa.

Bursitis Inflammation of a bursa.

Canal A tubular passage, e.g. adductor canal of the thigh.

Cancer A tumour arising due to abnormal and uncontrolled cell division that may spread to other tissues.

Carcinoma Cancer of epithelial origin (rather than connective tissue).

Cardia Heart (adjective cardiac).

Cerebellum Part of the brain that controls coordinated movement, balance and muscle tone (adjective cerebellar).

Cerebrum Largest part of the brain that comprises the cerebral hemispheres (adjective cerebral).

Cerebrospinal fluid CSF fluid that surrounds the central nervous system and fills the internal ventricles.

Cerebrovascular accident (CVA), see stroke.

Cervix The neck, also the narrow part or 'neck' of an organ (cervix of the uterus) (adjective cervical).

Chondro- Relates to cartilage, e.g. chondrocytes – cartilage cells.

Coeliac disease A condition of the small intestine in which loss of villi is caused by sensitivity to gliadin protein.

Collateral Accessory or secondary, e.g. collateral circulation is an accessory route of blood flow to an organ.

Colon Main part of the large intestine (adjective colic).

Condyle Literally means knuckle. Rounded articular surface, e.g. femoral condyles.

Connective tissue A tissue that supports or separates more specialized tissues, e.g. muscle.

Contrast studies A procedure that allows structures to become visualized in X-rays.

Coronary Encircling like a crown, e.g. coronary arteries, arteries that encircle the heart supplying it.

Cortex Outer part of a structure, e.g. cortex of the kidney (adjective cortical); see also medulla.

Costa Rib (adjective, costal), e.g. intercostal muscles lie between the ribs.

Cranial nerves 12 pairs of nerves that do not emerge from the spinal cord, e.g. the optic nerve (CN II).

Cranial venous sinuses Venous spaces lying between endocranium and dura within the cranium, e.g. superior sagittal sinus.

Cranium The section of the skull containing the brain.

Crohn's disease A disease of the gastrointestinal tract characterized by inflammation and ulceration of the bowel wall.

Cruciate Structures arranged like a cross, e.g. the cruciate ligaments.

CT scan Computed tomography or computed axial tomography (CAT scan). Imaging method that uses X-rays to create cross sectional views of the body.

Cusp Leaflet of a valve. Hence bicuspid valve means a valve comprising two leaflets.

Cutaneous Relating to the skin.

Cystic fibrosis An hereditary disease in which thick mucus secretion obstructs the intestines, ducts of glands and lungs.

Dendrite A short branch of the neuron cell body that forms synapses with other neurons.

Dental Related to teeth (dens tooth-shaped structure).

Depolarization A surge of charged particles across the nerve or muscle membrane due to a physiochemical change in that membrane.

Dermatome An area of skin supplied by a single spinal segment.

Dermis Deep connective tissue layer of the skin. Epidermis lies superficial to the dermis literally on the dermis (adjective is dermal).

Diastole Relaxation phase of the cardiac cycle (adjective diastolic).

Discharge The release of fluid or pus from its site of production, e.g. an infected wound.

Dislocate Joint displacement where the contact between the articular surface of bones is lost.

Duodenum First part of the small intestine.

Dura Outer tough layer of the meninges (dura mater).

DVT Deep vein thrombosis is the formation of a venous blood clot that causes obstruction.

ECG Electrocardiogram records the electrical activity of the heart.

Efferent Carrying away from. Efferent (i.e. motor) nerve impulses are carried away from the central nervous system.

Endo- Within or inner part of a structure, e.g. endocardium innermost layer of the heart.

Epi- Above or on the surface of a structure, e.g. epidermis outermost layer of the skin, epigastric relates to the area of the abdomen just below the sternum; literally means on the belly epicondyle projection on or above a condyle.

Epithelium One of the four basic tissue types. It forms glands, covers all surfaces and lines the body cavities (adjective epithelial).

Erythema Reddening of the skin due to dermal capillary dilatation.

Eversion Turning the sole of the foot outwards (laterally).

ex- extra- Out, e.g. expiration – to breathe out, extracapsular – outside a joint capsule.

Facet A flat articular surface of a bone, e.g. facet joints of the vertebra.

Fascia Connective tissue. Superficial fascia is loose connective tissue found immediately beneath the skin. Deep fascia forms fairly tough sheets or sheaths around muscles and neurovascular bundles, e.g. carotid sheath.

Fissure A groove or cleft, e.g. oblique fissure of the left lung separates upper and lower lobes.

Foramen Opening or passage through a bone, e.g. foramen magnum through which the spinal cord passes (plural foramina).

Fossa Literally means a ditch, therefore depression, hollow or pit (antecubital fossa of the elbow).

Fracture A break in the continuity of a bone.

Fundus Base of a hollow organ or the part furthest from the opening (stomach, uterus).

Ganglion A swelling. In the nervous system, it is a collection of nerve cell bodies outside the CNS, e.g. a sensory ganglion (without synapses), or an autonomic ganglion (with synapses). See nucleus.

Gastr-, gastro- Relates to the belly or gastrum which usually means the stomach, e.g. gastric artery, gastro-intestinal (GI) tract, gastroscopy.

Genicular Relates to the knee joint, e.g. genicular arteries that supply the knee.

Glosso- Relates to the tongue. The hypoglossal nerve lies below the tongue.

Glottis Gap between the vocal folds (adjective glottal).

Gonads Sex organs – female ovaries and male testes (adjective gonadal).

Greater sac General peritoneal cavity.

Gyrus Raised area of the cerebral cortex (pleural gyri). See sulcus.

Haemo- Relates to blood, e.g. haematology is the study of blood, haematoma (bruising) is the swelling caused by bleeding into the tissues.

Hemi- Denotes one half of the body or a structure, e.g. hemi-diaphragm.

Hepato- Relates to the liver, e.g. hepatic artery, hepatitis – inflammation of the liver.

Hernia Protrusion of an organ or tissue through the wall of a cavity which normally encloses it, e.g. femoral and inguinal hernias.

Hiatus An opening, e.g. adductor hiatus of adductor canal.

Hilum Place where vessels and nerves enter or leave an organ, e.g. hilum of the lung (adjective hilar).

Hyper- Literally above, or excessive, e.g. hyperextension – forced extension of a joint beyond normal limits, hypertrophy – increase in size.

Hypo- Literally below or depressed, e.g. hypochondrium – below the costal cartilages, hypoglossal – below the tongue.

Ileum Last part of the small intestine (e.g. ilio-colic junction).

Ilium Makes up the hip bone with the pubis and ischium (adjective iliac).

Infra- Below or lower, e.g. infraorbital, below the orbit of the skull, infrahyoid below the hyoid bone.

Infundibulum A funnel-shaped passage.

Inguinal Relates to the groin where the lower limb meets the trunk, e.g. inguinal hernia.

Insertion Relates to the more distal attachment of a muscle, which moves on contraction of the muscle.

Inter- Between, e.g. interosseous membrane lies between the bones, intercostal between the ribs.

Intra- Inside, e.g. an intracapsular tendon lies inside the capsule of the joint (see extra-).

Intraperitoneal A viscus suspended from the posterior abdominal wall by a mesentery, e.g. the ileum and jejunum.

Intervertebral discs Secondary cartilaginous joints between vertebrae.

Ischaemia Reduction of blood flow due to obstruction causing inadequate flow to an organ.

Isthmus Narrow region connecting two parts, e.g. isthmus of the thyroid gland.

-itis Inflammation, e.g. gastritis – inflammation of the stomach, arthritis – inflammation of joints.

Jejunum Second part of the small intestine (adjective jejunal).

Labium Lip (pleural labia, adjective labial).

Labrum Lip or a lip-like structure, e.g. glenoid labrum of the glenoid fossa of the shoulder joint.

Larynx That part of the airway, between the pharynx and trachea contains the vocal cords (adjective laryngeal, hence laryngoscope, laryngitis).

Lesser sac Diverticulum of peritoneum behind the stomach.

Ligament Tough connective tissue bands that tie together two or more structures, most commonly bones (adjective ligamentous).

Lingula Tongue (adjective lingual).

Loculus A small cavity or space (plural loculi).

Lumen Central cavity of a tube, e.g. artery, vein, intestine, etc. (adjective luminal).

Macro- Indicates the large size of a structure.

Mast- Relating to the breast, e.g. mastectomy – removal of the breast, mastitis – inflammation of the breast.

Mediastinum The space within the thorax between the two pleural cavities.

Medulla Inner part of a solid organ (adjective medullary), e.g. medulla of the kidney, see also cortex.

Meninges Three layers of connective tissue that surround the central nervous system (pia, arachnoid and dura) adjective meningeal.

Mesentery Double layer of peritoneum that attaches viscera to the posterior abdominal wall (adjective mesenteric).

Metastasis The spread of a cancerous lesion to distant sites, e.g. breast carcinoma to axillary lymph nodes.

Metro- Relating to the uterus, e.g. myometrium, uterine muscle, endometrium, uterine lining.

Mitral Relates to the valve between the left atrium and left ventricle, left AV valve.

Motor Relates to structures or activities that involve transmitting nerve impulses away from the CNS, see also efferent.

Motor endplate The enlarged end of a motor neuron that forms a synapse with part of the muscle membrane.

MRC Medical Research Council is an organization which funds medical research.

MRI Magnetic resonance imaging is a non-invasive imaging technique that depends upon the detection of nuclear movement caused by exposure to radio waves in a powerful magnetic field.

Mucus A thick glycoprotein secretion produced by glands (adjective mucous).

Myo- Relating to muscle, e.g. myocardium – muscle of the heart, myometrium – uterine muscle, myalgia – muscle pain.

Necrosis Death of a tissue, e.g. of cardiac muscle resulting from a myocardial infarction.

Nerve A term that may be used rather loosely. Strictly it should refer to a large collection of nerve fibres that can be seen with the naked eye, e.g. the ulnar nerve. However, it may also refer to a single neuron or its axon.

Neuro- Relates to nerves, e.g. neurology – study of the nervous system.

NMJ Neuromuscular junction is a synapse between a neuron and the muscle cell membrane.

Notch An indentation, e.g. the suprasternal notch of the sternum.

Noxious Harmful, e.g. a substance that causes damage to cells.

Nucleus In terms of the CNS, a nucleus is a collection of nerve cell bodies that share a similar function. See also ganglion.

Orifice An opening to a cavity.

Oss-, Osteo- Relates to bones, e.g. ossification – process of bone formation, osteoporosis – abnormal loss of bone density.

-oma Denotes a tumour, e.g. lymphoma (of the lymph nodes), carcinoma (of an epithelium).

Omentum Folds of peritoneum that link the stomach to other viscera, e.g. lesser omentum connects the stomach to the liver.

Omental bursa See lesser sac.

-ostomy Making a permanent opening, e.g. tracheostomy – permanent (or semipermanent) opening into the trachea.

-otomy Making a small, temporary opening, e.g. laparotomy, emergency opening of the abdomen.

Palpation Examination of the body by feeling with the hands (adjective palpable).

Palpebral Relates to the eyelids (palpebrae), e.g. the muscle that lifts the eyelids is levator palpebrae superioris.

Para- By the side of, e.g. paravertebral, alongside the vertebral column, para-aortic, beside the aorta, paranasal air sinuses.

Paraesthesia Abnormal sensation in the distribution of a peripheral nerve, e.g. pins and needles along the medial border of the forearm and medial one-and-a-half digits in ulnar nerve damage.

Paralysis Muscle weakness.

Parietal Relates to the surface of the inner walls of a body cavity, e.g. parietal pleura. Also relates to the parietal bone of the skull.

Pectoral (adj) Relating to the chest.

Perforation The formation of a hiatus in an organ or tissue, usually through a disease process.

Peri- Around or near, e.g. periosteum, membrane covering the surface of bone.

Perineum The region lying around the anus and external genitalia, below the pelvic diaphragm and bounded by the pelvic outlet.

Peristalsis Motion by which intestinal contents are moved through the alimentary tract.

Peritoneum Membrane lining the abdominal cavity.

Phrenic Relates to the diaphragm.

Pia Inner vascular layer of the meninges.

Pleura The epithelial covering of the lungs.

Plexus Network, e.g. brachial plexus is the network of nerves that supply the upper limb.

Pneumothorax A condition in which there air within the pleural cavity around the lungs.

Portal system Venous system that carries blood through a second capillary bed before returning blood to the heart, e.g. hepatic portal vein delivers blood from the GI tract to the capillaries of the liver before it is returned to the right atrium via the hepatic vein and the inferior vena cava.

Post- After or following, e.g. postganglionic describes a neuron that leaves a ganglion and terminates in an effector (muscle or gland).

Pre- Preceding or before, e.g. preganglionic describes a neuron that leaves the spinal cord and terminates in a ganglion.

Process A thin prominence or protuberance, e.g. spinous process of vertebrae.

Prominence A projection of bone.

Prone Patient lying face down.

Protuberance A rounded projection of bone.

Proprioception Ability to sense the position of the body in space. Proprioceptors are present in muscles and tendons and register mechanical changes in position.

Pulmonary circulation Vessels that carry blood from the right side of the heart to the alveolar capillaries of the lungs and back to the left side of the heart. In the process, gaseous exchange occurs with oxygen entering the blood and carbon dioxide leaving it.

Radiolucent A structure that does not absorb X-rays and appears dark on an X-ray film.

Radiopaque The ability to absorb X-rays and appear white on an X-ray film.

Raphe Literally, a seam. A line of union between two muscles such as is found in the pharyngeal constrictors.

Recess A depression or hollow cavity of an organ.

Reflex An unconscious, autonomic and involuntary action, e.g. muscle contraction through a neuronal circuit.

Regurgitation The backflow of a liquid against its normal direction, e.g. blood flows from the left ventricle to left atrium through a defective mitral valve.

Renal Relating to the kidneys, e.g. renal artery.

Retinaculum A thickened connective tissue band that holds other tissue in position, e.g. extensor tendons held by the extensor retinaculum in the forearm.

Retro- At the back or behind a structure, e.g. retroperitoneal.

Retroperitoneal A viscus lying against the posterior abdominal wall and covered by peritoneum only on its anterior surface, e.g. pancreas.

Sarcoma Cancer of connective tissue origin.

Sclerosis Is the hardening of a tissue.

Sensory Relates to structures or activities that involve transmitting nerve impulses towards the CNS from the periphery, see also afferent.

Septum A walled partition that divides an anatomical structure (interventricular septum – between the ventricles).

Serous Thin, watery secretion such as is secreted by a serous membrane like the pleura (see mucous).

Sesamoid An oval or round shaped bone within a tendon that slides over another bone, e.g. the patella over the patellar surface of the femur.

Sheath A connective tissue envelope that surrounds anatomical structures, e.g. nerve, muscle or tendon.

Sinus Cavity or channel; has many meanings, e.g. paranasal sinus, hepatic sinus, dural venous sinus.

Somatic Relates to the structures that make up the body wall or its primitive divisions known as somites.

Sphincter Muscular valve that controls the diameter of a tube, e.g. the pyloric sphincter lies between the stomach and duodenum.

Sphygmomanometer The instrument that measures arterial blood pressure.

Splanchnic Equivalent to visceral – splanchnic is derived from Greek, visceral from Latin.

Squamous Flattened, scale-like cells, e.g. squamous epithelium consists of very flattened cells.

Stroke Sudden onset of weakness due to interruption of blood flow to the brain.

Sub- Below or underlying, e.g. subcostal denotes below the ribs.

Sulcus Gutter, depression (plural sulci) particularly used in relation to the surface of the cerebrum where sulci lie between the gyri, e.g. central sulcus of the cerebral cortex.

Supine Patient lying on their back, face up.

Supra- Above, e.g. supraorbital nerve.

Synapse Junction between two neurons or between a nerve and an effector.

Synovial Such joints are freely movable. Literally, synovial means like an egg. Synovial fluid secreted by synovial membrane has the consistency of egg white and lubricates and nourishes the joint surfaces.

Systemic circulation Vessels that carry blood from the left side of the heart to the capillary beds of the entire body (except the lungs) and back to the right side of the heart. In the process gaseous exchange occurs with oxygen leaving the blood and carbon dioxide entering it.

Systole Contraction phase of the cardiac cycle (adjective systolic) see also diastole.

Tamponade An abnormal pressure on a body part, e.g. the presence of fluid within the pericardial cavity that compresses the heart.

Tendon The tough extension of the connective tissue associated with muscles that form the attachment of muscle to bone.

Thermoregulation Regulation of body temperature through shivering or peripheral capillary dilatation and sweating.

Thoraco- Relating to the thorax.

Thrombus A blood clot.

Tissue Similar cells that perform specialized functions. There are four basic types: epithelia, muscle, nerve and connective tissues.

Transverse A plane that divides a structure into superior and inferior parts.

Tubercle A small rounded bony protuberance, e.g. lesser tubercle of the humerus.

Tuberosity A large rounded bony protuberance, e.g. the greater tuberosity of the femur.

Tunica A layer of an anatomical structure, e.g. tunica media – the smooth muscle layer of an artery.

Umbilicus Abdominal site of attachment of the umbilical cord.

Ureter The muscular tube that carries urine between the kidney and bladder.

Urethra The muscular tube that carries urine from the bladder to the exterior.

Varicose Enlarged and twisted superficial veins, especially in the lower limb.

Vaso- Relating to vessels, e.g. vasoconstriction physiological narrowing of blood vessels (plural vasa).

Venae comitantes Veins that closely accompany arteries, e.g. the deep veins of the limbs.

Venepuncture The puncture of a vein to either obtain a sample of blood or administering medication, e.g. antibiotics.

Ventricle Chamber, e.g. thicker walled chambers of the heart. There are also four ventricles in the brain.

Vinculae A connecting band of synovial tissue connecting the flexor tendons to the phalanges.

Visceral Relates to internal organs. Visceral nerves tend to be under involuntary control, and sensation tends to be vague and imprecisely perceptible or even imperceptible. See also somatic.

Viscus Internal organ, e.g. heart, spleen, etc. (plural viscera).

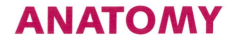

ANATOMY

Basic concepts of anatomy

Objectives

In this chapter you will learn to:

- Describe the anatomical position.
- Describe the anatomical planes.
- Define the anatomical terms used in anatomy and clinical practice.
- Describe the terms of movement, including those of the thumb.
- Understand the structure of bone.
- List the factors that contribute to joint stability.
- Describe the classification of muscles according to their actions.
- Describe the organization and function of muscle.
- Draw a diagram of the components of a spinal nerve.
- Describe the layers of a blood vessel wall.
- Describe factors causing lymphatic fluid movement and functions of lymph.
- Outline the layout of the gastrointestinal system and general functions.
- Outline the layout of the urinary system and general functions.

DESCRIPTIVE ANATOMICAL TERMS

The anatomical position

This is a standard position used in anatomy and clinical medicine to allow accurate and consistent description of one body part in relation to another (Fig. 1.1):

- The head is directed forwards with eyes looking into the distance.
- The body is upright, legs together, and directed forwards.
- The palms are turned forward, with the thumbs laterally.

Anatomical planes

These comprise the following (Fig. 1.2):

- The median sagittal plane is the vertical plane passing through the midline of the body from the front to the back. Any plane parallel to this is termed paramedian or sagittal.
- Coronal (or frontal) planes are vertical planes perpendicular to the sagittal planes.
- Horizontal or transverse planes lie at right angles to both the sagittal and coronal planes.

Such anatomical planes are frequently used in computer tomography (CT) scans and magnetic resonance imaging (MRI), to visualize muscle, bone, lung and other soft tissues as well as pathologies, for example pancreatic cancer or a brain abscess.

Terms of position

The terms of position commonly used in clinical practice and anatomy are illustrated in Figure 1.3.

Terms of movement

Various terms are used to describe movements of the body (Fig. 1.4):

- Flexion—forward movement in a sagittal plane which in general reduces the angle at the joint, e.g. bending the elbow. Exceptions are at the ankle joint (when the angle is increased) and the shoulder joint (when the angle between the upper limb and trunk is increased).
- Extension—backward movement in a sagittal plane which in general increases the angle at joints except at the ankle joint (when the angle is decreased) and the knee joint due to lower limb rotation during embryonic development.

Fig. 1.1 Anatomical position and regions of the body.

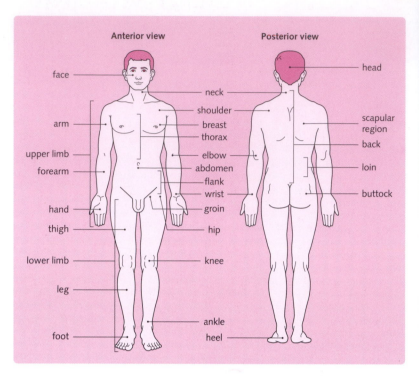

Anterior view — Posterior view

face, arm, upper limb, forearm, hand, thigh, lower limb, leg, foot

neck, shoulder, breast, thorax, elbow, abdomen, flank, wrist, groin, hip, knee, ankle, heel

head, scapular region, back, loin, buttock

- Abduction—movement away from the median plane.
- Adduction—movement towards the median plane.
- Supination—lateral rotation of the forearm, causing the palm to face anteriorly.
- Pronation—medial rotation of the forearm, causing the palm to face posteriorly.
- Eversion—turning the sole of the foot outwards.
- Inversion—turning the sole of the foot inwards.
- Rotation—movement of part of the body around its long axis.
- Circumduction—a combination of flexion, extension, abduction, and adduction.

The terms used to describe movements of the thumb are perpendicular to the movements of the body, e.g. flexion of the thumb is at 90° to that of flexion of the fingers (Fig. 1.5).

To differentiate supination from pronation remember that you hold a bowl of soup with a supinated forearm.

BASIC STRUCTURES OF ANATOMY

Skin

The skin completely covers the body surface and is the largest organ of the body. The functions of the skin include:

- Protection from ultraviolet light and mechanical, chemical, and thermal insults.
- Sensations including pain, temperature, touch and pressure.
- Thermoregulation.
- Metabolic functions, e.g. vitamin D synthesis.

The skin is composed of the following (Fig. 1.6):

- The epidermis forms a protective waterproof barrier. It consists of keratinized stratified squamous epithelium, which is continuously being shed and replaced. It is avascular.
- The dermis supports the epidermis and it has a rich network of vessels and nerves. It is composed mainly of collagen fibres with elastic fibres giving the skin its elasticity.
- The hypodermis or superficial fascia. It consists of fatty tissue which provides thermal insulation and protection for underlying structures.

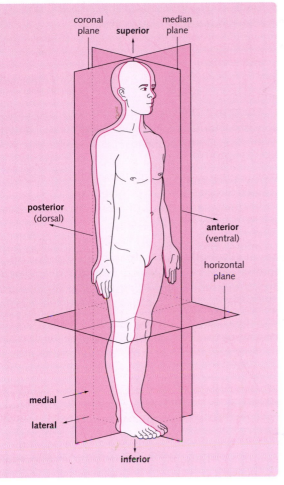

Fig. 1.2 Anatomical planes.

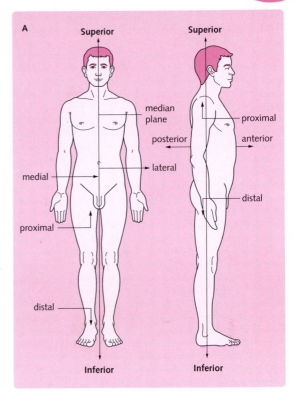

Fig. 1.3 Relationship and comparison (A) and classification (B) of terms of position commonly used in anatomy and clinical practice.

Position	Description
Anterior	In front of another structure
Posterior	Behind another structure
Superior	Above another structure
Inferior	Below another structure
Deep	Further away from body surface
Superficial	Closer to body surface
Medial	Closer to median plane
Lateral	Further away from median plane
Proximal	Closer to the trunk or origin
Distal	Further away from the trunk or origin
Ipsilateral	The same side of the body
Contralateral	The opposite side of the body

Dermatology

A genetic mutation in collagen synthesis affects the protein's function. Dermal collagen is normally resistant to stretch, preventing excessive elasticity. However, this is lost in Ehlers–Danlos syndrome where individuals have very elastic skin as well as other features due to collagen in joints (are hyperextendable) or heart valves (mitral valve regurgitation).

The skin appendages include:

- Hairs—highly modified, keratinized structures.
- Sweat glands—produce sweat, which plays a role in thermoregulation.
- Sebaceous glands—produce sebum, which lubricates the skin and hair.

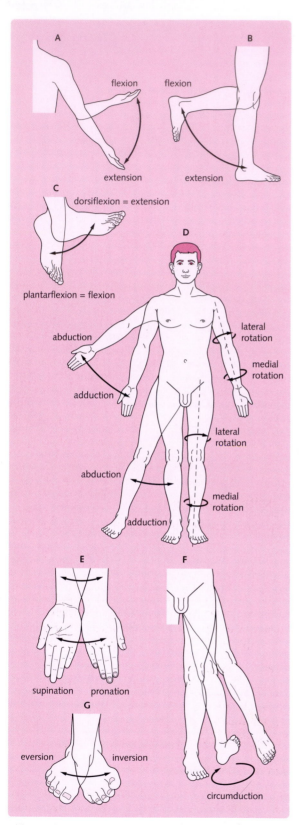

- Nails—highly specialized appendages found on the dorsal surface of each digit.

Fascia

The fascia of the body may be divided into superficial and deep layers.

The superficial fascia (subcutaneous fatty tissue) consists of loose areolar tissue that unites the dermis to the deep fascia. It contains cutaneous nerves, blood vessels and lymphatics that supply to the dermis. Its thickness varies at different sites within the body and women have a thicker layer than men.

In some places sheets of muscle lie in the fascia, e.g. muscles of facial expression.

The deep fascia forms a layer of fibrous tissue around the limbs and body and the deep structures. Intermuscular septa extend from the deep fascia, attach to bone, and divide limb musculature into compartments. The fascia has a rich nerve supply and it is, therefore, very sensitive. The thickness of the fascia varies widely: e.g. it is thickened in the iliotibial tract but very thin over the rectus abdominis muscle and absent over the face. The arrangement of the fascia determines the pattern of spread of infection as well as blood due to haemorrhaging into tissues.

Bone

Bone is a specialized form of connective tissue with a mineralized extracellular component.

The functions of bone include:

- Locomotion (by serving as a rigid lever).
- Support (giving soft tissue permanent shape).
- Attachment of muscles.
- Calcium homeostasis and storage of other inorganic ions.
- Production of blood cells (haematopoiesis).

Fig. 1.4 Terms of movement.

(A) Flexion and extension of forearm at elbow joint.
(B) Flexion and extension of leg at knee joint.
(C) Dorsiflexion and plantarflexion of foot at ankle joint.
(D) Abduction and adduction of right limbs and rotation of left limbs at shoulder and hip joints, respectively.
(E) Pronation and supination of forearm at radioulnar joints.
(F) Circumduction (circular movement) of lower limb at hip joint.
(G) Inversion and eversion of foot at subtalar and transverse tarsal joints.

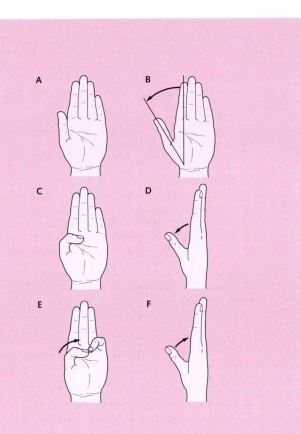

Fig. 1.5 Terms of movement for the thumb. (Adapted from *Crash Course: Musculoskeletal System* by SV Biswas and R Iqbal. Mosby.)

(A) Neutral hand position.
(B) Extension (radial abduction).
(C) Flexion (transpalmar adduction).
(D) Abduction (palmar abduction).
(E) Opposition.
(F) Adduction.

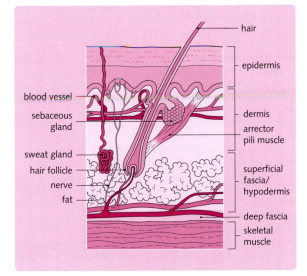
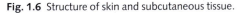

Fig. 1.6 Structure of skin and subcutaneous tissue.

Classification of bone

Bones are classified according to their position and shape.

The position can be described as:

- Axial skeleton, consists of the skull, vertebral column including the sacrum, ribs, and sternum.
- Appendicular skeleton, consists of the pelvic girdle, pectoral girdle, and bones of the upper and lower limbs.

Types of shape include:

- Long bones, e.g. femur, humerus.
- Short bones, e.g. carpal bones.
- Flat bones, e.g. skull vault.
- Irregular bones, e.g. vertebrae.

General structure of bone

Bone is surrounded by a connective tissue membrane called the periosteum (Fig. 1.7). This is continuous with muscle attachments, joint capsules and the

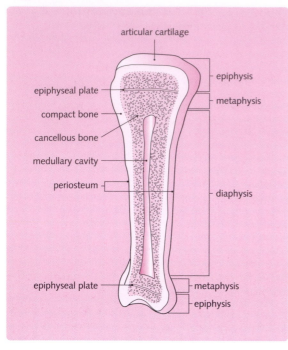

articular cartilage

epiphysis

metaphysis

epiphyseal plate

compact bone

cancellous bone

medullary cavity

periosteum

diaphysis

epiphyseal plate

metaphysis

epiphysis

Fig. 1.7 Long bone and its components.

Orthopaedics

As an individual ages their bone density is reduced (osteopenia). The cortical bone becomes thinner and the trabeculae decrease in number. As a result, bone structure is weaker and predisposes to fractures, especially in osteoporotic postmenopausal women. Fractures tend to occur where, in normality, there is a greater amount of trabecular bone to cortical bone, e.g. radius (Colles fracture), femoral neck and vertebral body. Fractures occurring secondary to another process, e.g. osteoporosis, are known as pathological fractures.

Blood supply of bones

There are two main sources of blood supply to bone:

- A major nutrient artery that supplies the marrow.
- Vessels from the periosteum.

The periosteal supply to bone assumes greater importance in the elderly. Extensive stripping of the periosteum, e.g. during surgery or following trauma, may result in bone death.

Joints

These are unions between bones of which there are three major types (Fig. 1.8).

Synovial joints

These are moveable joints and have the following features:

- The bone ends are covered by hyaline articular cartilage.
- The joint is surrounded by a fibrous capsule.
- A synovial membrane lines the inner aspect of the joint and its capsule, except where there is cartilage and it secretes synovial fluid. This lubricates the joint and transports nutrients, especially to the cartilage.
- Some synovial joints, e.g. the temporomandibular joints, are divided into two cavities by an articular disc.

Blood supply of joints

A vascular plexus around the epiphysis provides the joint with a very good blood supply.

deep fascia. There is an outer fibrous layer and an inner cellular layer. The inner layer is vascular, and it provides the underlying bone with nutrition. The periosteum is an osteogenic layer consisting of osteoproginator cells that can differentiate into osteoblasts, e.g. at a fracture site and cause formation of a bone cuff (callus) which stabilizes the fracture.

Bone includes the following components:

- The outer compact layer or cortical bone provides great strength and rigidity.
- The cancellous or spongy bone consists of a network of trabeculae arranged to resist external forces.
- The medullary cavity of long bones and the interstices of cancellous bone are filled with bone marrow. At birth virtually all the bone marrow is red (haematopoietic), but this is replaced by yellow (fatty) marrow—only the ribs, sternum, vertebrae, clavicle, pelvis, and skull bones contain red marrow in adult life.
- The endosteum is a single layer of osteogenic cells lining the inner surface of bone.

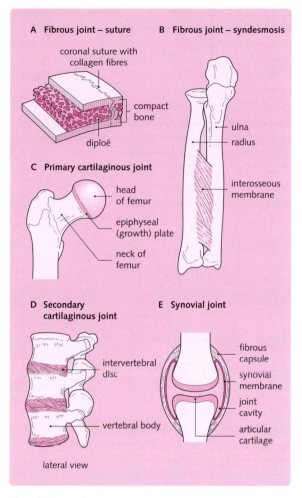

A **Fibrous joint – suture**

coronal suture with collagen fibres

compact bone

diploë

B **Fibrous joint – syndesmosis**

ulna

radius

interosseous membrane

C **Primary cartilaginous joint**

head of femur

epiphyseal (growth) plate

neck of femur

D **Secondary cartilaginous joint**

intervertebral disc

vertebral body

lateral view

E **Synovial joint**

fibrous capsule

synovial membrane

joint cavity

articular cartilage

Fig. 1.8 Types of joints.

(A) Fibrous joint—sutural (bones are united by fibrous tissue, as in sutures of the skull).

(B) Fibrous joint—syndesmosis (bones are joined by a sheet of fibrous tissue).

(C) Primary cartilaginous joint (where bone and hyaline cartilage meet).

(D) Secondary cartilaginous joint (articular surfaces are covered by a thin lamina of hyaline cartilage; the hyaline laminae are united by fibrocartilage).

(E) Synovial joint.

Nerve supply of joints

According to Hilton's law, the motor nerve to a muscle tends also to give a sensory branch to the joint that the muscle moves and another branch to the skin over the joint. The capsule and ligaments are supplied by afferent nerve endings, including pain fibres. Innervation of a joint and the muscles that move that joint allow proprioception to occur. This is the sensation of joint position and it is necessary for motor control and posture.

Stability of joints

Stability is achieved by the following components:

- Bony—e.g. in a firm ball-and-socket joint such as the hip joint, bony contours contribute to stability.
- Ligaments—these are important in most joints, and they act mainly to prevent excessive movement.
- Muscles—these are an important stabilizing factor in most joints.

Muscles and tendons

Skeletal muscles are aggregations of contractile fibres that move the joints of the skeleton.

Muscles are usually joined to bone by tendons at their origin and insertion.

Muscle action

Muscles can be classified according to their action:

- Prime mover—the muscle is the major muscle responsible for a particular movement, e.g. brachialis is the prime mover in flexing the elbow.
- Antagonist—any muscle that opposes the action of the prime mover: as the primer mover contracts the antagonist relaxes, e.g. triceps brachii relaxes during elbow flexion.
- Fixator—prime mover and antagonist acting together to 'fix' a joint, e.g. muscles holding the scapula steady when deltoid moves the humerus.
- Synergist—prevents unwanted movement in an intermediate joint, e.g. extensors of the carpus contract to fix the wrist joint, allowing the long flexors of the fingers to function effectively.

In general, if a joint is very stable it has a reduced range of movement, e.g. the stable hip joint compared with the less stable shoulder joint; the latter has a greater range of movement.

Muscle design

Muscle fibres may be either parallel or oblique to the line of pull of the whole muscle.

Parallel fibres allow maximal range of movement. These muscles may be quadrangular, fusiform, or strap shaped, e.g. sartorius and sternocleidomastoid.

Oblique fibres increase the force generated at the expense of a reduced range of movement. These muscles may be unipennate (e.g. flexor pollicis longus), bipennate (e.g. dorsal interossei), multipennate (e.g. deltoid) or triangular (e.g. deltoid).

Muscle organization and function

Motor nerves control the contraction of skeletal muscle. Each motor neuron together with the muscle fibres it supplies constitutes a motor unit.

The size of motor units varies considerably: where fine precise movements are required, a single neuron may supply only a few muscle fibres, e.g. the extrinsic eye muscles; conversely, in the large gluteus maximus muscle, a single neuron may supply several hundred muscle fibres. The smaller the size of the motor unit, the more precise are the possible movements. If powerful contractions are required then larger motor units are recruited (activated) which cause contraction of larger muscles.

Clinical examination

During a neurological and musculoskeletal examination muscle power is assessed by asking the patient to perform movements against resistance, e.g. asking the patient to flex the elbow while the examiner tries to prevent this by holding the wrist and supporting the patient's elbow. The power is graded (5 to 0) by the UK Medical Research Council (MRC) scale:

Grade 5: Full power
Grade 4: Contraction against resistance
Grade 3: Contraction against gravity
Grade 2: Contraction with gravity eliminated
Grade 1: Flicker of muscle contraction
Grade 0: No muscle contraction

Muscle weakness is seen in myasthenia gravis when autoantibodies are produced that attack the receptors on the neuromuscular junction (NMJ). Rapid repeated movements cause muscle fatigue.

The force generated by a skeletal muscle is related to the cross-sectional area of its fibres. For a fixed volume of muscle, shorter fibres produce more force but less shortening.

In muscles, there is an optimum length of muscle filaments, which produces optimum tension and contraction. Optimum tension is reduced if the muscle becomes stretched beyond this length or is compressed. This is a property of the muscle length–tension relationship.

Muscle attachments

The ends of muscles are attached to bone, cartilage and ligaments by tendons. Some flat muscles are attached by a flattened tendon, an aponeurosis or fascia.

When symmetrical halves of a muscle fuse to form a seam like intersection, e.g. in mylohyoid muscle, a raphe is formed.

When tendons cross joints they are often enclosed and protected by a synovial sheath, a layer of connective tissue lined by a synovial membrane and lubricated by synovial fluid.

Bursae are sacs of connective tissue filled with synovial fluid, which lie between tendons and bony areas, acting as cushioning devices.

Nerves

The nervous system is divided into the central nervous system and the peripheral nervous system: the central nervous system is composed of the brain and spinal cord; the peripheral nervous system consists of the cranial and spinal nerves, and their distribution. The nervous system may also be divided into the somatic and autonomic nervous systems.

The conducting cells of the nervous system are termed neurons. A typical motor neuron consists of a cell body which contains the nucleus and gives off a single axon and numerous dendrites (Fig. 1.9). The cell bodies of most neurons are located within the central nervous system, where they aggregate to form nuclei. Cell bodies in the peripheral nervous system aggregate in ganglia.

Axons are nerve fibres that conduct action potentials generated in the cell body to influence other neurons or affect organs. They may be myelinated or non-myelinated.

Most nerves in the peripheral nervous system are bundles of motor, sensory and autonomic axons. The head is largely supplied by the 12 cranial nerves. The

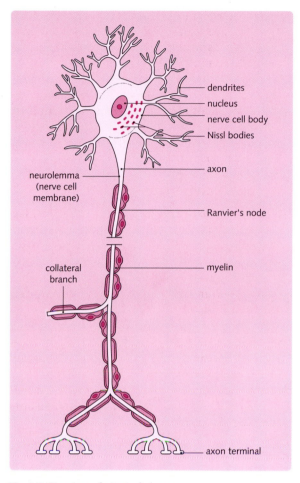

Fig. 1.9 Structure of a typical neuron.

dendrites
nucleus
nerve cell body
Nissl bodies
neurolemma (nerve cell membrane)
axon
Ranvier's node
collateral branch
myelin
axon terminal

Clinical examination/neurology

When testing reflexes the reflex arc is being assessed at a particular spinal cord level. On striking a tendon with a hammer it stretches the tendon and a receptor within the muscle (a muscle spindle). This receptor monitors muscle length and prevents over-stretching by initiating a reflex arc and causing muscle contraction to counter the stretching. This is witnessed as a jerk of the limb; for example, on striking the patella tendon the quadriceps muscle contracts, causing knee extension. The common limb reflexes and their spinal cord segment levels, which are tested, are:

- Biceps brachii (C5–6)
- Triceps brachii (C7–8)
- Brachioradialis (C6–7)
- Quadriceps femoris (L3–4)
- Gastrocnemius (S1–2)

the structural basis of a reflex arc (Fig. 1.10). The reflex arc is an involuntary protective mechanism that occurs unconsciously although higher centres can influence its activity, i.e. increase or decrease activity. In a stroke the inhibitory input of higher centres that dampens the reflex arc activity is lost and hyper-reflexia (exaggerated limb reflexes) occurs.

Autonomic nerves are either sympathetic or parasympathetic. Sympathetic preganglionic fibres arise from the thoracic and upper two lumbar segments of the spinal cord. The preganglionic fibres synapse in a ganglion of the sympathetic chain which runs either side of the vertebral column. The post-ganglionic fibres that arise from the sympathetic chain ganglia can either enter a spinal nerve to supply the limbs or body wall. Some preganglionic fibres do not synapse in the sympathetic chain. Instead they pass through the chain and synapse in a prevertebral ganglion, e.g. coeliac ganglion. Postganglionic fibres arise from prevertebral ganglia and supply viscera, e.g. stomach. Parasympathetic preganglionic fibres arise from cranial nerves and sacral nerves (S2–S4). They synapse in ganglia associated with organs, e.g. a pulmonary ganglion, to form postganglionic fibres that innervate an organ, e.g. lung.

Spinal nerves

There are 31 pairs of spinal nerves: 8 cervical, 12 thoracic, 5 lumbar, 5 sacral, and the coccygeal nerve.

trunk and the limbs are supplied by the segmental spinal nerves.

Motor nerves originate in the ventral (anterior) horn of the spinal cord (Fig. 1.10) and synapse with the sarcolemma (plasma membrane) of muscle to form a structure called the motor endplate. A nerve impulse reaches the end of the nerve fibre causing the release of neurotransmitter. This leads to depolarization of the sarcolemma and initiation of muscle contraction.

Sensory nerves carry impulses from receptors in skin, muscle or viscera to the dorsal (posterior) horn of the spinal cord. Receptors respond to specific stimuli, e.g. stretch, noxious substances or pressure. Sensory neurons synapse with neurons, which ascend in the spinal cord and travel to higher centres, e.g. cerebral cortex or cerebellum. They also synapse with motor neurons directly or via an interneuron. This is

Fig. 1.10 Components of a typical spinal nerve.

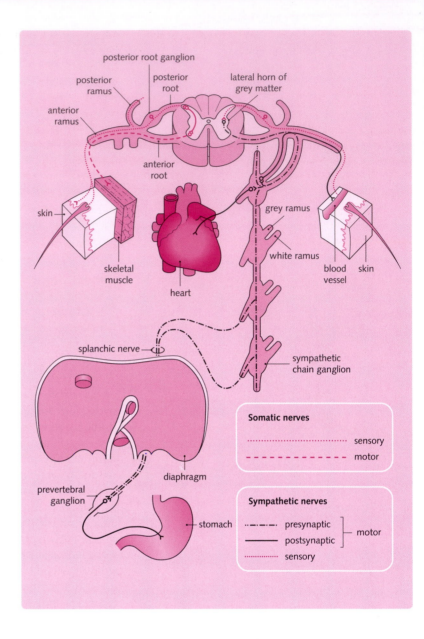

The spinal cord ends at the lower border of the first lumbar vertebra in the adult. Below this, the nerve roots of the cord form a vertical bundle: the cauda equina.

Each spinal nerve is formed by the union of the anterior and posterior roots (Fig. 1.10):

- The anterior root contains motor fibres for skeletal muscles. Those from T1 to L2 also contain preganglionic sympathetic fibres; S2 to S4 also contain preganglionic parasympathetic fibres.
- The posterior root contains sensory fibres whose cell bodies are in the posterior root ganglion.

Immediately after formation, the spinal nerve divides into anterior and posterior rami. The great nerve plexuses, e.g. the brachial, lumbar and sacral, are formed by anterior rami. The posterior rami supply the erector spinae muscles and skin that cover them.

The spinal nerves each supply an area of skin called a dermatome (except the face, which is supplied by the fifth cranial nerve). The nerve supply of each dermatome overlaps above and below with adjacent dermatomes. Testing for loss of sensation over a dermatome indicates the level of a lesion within the spinal cord. Dermatomes of the limbs and trunk are illustrated in the relevant chapters.

Cardiovascular system

The cardiovascular system functions principally to transport oxygen and nutrients to the tissues and carbon dioxide and other metabolic waste products away from the tissues.

The right side of the heart pumps blood to the lungs via the pulmonary circulation. The left side of the heart pumps oxygenated blood through the aorta to the rest of the body via the systemic circulation (Fig. 1.11A).

Blood is distributed to the organs via the arteries and then arterioles, which branch to form capillaries where gaseous exchange occurs. Deoxygenated blood is eventually returned to the heart first by venules then by veins (Fig. 1.11A). Valves in the low-pressure venous system are required to prevent back-flow of blood. However, some veins have no true valves, e.g. venae cavae, vertebral, pelvic, head and neck veins.

The general structure of the blood vessel wall consists of three layers or tunicas (Fig. 1.11B). The contents of each vary with vessel type and its function. Arteries have a well-developed tunica media of smooth muscle. The walls of the largest arteries contain numerous elastic tissue layers; however, veins have relatively little smooth muscle and elastic tissue. Capillaries consist of an endothelial tube.

The larger vessels, e.g. aorta, also contain an additional external layer of blood vessels (vasa

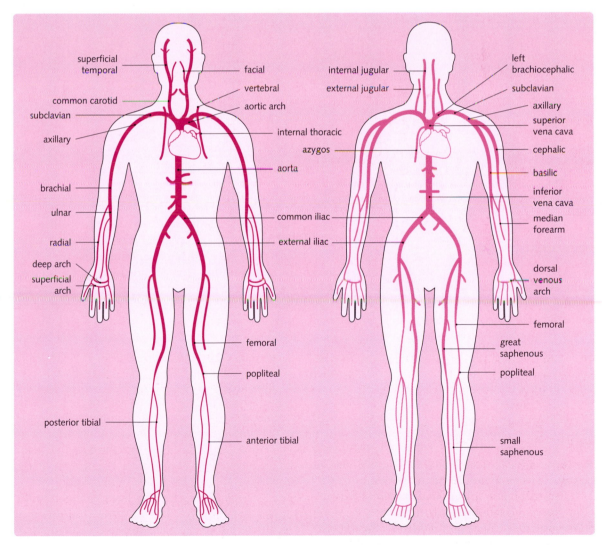

Fig. 1.11(A) The arterial tree (A) and venous tree (B) of the cardiovascular system.

Fig. 1.11(C) Cross section of vessel wall showing basic layers.

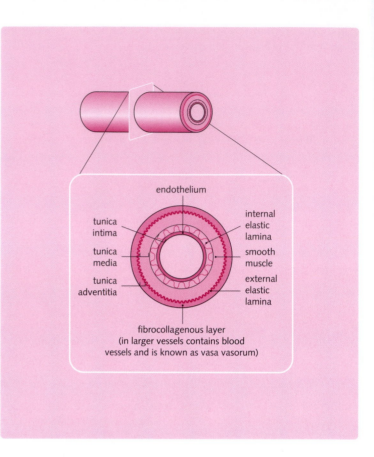

vasorum) and nerves (vasa nervosa) that supplies the wall.

Anastomosis

Not all blood traverses a capillary bed. Direct connections (anastomoses) between arterioles and venules (arteriovenous shunts) exist. Pre-capillary sphincters regulate flow through the capillary bed under sympathetic nerve control. In the skin such shunts are involved in thermoregulation. Capillary beds can be opened up or closed off depending on metabolic requirements, e.g. during exercise.

Direct communication between larger vessels can be advantageous. If an artery becomes occluded anastomoses maintain the circulation to an organ. When an artery is slowly occluded by disease, new vessels may develop (collaterals), forming an alternative pathway, e.g. coronary arteries.

When such communications are absent (e.g. the central artery of the retina) between arteries the vessel is known as an end artery. Occlusion in these vessels causes necrosis.

Lymphatics

Figure 1.12 illustrates the lymphatic system in man.

Fluid moves out of capillaries into tissues at the arterial end due to hydrostatic pressure, which is created by blood pressure. At the venous end of the capillary oncotic pressure acts to draw fluid back into the vessel. Oncotic pressure is created by proteins, e.g. albumin and cations (sodium ions). However, not all fluid is returned to the blood and excess within the tissues drains into the lymphatic system. Movement of lymphatic fluid through the vessels is the result of (i) muscle contraction, (ii) pulsation of an adjacent artery, (iii) a suction action by the negative intrathoracic pressure, and (iv) pressure within the lymphatic vessels.

The lymphatics on the right side of the head, neck, upper limb and thorax drain into the right lymphatic duct which enters the venous circulation at the junction of the right subclavian and right internal jugular veins. The rest of the body drains into the thoracic duct, which enters the venous circulation at the junction of the left subclavian and left internal jugular veins (Fig. 1.12).

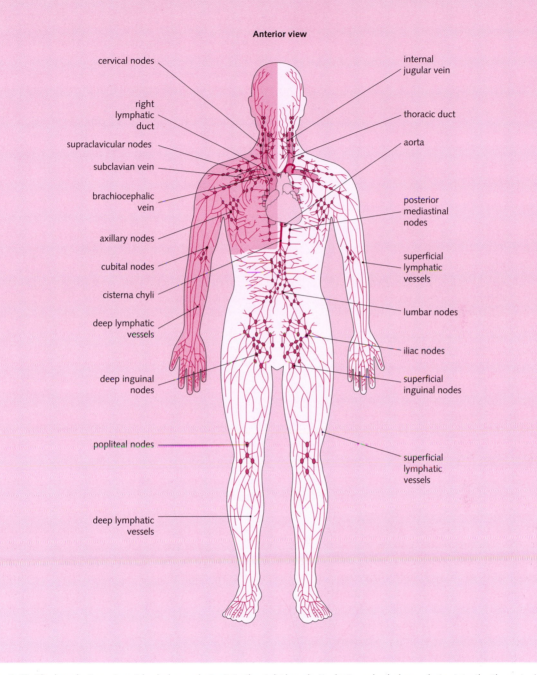

Anterior view

cervical nodes

internal jugular vein

right lymphatic duct

thoracic duct

supraclavicular nodes

aorta

subclavian vein

brachiocephalic vein

posterior mediastinal nodes

axillary nodes

superficial lymphatic vessels

cubital nodes

cisterna chyli

lumbar nodes

deep lymphatic vessels

iliac nodes

deep inguinal nodes

superficial inguinal nodes

popliteal nodes

superficial lymphatic vessels

deep lymphatic vessels

Fig. 1.12 The lymphatic system (shaded area drains into the right lymphatic duct; unshaded area drains into the thoracic duct).

Lymph carries foreign material (not recognized as self), which may be presented by special cells in the lymph nodes (antigen-presenting cells) to cells of the immune system to mount an immune response. The lymphatics also are involved in the absorption and transport of fats. Lacteals (end lymphatic vessels) of the intestinal villi contain chyle (a milky lymph fluid), which drains into larger lymphatic vessels and eventually into the thoracic duct.

Lymphatics are found in all tissues except the central nervous system, eyeball, internal ear, cartilage, bone, and the epidermis of the skin.

Oncology

Lymphatic drainage of organs provides one of the routes by which a cancer can spread to other anatomical sites (metastasis). In breast carcinoma, metastasis can be to the lymph nodes of the armpit (axilla), or in gastric carcinoma spread can be to the left supraclavicular nodes only and this is known as Troissier's sign.

Gastrointestinal system

The gastrointestinal system has three functions:

- Digestion of food material starting with mastication and continuing in stomach and duodenum.
- Absorption of the products of digestion in the small intestine.
- Absorption of fluid and formation of solid faeces in the large intestine.

The process of digestion begins in the mouth with enzyme secretion by the salivary glands and chewing (mastication). In the stomach, acid and enzyme secretion continue the process; then, in the second part of the duodenum, pancreatic enzymes, along with bile from the liver, complete this process. The majority of absorption occurs in the jejunum, which has an increased surface area due to plicae circularis (folds), villi (finger-like projections) and microvilli (microscopic projections on individual cells). Carbohydrates and proteins enter the portal circulation (see below) via the intestinal villi capillaries and fats enter the lacteals of the lymphatic system.

The portal circulation is a circulation consisting of two capillary beds. Capillaries originating in the intestine enter veins that eventually drain into the hepatic portal vein and this drains into the liver capillaries (sinusoids). Hepatic veins drain blood from the liver into the systemic circulation and it returns to the heart. The portal vein also receives tributaries from the stomach, spleen and pancreas. There are anastomoses with the systemic venous circulation at the gastro-oesophageal and recto-anal junctions (portosystemic anastomoses).

The general structure of the gastrointestinal tract wall is illustrated in Figure 1.13. Modifications to this denote its underlying function, e.g. there are more folds and villi in the jejunum than in the ileum or colon.

Respiratory system

The upper part of the respiratory tract, consisting of the nasal and oral cavities, pharynx, larynx and trachea, is responsible for conditioning the air by (i) humidifying and warming e.g. blood vessels in the nasal cavity, and on conchae that increase the surface area avaliable, (ii) trapping of foreign material e.g. hair in the nasal vestibule and mucus secretion. The lower respiratory tract consists of a series of branching tubes that form the bronchial tree (see Chapter 3), which ends in the alveolar sacs where gaseous exchange occurs.

The general structure of the respiratory tree wall changes with function, e.g. the bronchi walls contain cartilage whereas the bronchioles lack cartilage. The alveoli consist of a sphere of epithelium surrounded by a network of capillaries.

Respiratory epithelium of the trachea, bronchi and bronchioles consists of cells which contain cilia (small hairs) that beat rhythmically and propel trapped foreign particles (within mucus) towards the pharynx. Moreover, the alveoli consist of thin epithelial cells (pneumocytes) which reduce the distance that gases have to diffuse across between it and the capillaries of the lung. This increases gaseous exchange efficiency.

The functions of the respiratory system include:

- Gaseous exchange.
- Metabolism and activation or inactivation of some proteins, e.g. angiotensin-converting enzyme.
- Acting as a reservoir for blood.
- Phonation (vocal sound production).
- Olfactory function.

Urinary system

The urinary system is composed of the kidneys, ureters, bladder and urethra (Fig. 1.14). The kidneys filter the blood at the glomerulus, and along the length of the nephron unit selective absorption and secretion occurs. The urine that is formed from these processes enters the renal pelvis and the ureters. The latter empty into the bladder, which stores urea until such time that it may be voided (micturation). The functions of the kidneys are:

- Excretion of waste products, e.g. urea (produced in the liver).
- Absorption of filtered substances, e.g. glucose, ions, proteins.

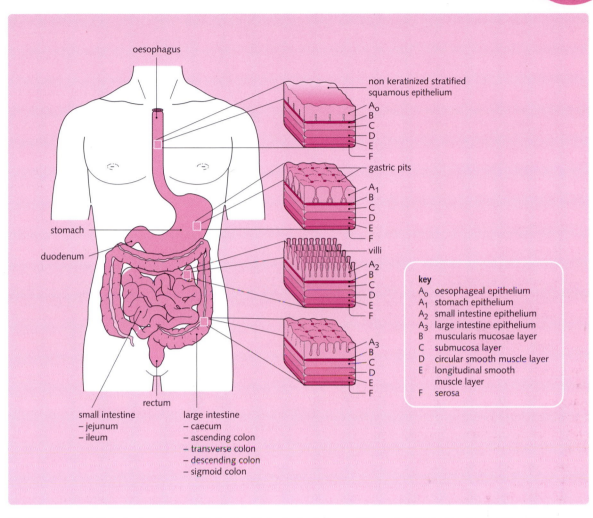

oesophagus

non keratinized stratified
squamous epithelium

A_o
B
C
D
E
F

gastric pits

A_1
B
C
D
E
F

villi

A_2
B
C
D
E
F

stomach

duodenum

key
A_o oesophageal epithelium
A_1 stomach epithelium
A_2 small intestine epithelium
A_3 large intestine epithelium
B muscularis mucosae layer
C submucosa layer
D circular smooth muscle layer
E longitudinal smooth
   muscle layer
F serosa

A_3
B
C
D
E
F

rectum

small intestine
– jejunum
– ileum

large intestine
– caecum
– ascending colon
– transverse colon
– descending colon
– sigmoid colon

Fig. 1.13 The gastrointestinal system. The illustration shows the basic layers of the gastrointestinal tract wall with epithelial adaptions, which dictate function.

- Metabolism of vitamin D.
- Blood pressure and sodium regulation (renin secretion).
- Rate of red blood cell production, e.g. erythropoietin secretion.

The ureters and bladder have a muscular wall and are lined by urothelium (transitional epithelium). This is a specialized stratified epithelium allowing distension, especially of the bladder to accommodate large volumes of fluid.

RADIOLOGICAL ANATOMY

Introduction

The use of plain radiography is frequently requested to detect and aid the diagnosis of disease within the thorax, abdomen or in bones. Using contrast studies to distinguish adjacent structures of similar lucency on a film can enhance the clinical usefulness of this investigation, especially in the gastrointestinal tract to detect a perforation of the bowel wall or a lesion. A contrast study uses a substance, e.g. barium, which appears radio-opaque (white) on an X-ray film and allows internal anatomical structures not normally seen to be visualized. The contrast study can be single

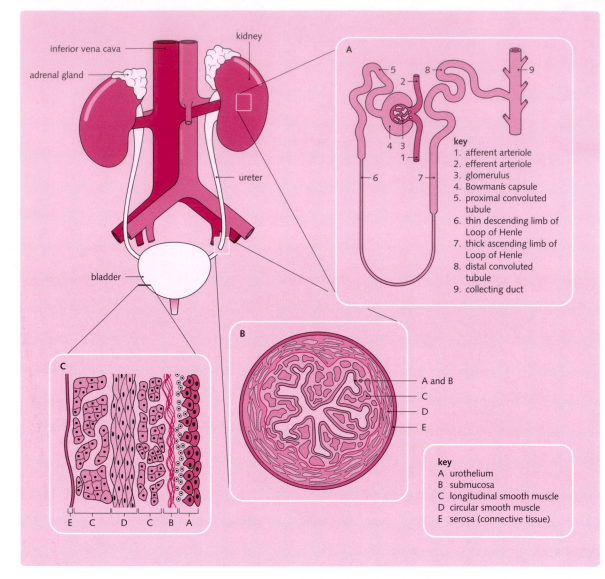

Fig. 1.14 Components of the urinary tract. Inset A shows the structure of a nephron, inset B shows the structure of the ureter and inset C shows the structure of the bladder wall.

(when only barium is used) or double when both barium and air are introduced into the intestines.

Angiography is a procedure in which a contrast medium is injected into an artery or vein via a percutaneous catheter. It is used to assess vascular disease such as atherosclerosis (fatty plaques) in the coronary arteries or an aneurysm (a balloon-like swelling) in the abdominal aorta.

The following chapters will introduce normal radiographic anatomical structures and give a method for reading X-rays because they will be presented to you not only in your anatomy studies but also in the clinical years. The pre-registration house officer will usually be expected to perform the initial interpretation of an X-ray.

The upper limb

2

Objectives

In this chapter you will learn to:

- Describe the superficial veins of the upper limb and common venepuncture sites.
- Describe the lymphatic drainage of the upper limb.
- Describe the bones and joints of the pectoral girdle.
- Understand the anatomy of the shoulder joint.
- Describe components and actions of the rotator cuff muscles.
- List the movements of the shoulder joint and know the muscles causing them.
- State the boundaries and know contents of the axilla.
- Describe the formation of the brachial plexus between the neck and axilla.
- Name the muscles and their nerve supply that are involved in elbow flexion and extension.
- Describe the vessels of the arm and their branches.
- State the boundaries and know contents of the cubital fossa.
- Understand the anatomy of the elbow joint.
- Name the muscles involved in wrist and digit movement.
- Outline the boundaries and contents of the anatomical snuffbox.
- Outline the cutaneous nerve supply of the hand.
- Discuss the synovial sheaths of the flexor tendons.
- Outline the carpal tunnel and the structures passing through it.
- Describe the intrinsic muscles of the hand.
- Describe a dorsal digital expansion.
- Describe the long flexor tendons within the hand and their sheaths.
- Recognize the bony features of a normal radiograph of the upper limb.
- Have a method for reviewing an upper limb X-ray.

REGIONS AND COMPONENTS OF THE UPPER LIMB

The upper limb is joined to the trunk by the pectoral girdle. The shoulder region is the area around the shoulder joint and pectoral girdle. The arm lies between the shoulder and the elbow. The forearm lies between the elbow and the wrist (radiocarpal joint). The hand is distal to the radiocarpal joint.

The pectoral girdle is composed of the scapula and clavicle, which articulate at the acromioclavicular joint. The sternoclavicular joint is the only joint between the pectoral girdle and the axial skeleton. All the remaining attachments to the axial skeleton are muscular. The humerus lies in the arm. It articulates proximally with the glenoid fossa of scapula to form the glenohumeral joint and distally with the ulna and radius at the elbow joint. The radius articulates with the carpal bones at the radiocarpal joint.

The subclavian artery is the major arterial supply of the upper limb. It arises from the brachiocephalic trunk on the right side and directly from the aorta on the left side. It continues as the axillary artery and then as the brachial artery within the arm. In the cubital fossa (anterior to the elbow joint) it divides into the radial and ulnar arteries that supply the forearm and hand.

Blood is returned to the axillary vein, which becomes the subclavian vein. Superficial veins drain into the axillary vein.

The nerve supply to the upper limb is derived from the brachial plexus: the median, musculocutaneous and ulnar nerves supply the anterior compartment; the posterior compartment is supplied by the radial nerve.

Surface anatomy

Surface anatomy of the shoulder region is shown in Figure 2.1.

Clavicle

The shape of the bone is like an italic letter *f*. It is palpable along its length. The medial two-thirds are convex anteriorly and its sternal end articulates with the superior border of the sternum at the suprasternal notch. Medially the attachments of the pectoralis major and sternocleidomastoid muscles obscure the bone.

The lateral third is concave anteriorly, its acromial end articulating with the acromial process of the scapula to form the acromioclavicular joint.

Scapula

The tip of the coracoid process can be felt on deep palpation in the lateral part of the deltopectoral

triangle—a small depression situated below the outer third of the clavicle, bounded by the pectoralis major and deltoid muscles. The deltoid muscle forms the smooth round curve of the shoulder.

The acromion process is easily located in its subcutaneous position forming the point of the shoulder.

The spine of the scapula may be palpated (felt) and followed to its medial border. Inferiorly, the medial (vertebral) border of the scapula can be traced to the inferior angle of the scapula (opposite the T7 vertebral spine).

Axilla and axillary folds

The anterior and posterior axillary folds may be palpated. The anterior fold contains the pectoralis major muscle. The posterior fold contains the teres major and latissumus dorsi muscles. The head of the humerus can be palpated through the floor of the axilla (armpit).

Elbow region

The medial and lateral epicondyles of the humerus and the olecranon process of the ulna can be palpated. The head of the radius can be palpated in a depression on the posterior aspect of the extended elbow, distal to the lateral epicondyle. The cubital fossa lies anterior to the elbow joint. The biceps brachii tendon is palpable as it enters the fossa.

The brachial artery may be palpated as it passes down the medial aspect of the arm as well as in the cubital fossa, medial to the biceps brachii tendon.

Wrist and hand

The styloid processes of the radius and ulna may be palpated at the wrist. The radial artery can be palpated laterally on the anterior surface of the wrist.

The anatomical snuffbox is seen on the lateral part of the wrist and is a depression between forearm extensor compartment muscle tendons to the thumb (pollux).

Anteriorly at the wrist, the scaphoid tuberosity and the pisiform bone can be seen and palpated laterally and medially respectively. The majority of the anterior surface of the carpus is covered by the long flexor tendons of the forearm muscles and intrinsic hand muscles.

On the posterior aspect of the hand, the metacarpal bones can be palpated and the extensor tendons that

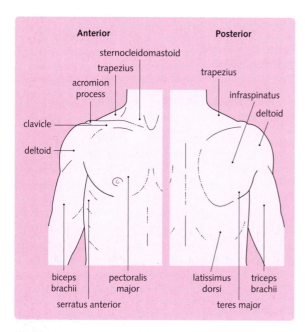

Fig. 2.1 Surface anatomy of the anterior and posterior views of the shoulder region.

cover them are seen. The metacarpal heads form the knuckles of a clenched fist. Anteriorly the metacarpal heads are hidden by an overlying aponeurosis, intrinsic muscles and long flexor tendons.

Musculature

The anterior border of trapezius runs from medial to lateral above the clavicle. The superior fibres of the trapezius muscle attach to the lateral third of the clavicle. The lateral border of latissimus dorsi may be traced superiorly and forms the posterior axillary fold.

The pectoralis major muscle covers a large part of the anterior chest wall and is traced laterally, forming the anterior axillary fold. The serratus anterior muscle can be seen laterally on the chest wall as six serrations during arm abduction, as it rotates the scapula and allows the arm to be raised above the shoulder joint.

In the arm, biceps brachii is seen as a rounded mass on contraction. The tendon of the long head of biceps brachii is palpable in the intertubercular groove (between the greater and lesser tubercles). At rest in the lower part of the arm, brachialis is seen either side of biceps brachii. Posteriorly triceps brachii emerges from under deltoid.

Individual forearm muscles appear as one mass proximally. However, identifiable tendons over the anterior aspect of the radiocarpal joint include (from medial to lateral) flexor carpi ulnaris, flexor digitorum superficialis, palmaris longus and flexor capri radialis. Over the lateral aspect of the radiocarpal joint abductor pollicis longus, extensor pollicis brevis and longus forming the borders of the anatomical snuffbox.

The intrinsic muscles of the palm of the hand form the thenar eminence laterally and the hypothenar eminence medially. On the dorsal surface, the dorsal interossei are localized masses between metacarpal bones.

Superficial venous drainage

The dorsal and the palmar veins of the hand drain into the dorsal venous network (Fig. 2.2). From this the medial basilic and lateral cephalic veins arise, and they ascend in the forearm to the arm. The basilic vein, halfway up the arm, pierces the deep fascia, and drains into the brachial vein. The cephalic vein passes onto the anterolateral aspect of the forearm, and communicates anterior to the cubital fossa with the basilic vein via the median cubital vein—this last vein is usually easy to identify and it is frequently used for

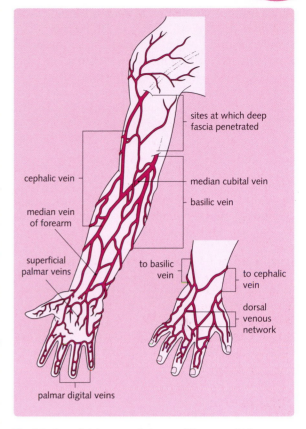

Fig. 2.2 Superficial venous drainage of the upper limb.

venepuncture. The cephalic vein continues laterally up the arm to the deltopectoral groove before piercing the deep fascia in the infraclavicular fossa, and drains into the axillary vein.

Lymphatic drainage

Lymphatics in the hand coalesce to form trunks that ascend the forearm and the arm with the cephalic and basilic veins and the deep veins. Vessels accompanying the cephalic vein drain into the infraclavicular nodes or the axillary nodes. Some vessels along the basilic vein

General practitioner

Venepuncture is a procedure that allows blood to be taken or the administration of medication via an intravenous catheter. A common site is the median cubital vein within the cubital fossa. A tourniquet is applied above the cubital fossa to hinder venous return and make the vein more prominent.

are interrupted at the elbow by a supratrochlear node, but ultimately they all drain into the axillary nodes. Lymph from the axillary nodes drains to the apical then supraclavicular nodes and finally into the subclavian trunk. This is joined by the jugular trunks (containing lymph from head and neck) and drain either to the right lymphatic trunk or thoracic duct before emptying into the subclavian vein.

Cutaneous innervation of the upper limb

Figures 2.3 and 2.4 illustrate the dermatomes and cutaneous innervation of the upper limb, respectively. This knowledge aids a differential diagnosis of the level of a spinal nerve injury or lesion from peripheral nerve damage and sensory loss.

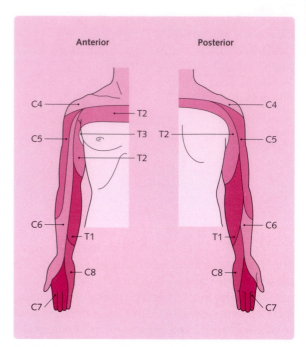

Fig. 2.3 Dermatomes of the upper limb.

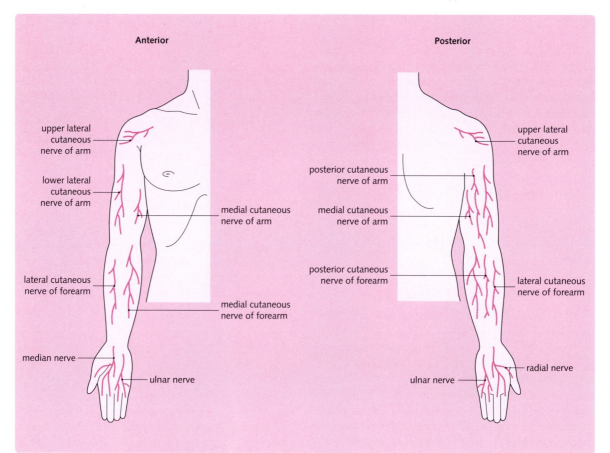

Fig. 2.4 Cutaneous innervation of the upper limb.

THE SHOULDER REGION AND AXILLA

Pectoral girdle

The pectoral girdle (clavicle and scapula) suspends the upper limb and holds the upper limb away from the trunk (Fig. 2.5). The girdle itself is suspended from the head and neck by the trapezius muscle. It articulates directly with the axial skeleton only via the sternoclavicular joint; the remaining attachments are muscular. This partly accounts for the great mobility of the shoulder girdle.

Clavicle

The clavicle is subcutaneous, and it articulates with the sternum medially and with the acromion process of the scapula laterally (Fig. 2.6). It has a longitudinal groove on its inferior surface for insertion of the subclavius muscle and laterally there is a roughened

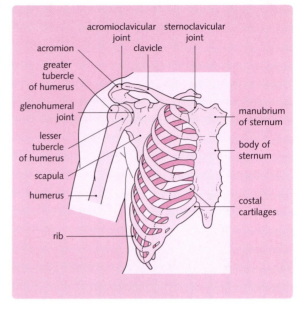

Fig. 2.5 Skeleton of the pectoral girdle.

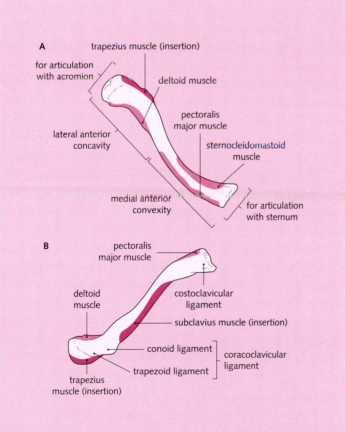

Fig. 2.6 Superior (A) and inferior (B) aspects of the right clavicle and its muscular attachments.

area for attachment of the trapezoid part of the coracoclavicular ligament. A conoid tubercle provides attachment for the conoid part of the coracoclavicular ligament. Medially at the sternal end, a roughened area is the site of attachment for the costoclavicular ligament. These strong ligaments prevent joint dislocation.

Joints of the pectoral girdle

Sternoclavicular joint

This is an atypical synovial joint because the articular surfaces are covered by fibrocartilage, not hyaline cartilage. A capsule surrounds the joint and is reinforced by anterior and posterior sternoclavicular ligaments. These ligaments are attached to the clavicle and the manubrium of the sternum. The costoclavicular ligament running between the clavicle and the first rib strengthens the joint. An articular disc is attached to the capsule, dividing the joint into two cavities, preventing the clavicle from overriding the sternum.

As the lateral end of the clavicle moves, its medial end moves in the opposite direction, moving around the axis of the coracoclavicular ligaments.

The joint is supplied by the medial supraclavicular nerve (C3–C4) from the cervical plexus.

Acromioclavicular joint

This is where the lateral end of the clavicle articulates with the medial border of the acromion. It is an atypical synovial joint, the articular surfaces being fibrocartilage.

A weak capsule surrounds the articular surfaces. It is reinforced by the acromioclavicular ligament superiorly. The coracoclavicular ligament is very strong. It is composed of a conoid and a trapezoid part, which run between the inferior surface of the

clavicle and the coracoid process. This is the major factor in joint stability.

Movements are passive as no muscle connects the bones to move the joint. Scapular movements involve movement at both ends of the clavicle.

The joint is supplied by the lateral supraclavicular nerve (C3–C4).

Scapula

The scapula is a triangular flat bone lying on the posterior thoracic wall. It has superior, medial, and lateral borders, and superior and inferior angles (Fig. 2.7). The glenoid cavity articulates with the head of the humerus. The coracoid process projects upwards and forwards anterior to the glenoid cavity, and it provides attachment for muscles and ligaments.

The subscapular fossa lies on the anterior surface; the supraspinous and infraspinous fossae are on the posterior surface, divided by the spine of the scapula, which expands laterally as the acromion above the glenoid cavity. The scapula is attached medially to the vertebral column by muscles, e.g. levator scapulae, trapezius and rhomboideus major and minor. Laterally it attaches to the humerus via the rotator cuff, and deltoid muscles.

Humerus

The upper end of the humerus is shown in Figure 2.8. The head articulates with the glenoid cavity of the scapula. The surgical neck is a common fracture site and is related to the axillary nerve. The spiral groove of the humerus is related to the radial nerve.

Shoulder joint

At the shoulder (glenohumeral) joint, the humeral head articulates with the glenoid cavity of the scapula (Fig. 2.9). It is a multiaxial, ball-and-socket synovial joint. A rim of fibrocartilage is attached to the margins

Fig. 2.7 Anterior (A), posterior (B), and lateral (C) aspects of the right scapula and its muscular attachments.

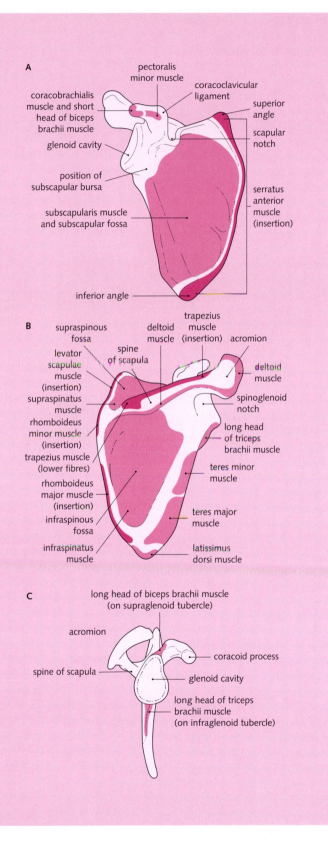

A

pectoralis minor muscle

coracoclavicular ligament

coracobrachialis muscle and short head of biceps brachii muscle

superior angle

scapular notch

glenoid cavity

position of subscapular bursa

serratus anterior muscle (insertion)

subscapularis muscle and subscapular fossa

inferior angle

B

supraspinous fossa

deltoid muscle

trapezius muscle (insertion)

acromion

spine of scapula

levator scapulae muscle (insertion)

deltoid muscle

supraspinatus muscle

spinoglenoid notch

rhomboideus minor muscle (insertion)

long head of triceps brachii muscle

trapezius muscle (lower fibres)

teres minor muscle

rhomboideus major muscle (insertion)

infraspinous fossa

teres major muscle

infraspinatus muscle

latissimus dorsi muscle

C

long head of biceps brachii muscle (on supraglenoid tubercle)

acromion

coracoid process

spine of scapula

glenoid cavity

long head of triceps brachii muscle (on infraglenoid tubercle)

Fig. 2.8 (A) Anterior and (B) posterior views of the upper end of the humerus and its muscle attachments.

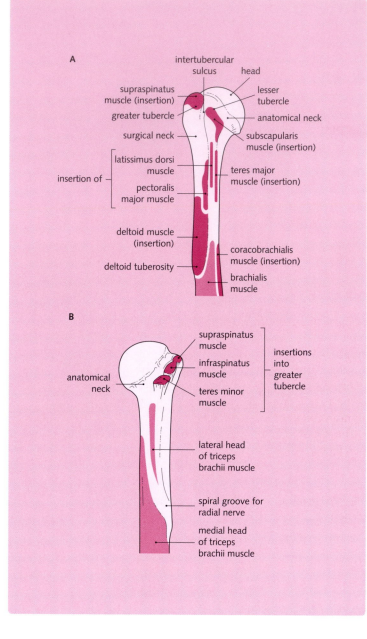

of the glenoid cavity; it is called the glenoid labrum, which deepens the shallow glenoid fossa.

A fibrous capsule surrounds the joint, which is attached to the margins of the glenoid labrum and to the humerus around the anatomical neck. The capsule is strong but loose, allowing great mobility. It is strengthened by the tendons of the rotator cuff. The long tendon of biceps brachii passes into the capsule to attach to the supraglenoid tubercle and is therefore intracapsular. The synovial membrane lines the capsule and part of the neck of the humerus. It communicates anteriorly with the subscapular bursa through a defect in the joints fibrous capsule and invests the long head of biceps brachii in a tubular synovial sheath.

The glenohumeral ligaments are three thickenings that strengthen the capsule anteriorly. The capsule is also reinforced superiorly by the strong coracohumeral ligament. The coracoacromial ligament forms an arch above the joint, and it prevents superior dislocation.

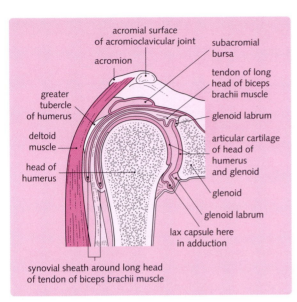

Fig. 2.9 Shoulder joint and related structures.

The shoulder joint is inherently unstable owing to the very large head of the humerus compared with the shallow glenoid cavity. Factors stabilizing the shoulder joint are the glenoid labrum, all the ligaments, and the rotator cuff muscles. The nerve supply to the joint is from the lateral pectoral nerve, the suprascapular nerve, and the axillary nerve.

The movements at the shoulder joint, and the muscles performing them, are described in Figure 2.10.

Fig. 2.10 Movements of the shoulder joint and the muscles performing them

Movement	Muscles
Flexion	Pectoralis major, anterior fibres of deltoid
Extension	Posterior fibres of deltoid, latissimus dorsi, teres major
Abduction	Deltoid, supraspinatus
Adduction	Pectoralis major, latissimus dorsi, subscapularis, teres major, infraspinatus
Lateral rotation	Infraspinatus, teres minor, posterior fibres of deltoid
Medial rotation	Pectoralis major, anterior fibres of deltoid, latissimus dorsi, teres major, subscapularis
Circumduction	Varying combinations of flexion, extension, abduction, and adduction muscles

The movement of abduction deserves special mention: a maximum of 120° of abduction is possible at the glenohumeral joint. Further movement is obtained by rotating the inferior angle of the scapula laterally and anteriorly, turning the glenoid fossa upwards. This is achieved by serratus anterior and trapezius.

Rotator cuff

The rotator cuff consists of the subscapularis, supraspinatus, infraspinatus and teres minor. The tendons of these muscles surround the shoulder joint on all sides except inferiorly, and they blend with the capsule. They help to keep the large humeral head applied to the shallow glenoid cavity.

Muscles of the upper limb

Figure 2.11 outlines the major muscles of the upper limb.

Axilla

This pyramidal shaped space between the upper part of the humerus and thoracic wall contains the major vessels and nerves from the neck, which supply the upper limb. They enter through the apex of the axilla and then pass distally into the arm. The boundaries of the axilla are:

- Anteriorly: clavipectoral fascia, pectoralis major and minor muscles.
- Posteriorly: subscapularis, latissimus dorsi, and teres major muscles.
- Medially: the upper four ribs, intercostal, and serratus anterior muscles.
- Laterally: intertubercular sulcus, coracobrachialis, and biceps brachii muscles.
- The apex communicates with the root of the neck between the clavicle, first rib and the superior border of the scapula.
- The base is composed of skin and axillary fascia.

The clavipectoral fascia is a strong sheet of connective tissue that attaches to the clavicle and encloses the subclavius muscle. Below, it splits to enclose pectoralis minor and continues as the suspensory ligament of the axilla.

The following structures pass through the clavipectoral fascia:

- Cephalic vein.
- Thoracoacromial artery.

Fig. 2.11 Major muscles of the upper limb

Name of muscle (nerve supply)	Origin	Insertion	Action
Latissimus dorsi (thoracodorsal nerve)	Iliac crest, lumbar fascia, spinal processes of lower six thoracic vertebrae, lower ribs, scapula	Floor of intertubercular sulcus of humerus	Extends, adducts, and medially rotates arm
Levator scapulae (C3 and C4 and dorsal scapular nerve)	Transverse processes of C1–C4	Medial border of scapula	Elevates scapula
Rhomboideus minor (dorsal scapular nerve)	Ligamentum nuchae, spines of C7 and T1	Medial border of scapula	Elevates and retracts medial border of scapula
Rhomboideus major (dorsal scapular nerve)	Spines of T2–T5	Medial border of scapula	Elevates and retracts medial border of scapula
Trapezius (spinal part of XI nerve and C2 and C3)	Occipital bone, ligamentum nuchae, spinous processes of thoracic vertebrae	Lateral third of clavicle, acromion, spine of scapula	Elevates scapula, pulls scapula medially and pulls medial border of scapula downward
Subclavius (nerve to subclavius)	First costal cartilage	Clavicle	Depresses and stabilizes the clavicle
Pectoralis major (medial and lateral pectoral nerves)	Clavicle, sternum, upper six costal cartilages	Lateral lip of intertubercular sulcus of humerus	Adducts arm, rotates it medially, and flexes humerus
Pectoralis minor (medial pectoral nerve)	Third, fourth, and fifth ribs	Coracoid process of scapula	Depresses point of shoulder protracts shoulder
Serratus anterior (long thoracic nerve)	Upper eight ribs	Medial border and inferior angle of scapula	Pulls scapula forwards and rotates it
Deltoid (axillary nerve)	Clavicle, acromion, spine of scapula	Lateral surface of humerus (deltoid tubercle)	Abducts, flexes and medially rotates, extends, and laterally rotates arm
Supraspinatus (suprascapular nerve)	Supraspinous fossa of scapula	Greater tubercle of humerus, capsule of shoulder joint	Initiates abduction of the arm
Subscapularis (upper and lower subscapular nerves)	Subscapular fossa	Lesser tubercle of humerus	Medially rotates arm
Teres major (lower subscapular nerve)	Lateral border of scapula	Medial lip of intertubercular sulcus of humerus	Medially rotates and adducts arm
Teres minor (axillary nerve)	Lateral border of scapula	Greater tubercle of humerus, capsule of shoulder joint	Laterally rotates arm
Infraspinatus (suprascapular nerve)	Infraspinous fossa of scapula	Greater tubercle of humerus, capsule of shoulder joint	Laterally rotates arm

- Lymphatic vessels from the infraclavicular nodes.
- Lateral pectoral nerve.

The contents of the axilla are shown in Figure 2.12 and include:

- Axillary artery.
- Axillary vein.

- Brachial plexus.
- Axillary lymph nodes.

Axillary artery

The axillary artery is a continuation of the third part of the subclavian artery, and it commences at the outer

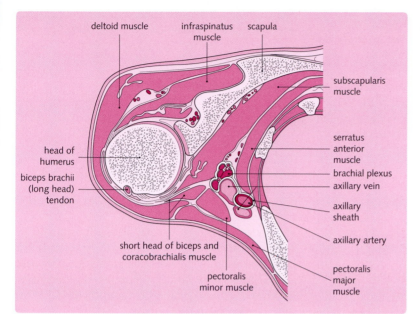

Fig. 2.12 A horizontal cross-section demonstrating the contents and muscular boundaries of the axilla.

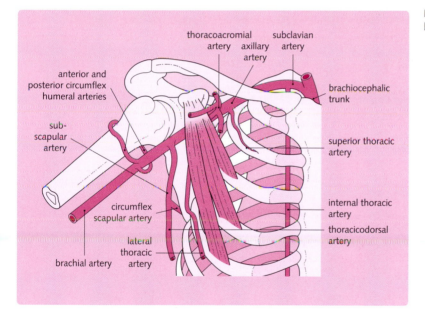

Fig. 2.13 Axillary artery and its branches.

border of the first rib. It is invested in fascia (axillary sheath), with the brachial plexus, derived from the prevertebral fascia (part of the deep cervical fascia of the neck). The axillary artery becomes the brachial artery at the lower border of teres major. It is divided into three parts by pectoralis minor (Fig. 2.13):

- The first part has one branch—the superior thoracic artery. This supplies both pectoral muscles and the thoracic wall.

- The second part has two branches—the thoracoacromial artery supplies the sternoclavicular joint, pectoral, and deltoid muscles. The lateral thoracic artery supplies serratus anterior, breast, and the axillary nodes.
- The third part has three branches—the subscapular artery supplies latissimus dorsi and forms part of a scapular anastomosis. The anterior and posterior circumflex humeral arteries supply the shoulder joint.

Axillary vein

The axillary vein is the continuation of the venae comitantes of the brachial artery, which are joined by the basilic vein. It commences at the lower border of teres major and ascends through the axilla medial to the axillary artery. At the outer border of the first rib, it becomes the subclavian vein. The axillary vein lies outside the axillary sheath. This allows expansion and increased venous return during exercise.

Brachial plexus

The brachial plexus is formed from the anterior rami of spinal nerves C5–C8 and T1. Figure 2.14 demonstrates that the plexus is divided into roots (deep to the scalene muscles), trunks (found in the posterior triangle of the neck), divisions (behind the clavicle)

Surgery

During breast surgery, involving the removal of axillary lymph nodes, conservation of nerves is paramount. The long thoracic nerve is at risk of damage as it crosses the thoracic wall from the brachial plexus to supply serratus anterior. Damage causes paralysis of this muscle and 'winging' of the scapula, demonstrated by pushing the affected arm against a wall. The patient has difficulty raising her arm above the head.

and cords (named with their respect to the axillary artery). Figure 2.15 tabulates the branches.

Axillary lymph nodes

These comprise (Fig. 2.16):

1. Lateral group.
2. Pectoral group.
3. Subscapular group.
4. Central group.
5. Infraclavicular group (receives lymph from upper limb).
6. Apical group.

These nodes receive lymph from the upper limb as well as from the lateral part of the breast. The lateral, pectoral and subscapular groups drain into the central group of nodes. The central and infraclavicular groups of nodes drain into the apical then into the supraclavicular nodes.

Quadrangular and triangular spaces

A number of spaces are formed by the muscles and bones in the axillary region (Fig. 2.17). The triangular space contains the circumflex scapular artery, a branch of the subscapular artery which, with the dorsal scapular and suprascapular arteries, forms a collateral circulation should the second part of the axillary artery be occluded. The quadrangular

Fig. 2.14 Brachial plexus showing the trunks, divisions, cords and branches.

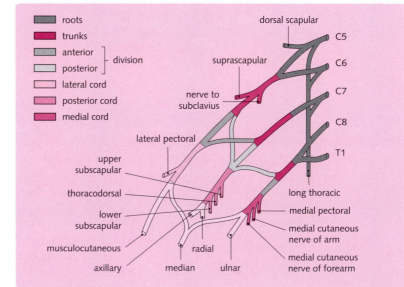

Fig. 2.15 Branches of the brachial plexus and their distribution

Branches	Distribution
Roots	
Dorsal scapular nerve (C5)	Rhomboid major, rhomboid minor, and levator scapulae muscles
Long thoracic nerve (C5–C7)	Serratus anterior muscle
Upper trunk	
Suprascapular nerve (C5, C6)	Supraspinatus and infraspinatus muscles
Nerve to subclavius (C5, C6)	Subclavius muscle
Lateral cord	
Lateral pectoral nerve (C5–C7)	Pectoralis major muscle
Musculocutaneous nerve (C5–C7)	Coracobrachialis, biceps brachii, brachialis muscles, and the skin along the lateral border of the forearm (lateral cutaneous nerve of the forearm)
Lateral root of median nerve (C5–C7)	Joins the medial root (C8, T1) to form the median nerve (see below)
Posterior cord	
Upper subscapular nerve (C5–C6)	Subscapularis muscle
Thoracodorsal nerve (C6–C8)	Latissimus dorsi muscle
Lower subscapular nerve (C5–C6)	Subscapularis and teres major muscles
Axillary nerve (C5–C6)	Deltoid and teres minor muscles. Skin over the lower half of the deltoid muscle (upper lateral cutaneous nerve of arm)
Radial nerve (C5–C8, T1)	Triceps, brachialis, anconeus, and posterior muscles of forearm. Skin of the posterior aspects of arm, forearm, the lateral half of the dorsum of the hand, and dorsal surface of the lateral three and a half digits.
Medial cord	
Medial pectoral nerve (C8, T1)	Pectoralis major and minor muscles
Medial cutaneous nerve of the arm (C8, T1)	Skin of the medial side of the arm
Medial cutaneous nerve of the forearm (C8, T1)	Skin of the medial side of the forearm
Ulnar nerve (C8, T1)	Flexor carpi ulnaris and medial half of flexor digitorum profundus (in forearm). Hypothenar, adductor pollicis, third and fourth lumbrical, interossei, palmaris brevis muscles (in hand). Skin of the medial half of the dorsum and palm of hand, skin of the palmar, and dorsal surfaces of the medial one and a half digits (palmar and dorsal digital cutaneous branches).
Median nerve (C5–C8, T1)	(In forearm) pronator teres, flexor carpi radialis, flexor digitorum superficialis (median nerve). Flexor pollicis longus, lateral half of flexor digitorum profundus and pronator quadratus (anterior interosseous branch). (In hand) thenar muscles, first two lumbricals (median nerve). Skin of lateral half of palm and palmar surface of lateral three and a half digits (palmar and digital cutaneous branches).

space allows passage of the axillary nerve and posterior circumflex artery as it winds around the surgical neck of the humerus. The triangular interval (lower triangular space) contains the radial nerve and profunda brachii artery within the radial groove of humerus.

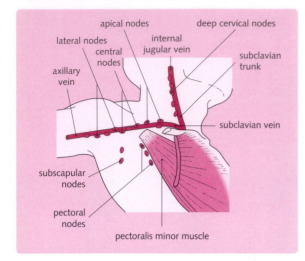
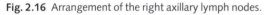

Fig. 2.16 Arrangement of the right axillary lymph nodes.

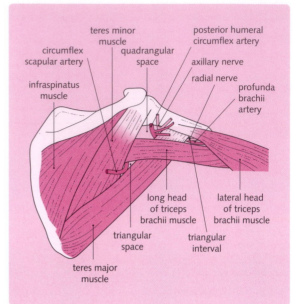

Fig. 2.17 Quadrangular and triangular spaces.

THE ARM

The arm lies between the shoulder and elbow joint. The anterior and posterior compartments are separated by the medial and lateral intermuscular septa. These septa arise from the deep fascia surrounding the arm. The lateral intermuscular septum extends from the lateral lip of the intertubercular sulcus to the lateral epicondyle of the humerus. The medial intermuscular septum extends from the medial lip of the intertubercular sulcus to the medial epicondyle of the humerus.

Flexor compartment of the arm

The bony skeleton of the arm and the muscle attachments of the anterior compartment are shown in Figure 2.18.

Muscles of the arm

The muscles of the arm are shown in Figure 2.19.

To remember the contents of the anterior arm compartment use the mnemonic B, B, C (biceps brachii, brachialis and coracobrachialis). All are innervated by the musculocutaneous nerve.

Vessels of the arm

Brachial artery

The brachial artery is a continuation of the axillary artery, commencing at the lower border of teres major (Fig. 2.20). It terminates at the neck of the radius by dividing into the radial and ulnar arteries. This artery and its profunda brachii branch supply the anterior and posterior compartments of the arm respectively. Collateral branches anastomose with recurrent radial and ulnar branches to form a collateral circulation around the elbow. The artery is very superficial throughout its course, being covered by skin and fascia only. It lies deep to the medial border of biceps brachii.

Brachial veins

Usually a pair of venae comitantes accompany the brachial artery. They are joined by tributaries that correspond to branches of the brachial arteries. The veins receive the basilic vein before becoming the axillary vein at the inferior border of the teres major muscle.

Nerves of the arm

Musculocutaneous nerve

After its formation, the musculocutaneous nerve passes through coracobrachialis and runs down

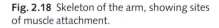

Fig. 2.18 Skeleton of the arm, showing sites of muscle attachment.

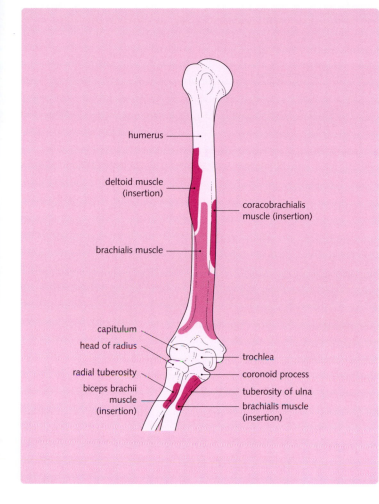

humerus

deltoid muscle (insertion)

coracobrachialis muscle (insertion)

brachialis muscle

capitulum
head of radius

trochlea

radial tuberosity

coronoid process

biceps brachii muscle (insertion)

tuberosity of ulna

brachialis muscle (insertion)

between biceps and brachialis to reach the lateral aspect of brachialis. It supplies the muscles of the anterior compartment, and it terminates by piercing the deep fascia to become the lateral cutaneous nerve of the forearm.

Median nerve

The median nerve enters the arm on the lateral side of the brachial artery and crosses in front of the artery to be on its medial side. It continues to the cubital fossa in this relationship, where it is crossed by the bicipital aponeurosis. The median nerve has a branch to pronator teres that arises above the elbow joint, i.e. in the arm.

Ulnar nerve

The ulnar nerve passes down the arm medial to the brachial artery. It pierces the medial intermuscular septum halfway down, and accompanied by the superior ulnar collateral artery, it enters the posterior compartment. It continues between the medial intermuscular septum and the medial head of triceps, then, on the posterior aspect of the medial epicondyle of the humerus, it enters the forearm between the heads of flexor carpi ulnaris muscle. The ulnar nerve has no branches in the arm.

Radial nerve

The radial nerve enters the posterior compartment of the arm by passing over the lower border of teres

Pressure on the ulnar nerve as it crosses behind the medial epicondyle results in a tingling sensation in the medial one and a half digits—this area is referred to as the 'funny bone'.

Fig. 2.19 Muscles of the upper arm. (Adapted from *Clinical Anatomy, An Illustrated Review with Questions and Explanations*, 2nd edn, by R S Snell Little Brown & Co)

Name of muscle (nerve supply)	Origin	Insertion	Action
Anterior fascial compartment			
Biceps brachii—long head (musculocutaneous nerve)	Supraglenoid tubercle of scapula	Tuberosity of radius and bicipital aponeurosis into deep fascia of forearm	Supinator of flexed forearm, flexor of elbow joint, weak flexor of shoulder joint
Biceps brachii—short head (musculocutaneous nerve)	Coracoid process of scapula	Tuberosity of radius and bicipital aponeurosis into deep fascia of forearm	Supinator of flexed forearm, flexor of elbow joint, weak flexor of shoulder joint
Coracobrachialis (musculocutaneous nerve)	Coracoid process of scapula	Shaft of humerus	Flexes and adducts shoulder joint
Brachialis (musculocutaneous nerve and radial nerve)	Anterior surface of humerus	Ulnar tuberosity and coronoid process	Flexes elbow joint
Posterior fascial compartment			
Triceps—long head (radial nerve)	Infraglenoid tubercle of scapula	Olecranon process of ulna	Extends elbow joint
Triceps—lateral head (radial nerve)	Posterior surface of humerus (upper part)	Olecranon process of ulna	Extends elbow joint
Triceps—medial head (radial nerve)	Posterior surface of humerus (lower part)	Olecranon process of ulna	Extends elbow joint

major through the triangular interval (Fig. 2.10). It runs, with the profunda brachii artery, in the spiral groove of the humerus. The nerve enters the anterior compartment of the arm and then passes into the forearm, deep to the brachioradialis muscle.

Branches in the axilla and arm comprise muscular branches to the three heads of triceps brachii and anconeus, and the posterior cutaneous nerve of the arm, the lower lateral cutaneous nerve of the arm, and the posterior cutaneous nerve of the forearm.

Branches at the level of the elbow joint comprise muscular branches to the lateral fibres of brachioradialis and extensor carpi radialis longus.

The radial nerve runs in the spiral groove, and it can be damaged by midshaft fractures of the humerus. This paralyses extensor muscles of the forearm, causing wrist drop. The triceps brachii muscle is unaffected due to its nerve supply originating proximally.

THE CUBITAL FOSSA AND ELBOW JOINT

Cubital fossa

The cubital fossa is a triangular region lying anterior to the elbow joint. Its boundaries are:

- Lateral—brachioradialis muscle.
- Medial—pronator teres.
- Base—an imaginary line drawn between the two epicondyles of the humerus.
- Floor—the supinator and brachialis muscles.
- Roof—skin, fascia, and the bicipital aponeurosis.

Figure 2.21 shows the contents of the cubital fossa. Note:

- The lateral cutaneous nerve of the forearm emerges between biceps and brachialis.
- The radial nerve enters the anterior compartment between brachialis and brachioradialis.
- The brachial artery crosses the tendon of biceps, and it lies deep to the bicipital aponeurosis.

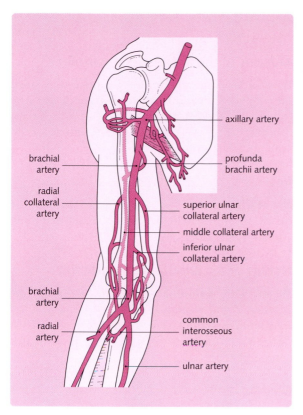

Fig. 2.20 Brachial artery and its branches.

- The median nerve lies medial to the brachial artery.
- The medial cutaneous nerve of the forearm lies superficial to pronator teres.
- Superficially, the median cubital vein lies between the basilic and cephalic veins.

Elbow joint

The elbow joint is a synovial hinge joint between the distal end of the humerus and the proximal end of the radius and the ulna (Fig. 2.22).

The articular surfaces comprise:

- Capitulum of the humerus and the head of the radius.
- Trochlea of the humerus and the trochlear notch of the ulna.

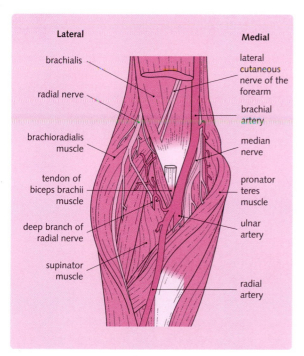

Fig. 2.21 Contents of the cubital fossa.

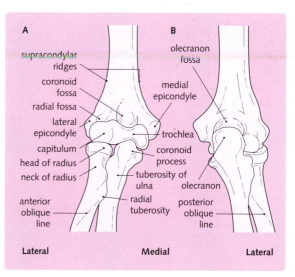

Fig. 2.22 Anterior (A) and posterior (B) aspects of the humerus and the upper end of the ulna and radius.

Movements of the elbow joint are limited to flexion and extension. Independent rotation of the radius occurs at the proximal radioulnar joint in the movements of pronation and supination of the forearm.

The capsule is lax anteroposteriorly, but it is strengthened medially and laterally by collateral ligaments.

Ligaments comprise:

- The ulnar collateral ligament—this triangular ligament consists of three bands, and it runs between the ulna and humerus.
- The radial collateral ligament—this is a band joining the lateral epicondyle of the humerus to the anular ligament.
- The anular ligament—this is attached to the margins of the radial notch of the ulna. It clasps the head and neck of the radius in the proximal radioulnar joint.

The nerve supply of the elbow joint consists of musculocutaneous, median, ulnar and radial nerves.

THE FOREARM

The forearm lies between the elbow and wrist joints. It is divided into anteriomedial and posteriolateral compartments (Fig. 2.23). The interosseous membrane is a thin strong membrane uniting the radius and ulnar bones at their interosseous borders. It provides attachments for muscles, and superiorly it is incomplete, allowing the posterior interosseus vessels to pass, while inferiorly it is pierced by the anterior interosseous vessels.

Remember that flexion and extension occur at the elbow joint; rotation occurs at the proximal and distal radioulnar joints.

Orthopaedics

A Colles fracture commonly occurs in postmenopausal osteoporotic women who fall onto an outstretched hand. Normally the radial styloid process is distal to the ulnar styloid process. In a Colles fracture the styloid processes are level. Other features include wrist (radial) abduction, posterior displacement of wrist, and dorsal angulation of hand. These features are seen on X-ray.

Anterior compartment of the forearm

Muscles of the anterior compartment

The muscles of the anterior compartment are divided into superficial and deep groups (Fig. 2.24). The superficial muscles arise from the medial supracondylar ridge and the medial epicondyle of the humerus (the common flexor origin).

Vessels of the anterior compartment

The brachial artery enters the forearm through the cubital fossa, and it divides into the radial and ulnar arteries (Fig. 2.25).

Nerves of the anterior compartment

The median and ulnar nerves pass through the anterior compartment, and they supply all the muscles in this compartment. The superficial branch of the radial nerve runs part of its course in this compartment.

Median nerve

This enters the forearm between the heads of pronator teres. It crosses the ulnar artery and then runs deep to flexor digitorum superficialis until just proximal to the wrist, where it appears between the tendon of this muscle and the tendon of flexor carpi radialis.

Branches of the median nerve in the forearm comprise:

- Anterior interosseous nerve. This leaves the median nerve as it passes through pronator teres. It joins the anterior interosseous artery and

Clinical examination

To check the patency of arterial supply to the hand, especially before performing an arterial blood gas procedure, it is prudent to perform Allen's test. Occlude both ulnar and radial arteries then get the patient to repeatedly flex fingers, causing an increase in venous return and the hand to become pale. Next, release one artery only and observe hand colour. If it goes pink again the artery is patent. Repeat again and release the other artery.

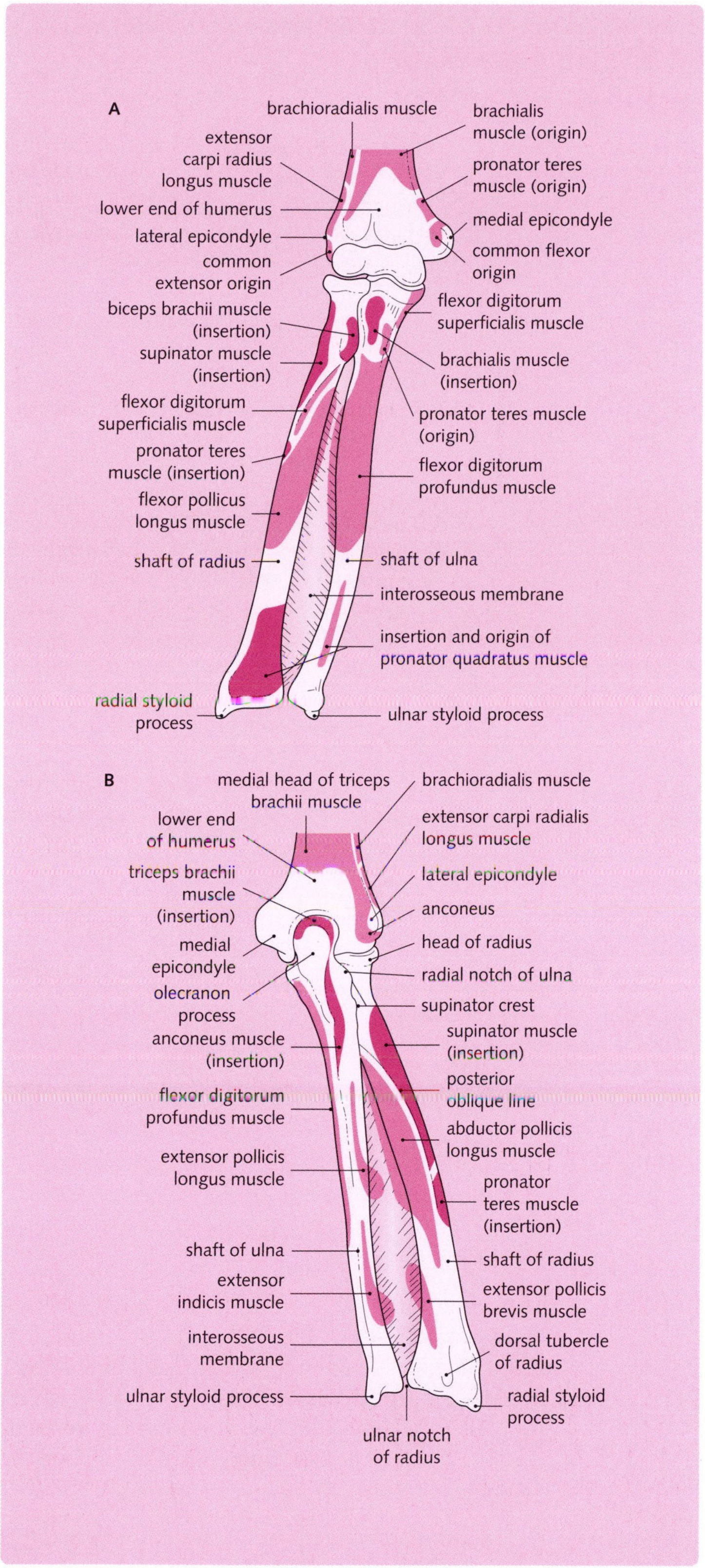

Fig. 2.23 Anterior (A) and posterior (B) aspects of the right radius and ulna, showing sites of muscular attachments.

A

brachioradialis muscle
brachialis muscle (origin)
extensor carpi radius longus muscle
pronator teres muscle (origin)
lower end of humerus
medial epicondyle
lateral epicondyle
common flexor origin
common extensor origin
biceps brachii muscle (insertion)
flexor digitorum superficialis muscle
supinator muscle (insertion)
brachialis muscle (insertion)
flexor digitorum superficialis muscle
pronator teres muscle (origin)
pronator teres muscle (insertion)
flexor digitorum profundus muscle
flexor pollicus longus muscle
shaft of radius
shaft of ulna
interosseous membrane
insertion and origin of pronator quadratus muscle
radial styloid process
ulnar styloid process

B

medial head of triceps brachii muscle
brachioradialis muscle
lower end of humerus
extensor carpi radialis longus muscle
triceps brachii muscle (insertion)
lateral epicondyle
anconeus
medial epicondyle
head of radius
olecranon process
radial notch of ulna
anconeus muscle (insertion)
supinator crest
supinator muscle (insertion)
flexor digitorum profundus muscle
posterior oblique line
extensor pollicis longus muscle
abductor pollicis longus muscle
pronator teres muscle (insertion)
shaft of ulna
shaft of radius
extensor indicis muscle
extensor pollicis brevis muscle
interosseous membrane
dorsal tubercle of radius
ulnar styloid process
radial styloid process
ulnar notch of radius

Fig. 2.24 Muscles of the anterior compartment of the forearm. (DIP, distal interphalangeal; PIP, proximal interphalangeal; MCP, metacarpophalangeal).

Name of muscle (nerve supply)	Origin	Insertion	Action
Superficial			
Flexor carpi radialis (median nerve)	Common flexor origin	Second and third metacarpal bones	Flexion and abduction of wrist joint
Flexor carpi ulnaris—humeral head (ulnar nerve)	Common flexor origin	Pisiform and through pisometacarpal ligament to fifth metacarpal bone	Flexion and abduction of wrist joint
Flexor carpi ulnaris—ulnar head (ulnar nerve)	Olecranon process and posterior border of ulna	Pisiform and through pisometacarpal ligament to fifth metacarpal bone	Flexion and abduction of wrist joint
Flexor digitorum superficialis— humeroulnar head (median nerve)	Common flexor origin and coronoid process of ulna	Middle phalanges of medial four digits	Flexion of PIP and MCP joints of the medial four digits and wrist joint
Flexor digitorum superficialis— radial head (median nerve)	Anterior oblique line of radius	Middle phalanges of medial four digits	Flexion of PIP and MCP joints of the medial four digits and wrist joint
Pronators teres—humeral head (median nerve)	Common flexor origin and medial supracondylar ridge	Lateral aspect of shaft of radius	Pronation of forearm and flexion of elbow
Pronator teres—ulnar head (median nerve)	Coronoid process of ulna	Lateral aspect of shaft of radius	Pronation of forearm
Palmaris longus (median nerve)	Common flexor origin	Palmar aponeurosis	Flexion of wrist joint
Deep			
Pronator quadratus (anterior interosseous nerve)	Anterior surface of ulna	Anterior surface of radius	Pronation of forearm
Flexor pollicis longus (anterior interosseous nerve)	Anterior surface of radius and interosseous membrane	Distal phalanx of thumb	Flexion of interphalangeal and MCP joints
Flexor digitorum profundus (medial half by ulnar nerve and lateral half by anterior interosseous nerve)	Anterior surface of ulna and interosseous membrane	Distal phalanges of medial four digits	Flexion of DIP, PIP, MCP, and wrist joint

passes down the forearm on the anterior surface of the interosseous membrane between flexor pollicis longus and flexor digitorum profundus. It supplies flexor pollicis longus, the lateral part of flexor digitorum profundus, and pronator quadratus, and it has articular branches to the distal radioulnar, wrist, and carpal joints.

- Muscular branches to the superficial muscles except flexor carpi ulnaris.
- Palmar cutaneous nerve. This is given off just proximal to the wrist joint. It supplies the skin over the thenar eminence and the central part of the palm of the hand.

- Articular branches to the elbow and proximal radioulnar joints.

Ulnar nerve

This enters the anterior compartment by passing between the heads of flexor carpi ulnaris. It runs with the ulnar artery between flexor carpi ulnaris and flexor digitorum profundus. In the lower half of the forearm, both artery and nerve become superficial on the lateral side of flexor carpi ulnaris.

Branches of the ulnar nerve comprise:

- Muscular branches to flexor carpi ulnaris and the medial half of flexor digitorum profundus.

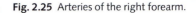

Fig. 2.25 Arteries of the right forearm.

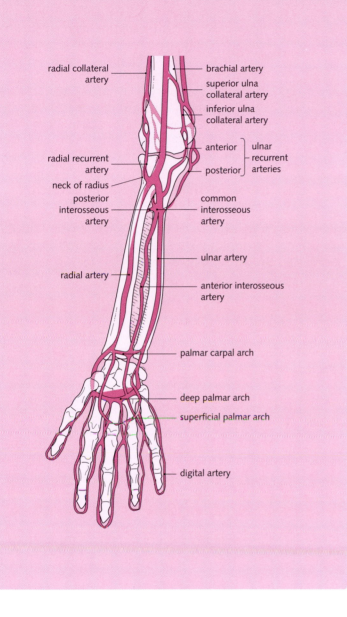

- radial collateral artery
- brachial artery
- superior ulna collateral artery
- inferior ulna collateral artery
- anterior | ulnar
- posterior | recurrent arteries
- radial recurrent artery
- neck of radius
- posterior interosseous artery
- common interosseous artery
- ulnar artery
- radial artery
- anterior interosseous artery
- palmar carpal arch
- deep palmar arch
- superficial palmar arch
- digital artery

- A palmar cutaneous branch, which supplies the skin over the medial part of the palm.
- A dorsal branch, which passes deep to flexor carpi ulnaris to reach the dorsal aspect of the hand and gives sensory innervation to the medial one and a half digits dorsally.

Radial nerve

This enters the forearm deep to the brachioradialis muscle. It immediately divides into a superficial and a deep branch. The deep branch passes laterally around the radius between the layers of supinator to enter the extensor compartment as the posterior interosseous nerve. The superficial branch continues distally in the forearm deep to brachioradialis, and it is joined by the radial artery. Both pass onto the dorsum of the hand. The radial nerve supplies the lateral three and a half digits dorsally except the nail beds, which are supplied by the median nerve.

Posterior compartment of the forearm

Muscles of the posterior compartment

The superficial group of muscles arise from the lateral epicondyle (the common extensor origin) and the supracondylar ridge of the humerus (Figs 2.23 and 2.26).

Vessels of the posterior compartment

The ulnar artery gives off the common interosseous artery near its origin. The latter divides into the anterior and posterior interosseous arteries, which both contribute to the supply for the extensor compartment.

The anterior interosseous artery passes down the anterior surface of the interosseous membrane. Branches pierce the membrane to supply the under-lying muscles. At the superior border of pronator quadratus the artery passes through the membrane to anastomose with the posterior interosseous artery, and then continues to the wrist to join the dorsal carpal arch. Anteriorly the anterior interosseus artery joins the palmar carpal arch.

The posterior interosseous artery passes posteriorly above the upper border of the interosseous membrane, and it accompanies the posterior interosseous nerve to supply the deep muscles of the extensor compartment.

Nerves of the posterior compartment

Brachioradialis and extensor carpi radialis longus are supplied directly by the radial nerve. All the other extensor muscles are supplied by the posterior interosseous nerve.

Name of muscle (nerve supply)	Origin	Insertion	Action
Brachioradialis (radial nerve)	Lateral supracondylar ridge of humerus	Styloid process of radius	Flexes elbow and rotates forearm
Extensor carpi radialis longus (radial nerve)		Base of second metacarpal bone	Extends and abducts hand at wrist joint
Extensor carpi radialis brevis (posterior interosseous nerve)	Common extensor origin	Base of third metacarpal bone	Extends and abducts hand at wrist joint
Extensor digitorum (posterior interosseous nerve)		Extensor expansion of middle and distal phalanges of the medial four digits	Extends the medial four fingers and hand at wrist joint
Extensor digiti minimi (posterior interosseous nerve)		Extensor expansion of little finger	Extends little finger
Extensor carpi ulnaris (posterior interosseous nerve)		Base of fifth metacarpal bone	Extends and adducts hand at the wrist
Anconeus (radial nerve)		Olecranon process and shaft of ulna	Extends and stabilizes the elbow joint
Supinator (posterior interosseous nerve)	Common extensor origin and supinator crest of ulna	Neck and shaft of radius	Supination of forearm
Abductor pollicis longus (posterior interosseous nerve)	Shafts of radius and ulna and interosseous membrane	Base of first metacarpal bone	Abducts thumb
Extensor pollicis brevis (posterior interosseous nerve)	Shaft of radius and interosseous membrane	Base of proximal phalanx of thumb	Extends metacarpophalangeal joint of thumb
Extensor pollicis longus (posterior interosseous nerve)	Shaft of ulna and interosseous membrane	Base of distal phalanx of thumb	Extends thumb
Extensor indicis (posterior interosseous nerve)		Extensor expansion of index finger	Extends index finger

Fig. 2.26 Muscles of the posterior compartment of the forearm

This nerve emerges from supinator and runs between the superficial and deep extensor muscles as far as the wrist joint, which it supplies.

Anatomical snuffbox

This is a depression proximal to the base of the first metacarpal and overlying the scaphoid and trapezoid bones when the thumb is actively extended.

In the anatomical position, the anterior margin is formed by the tendons of abductor pollicis longus and extensor pollicis brevis. The posterior margin is formed by the tendon of extensor pollicis longus. The radial artery runs on the floor of the anatomical snuffbox on its course to the dorsum of the hand. It lies on the scaphoid bone here.

Radioulnar joints

The movements of pronation and supination occur at the proximal and distal radioulnar joints. At the proximal radioulnar joint, the head of radius rotates in an osseofibrous ring formed by the radial notch of the ulna and the anular ligament. The radius also rotates around the ulna at the distal radioulnar joint.

Biceps brachii, brachioradialis and supinator cause supination, whereas pronator teres and pronator quadratus are responsible for pronation.

Orthopaedics

Tenderness in the anatomical snuffbox could be due to a fracture (Colles or scaphoid) or DeQuervain's tenosynovitis. The latter is due to inflammation of the tendon sheaths around abductor pollicis longus and extensor pollicis brevis because of excessive use of these muscles. Treatment is by steroid injection into the sheath.

A fracture of the radius proximal to pronator teres muscle insertion and distal to the biceps brachii tendon needs to be splinted in a supinated position if there is to be union of the fracture. This is due to the supination of the proximal fragment by biceps brachii.

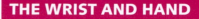

THE WRIST AND HAND

Figure 2.27 shows the skeleton of the wrist and hand.

Radiocarpal (wrist) joint

This is a synovial joint where the distal end of the radius articulates with the scaphoid, lunate and triquetral bones. An articular disc separates the joint cavity from the head of the ulna and the distal radioulnar joint (Fig. 2.28). The joint is strengthened by radiocarpal, ulnocarpal and collateral ligaments. The nerve supply to the joint is from anterior and posterior interosseous nerves.

Movements of the wrist joint are inseparable, functionally, from those at the midcarpal joint (synovial joints between the proximal and distal rows of carpal bones):

- The midcarpal joint participates mainly in flexion and abduction.
- The radiocarpal joint contributes mainly to extension and adduction.

Dorsum of the hand

The skin on the dorsum of the hand is thin and loose and the dorsal venous network of veins is usually visible. The veins drain into the cephalic and basilic veins.

The long extensor tendons of the forearm lie beneath the superficial veins. As the tendons cross the wrist joint they are surrounded by synovial sheaths and bound down by the extensor retinaculum. The attachments of the extensor retinaculum run from the radius to the pisiform and triquetral bones. The dorsal interossei are the only intrinsic muscles of the dorsum of the hand. The extensor tendons divide into three slips over the proximal phalanx: a central part that inserts into the middle phalanx, and two collateral bands that insert into the distal phalanx. These collateral bands receive a strong attachment from the interossei and lumbrical tendons. It is this attachment which forms the extensor expansion (Fig. 2.29).

Nerve supply to the dorsum of the hand

Figure 2.30 shows the cutaneous innervation of the hand. Note that the fingertips are supplied by palmar digital branches of the median and ulnar nerves.

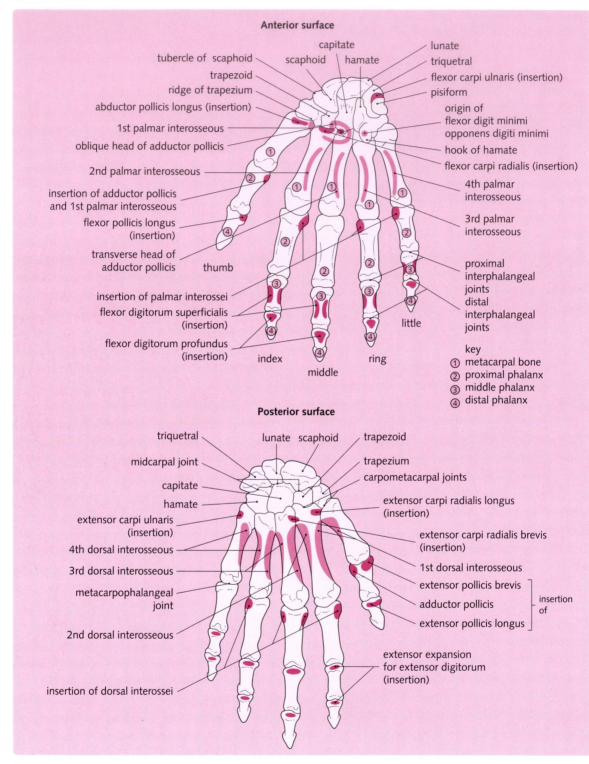

Fig. 2.27 Bones and joints of the wrist and hand.

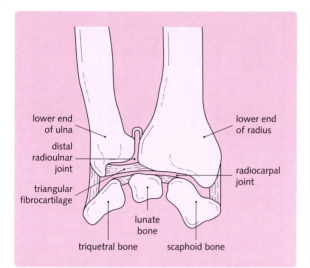

Fig. 2.28 Relationship of the distal radioulnar joint to the radiocarpal joint.

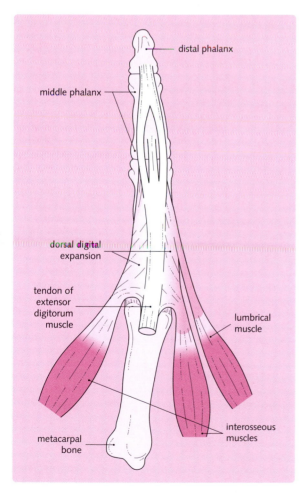

Fig. 2.29 Dorsal digital expansion and extensor tendon.

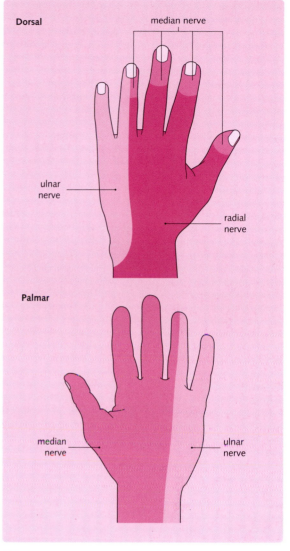

Fig. 2.30 Cutaneous innervation of the dorsal and palmar surfaces of the hand.

Vessels of the dorsum of the hand

Figure 2.31 shows the blood supply to the dorsum of the hand.

Palm of the hand

Skin

The skin is thick and hairless. Flexure creases and papillary ridges occupy the entire flexor surface, improving the gripping ability of the hand. Fibrous bands bind the skin down to the palmar aponeurosis and divide the subcutaneous fat into loculi, forming

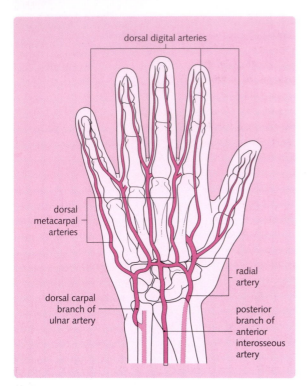

Fig. 2.31 Vessels of the dorsum of the hand.

a cushion capable of withstanding pressure. A small palmaris brevis muscle attaches the dermis of the skin to the palmar aponeurosis and flexor retinaculum. Its action of wrinkling the skin over the hypothenar eminence improves the ability to grip objects.

Palmar aponeurosis

Deep to the skin, the palmar aponeurosis forms a tough sheet lying between the thenar and hypothenar eminences, where it is continuous with the deep fascia. Distally it separates into four slips, which are joined by the superficial transverse metacarpal ligaments. At the base of each finger the four slips divide and fuse with the fibrous flexor sheaths, the

---

Orthopaedics

Dupuytren's contracture is a thickening of the palmar aponeurosis, which causes nodule-like lesions over the fourth and fifth digits. This thickening causes a fixed flexion deformity of these digits and interferes with hand function. Surgery may be required to release them.

---

capsule of the metacarpophalangeal joint, and the proximal phalanx.

Flexor retinaculum

The flexor retinaculum is a strong band of deep fascia that attaches the scaphoid and trapezium (laterally) to the pisiform and hook of the hamate (medially). Together with the concavity created by the carpal bones it forms an osseofibrous canal, called the carpal tunnel (Fig. 2.32). The flexor digitorum superficialis tendons enter the tunnel in two rows. The middle and ring finger tendons lie anterior to the index and little finger tendons. The flexor digitorum profundus tendons all lie in the same plane beneath the superficialis tendons. At the distal row of carpal bones the superficialis tendons all lie in the same plane. The remaining contents are the flexor pollicis longus tendon and median nerve.

The muscles of the thenar and hypothenar eminences arise from the flexor retinaculum and adjacent carpal bones.

Muscles of the hand

Thenar eminence

The thenar eminence is the prominent region between the base of the thumb and the wrist. It is composed of three muscles: abductor pollicis brevis, flexor pollicis brevis and opponens pollicis (Fig. 2.33). These muscles allow fine movements of the thumb, especially opposition and the pinch grip.

Hypothenar eminence

The hypothenar eminence lies between the base of the small finger and the wrist. It consists of the abductor

---

Orthopaedics

Carpal tunnel syndrome (CTS) is a common neuropathy that is the result of median nerve compression. Pain and paraesthesia over the cutaneous distribution of the median nerve are common symptoms. (Note that there is no paraesthesia over the palm due to the palmar branch arising proximal to the flexor retinaculum). If CTS is untreated it leads to wasting of the thenar eminence and weakness of pinch and precision grips, incapacitating the hand. Division of the retinaculum relieves the pressure.

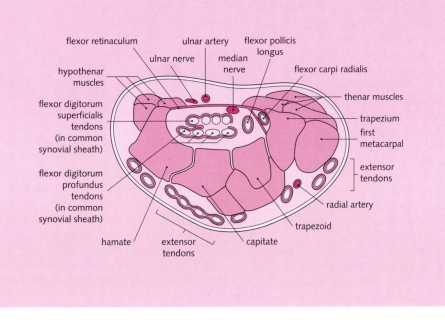

Fig. 2.32 Cross-section of the right carpal tunnel at the distal row of carpal bones showing its contents. (Adapted from *Gray's Anatomy*, 38th edn, edited by L H Bannister et al. Pearson Professional Ltd.)

digiti minimi, flexor digiti minimi and opponens digiti minimi (Fig. 2.33).

Other intrinsic hand muscles

These include adductor pollicis, four lumbricals, palmaris brevis, four dorsal and four palmar interosseous muscles (Fig. 2.33).

When dorsal and palmar interossei contract together as a group their individual actions, abduction and adduction respectively, cancel each other out. Instead, when all interossei and lumbrical muscles contract together their insertions into the dorsal digital expansion causes flexion at the metacarpophalangeal joints and assist extensor digitorum in extension of the interphalangeal joints.

Long flexor tendons in the hand

The following flexor tendons enter the hand: flexor carpi ulnaris, flexor carpi radialis, flexor digitorum superficialis and profundus, and flexor pollicis longus.

The muscle tendons are surrounded by synovial sheaths as they pass through the carpal tunnel beneath the flexor retinaculum, and as they enter the digits.

Synovial flexor tendon sheaths

There is a common synovial sheath for flexor digitorum superficialis and profundus, which is incomplete on its radial side. This sheath extends from just proximal of the flexor retinaculum to the palm around all digitorum tendons except for digitus minimus (the little finger). Here the sheath continues to the distal phalanx. For the second, third and fourth digit tendons, there is a bare area in the palm before the synovial sheath encloses them again as they enter the fibrous flexor sheaths of the digits. From this area the lumbrical muscles gain origin from flexor digitorum profundus.

The sheath around the flexor pollicis longus tendon extends from just proximal to the flexor

Use the mnemonics DAB and PAD to remember the actions of dorsal and palmar interossei: DAB-Dorsal, ABduct. PAD-Palmar, ADduct.

Penetrating hand injury can cause infection, especially if the thumb or fifth digit synovial sheaths are involved. The infection can track proximally to the palm and it can cause tendon necrosis due to loss of blood flow through the vinculae.

Fig. 2.33 The intrinsic muscles of the hand

Name of muscle (nerve supply)	Origin	Insertion	Action
Thenar eminence muscles			
Abductor pollicis brevis (recurrent branch of median nerve)	Scaphoid, trapezium and flexor retinaculum	Base of proximal phalanx	Abducts thumb at the MCP joint
Flexor pollicis brevis (recurrent branch of median nerve)	Trapezium and flexor retinaculum	Base of proximal phalanx	Flexes thumb at the MCP joint
Opponens pollicis (recurrent branch of median nerve)	Trapezium and flexor retinaculum	First metacarpal bone	Rotates metacarpal at carpometacarpal joint to oppose thumb
Hypothenar eminence muscles			
Abductor digiti minimi (deep branch of ulnar nerve)	Pisiform and flexor retinaculum	Base of proximal phalanx	Abducts little finger at the MCP joint
Flexor digiti minimi (deep branch of ulnar nerve)	Hook of hamate and flexor retinaculum	Base of proximal phalanx	Abducts little finger at the MCP joint
Opponens digiti minimi (deep branch of ulnar nerve)	Hook of hamate and flexor retinaculum	Fifth metacarpal bone	Assists in flexing the carpometacarpal joint, cupping the palm to assist gripping
Other intrinsic hand muscles			
Lumbricals (first and second: median nerve; third and fourth: deep branch of ulnar nerve)	Tendons of flexor digitorum profundus	Extensor expansion of the medial four digits	Extends the DIP and PIP joints of medial four digits. Flexes the MCP joint of the medial four digits
Palmar interossei (deep branch of ulnar nerve)	First, second, fourth and fifth metacarpal bones	Base of proximal phalanx and extensor expansion	Adduct the digits towards the middle finger. Flexes digit at MCP and extends interphalangeal joints
Dorsal interossei (deep branch of ulnar nerve)	Adjacent sides of the five metacarpal bones	Base of proximal phalanx and extensor expansion	Abduct the digits away from the middle finger. Flexes digit at MCP and extends interphalangeal joints
Adductor pollicis (deep branch of ulnar nerve)	Oblique head: capitate, trapezoid and second and third metacarpals. Transverse head: distal part of third metacarpal	Base of proximal phalanx	Adducts thumb
Palmaris brevis (superficial branch of the ulnar nerve)	Palmar aponeurosis and flexor retinaculum	Dermis of the skin on medial border of hand	Wrinkles the skin over the hypothenar eminence and improve the grip of the hand

retinaculum to the distal phalanx of the pollux (the thumb). See Figure 2.34.

Long flexor tendons in the digits

The tendon of flexor digitorum superficialis bifurcates before inserting into the middle phalanx, while that of flexor digitorum profundus runs between these slips to insert into the terminal phalanx. The tendons receive a blood supply via bands called vincula. Fibrous flexor sheaths bind the tendons down to the fingers. They are strong and thick over the phalanges but weak and loose over interphalangeal joints to allow movement (Fig. 2.35).

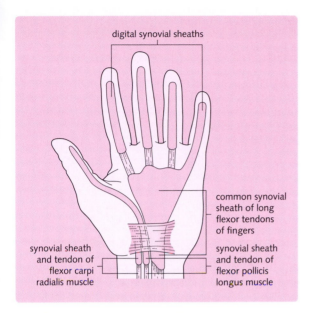

Fig. 2.34 Flexor synovial sheaths in the hand.

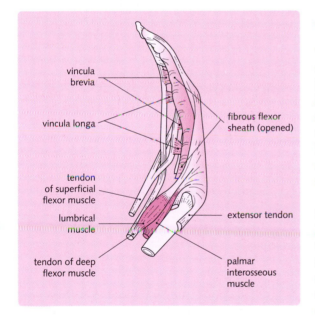

Fig. 2.35 Long flexor tendons of a finger and their vincula.

Nerves in the hand

Median nerve

The median nerve emerges from the carpal tunnel to enter the palm. Branches of the nerve in this region include:

- Recurrent branch to the muscles of the thenar eminence.

- Palmar digital nerves providing sensory innervation to the lateral three-and-a-half digits (including the nail bed and skin on the dorsum of the digit over the terminal phalanx) and motor supply to the first and second lumbricals.

Ulnar nerve

The ulnar nerve and artery pass into the hand together, superficial to the flexor retinaculum. The nerve divides into superficial and deep branches.

The superficial branch supplies palmaris brevis and palmar digital nerves to the medial one-and-a-half digits (including the skin over the dorsum of the distal phalanx).

The deep branch runs with the deep branch of the ulnar artery, and it supplies the hypothenar muscles, the two medial lumbricals, the interosseous muscles, and adductor pollicis.

See Figure 2.30 for the cutaneous innervation of the palmar and dorsal surfaces of the hand.

Vessels of the hand

The radial artery slopes across the anatomical snuffbox overlying the scaphoid and trapezium, and it passes between the two heads of the first dorsal interosseous. It appears deep in the palm of the hand, emerging between the two heads of adductor pollicis to form the deep palmar arch. Palmar metacarpal branches from the arch anastomose with the common palmar digital arteries of the superficial palmar arch.

The ulnar artery approaches the wrist between flexor digitorum superficialis and flexor carpi ulnaris. It enters the wrist with the ulnar nerve, superficial to the flexor retinaculum. In the hand it forms the superficial palmar arch from which common palmar digital arteries arise. The common digital arteries divide to form (proper) palmar digital arteries that enter the digits to supply the joints and phalanges.

Both the superficial and deep palmar arches form anastomoses between the radial and ulnar arteries. The radial artery gives off a superficial palmar branch to join the superficial palmar arch and the ulnar artery has a deep palmar branch that joins the deep palmar arch.

Palmar spaces

The intermediate palmar septum from the palmar aponeurosis to the third metacarpal divides the central part of the palm into two fascial spaces: the thenar space lies laterally and the midpalmar space lies medially.

The spaces communicate with the subcutaneous tissue of the webs of the fingers. Deep infections of the midpalmar space often spread to these sites.

Nails

These lie on the dorsal surface of the distal phalanges, and they are formed from modified skin tissue.

Clinical examination

Examination of the hands and nails is a part of the clinical examination because they are a source of clinical signs. Reddening of the palm (palmar erythema) over the hypothenar eminence indicates liver pathology. Bulbous shaped nails (clubbing) occurs in many pathological conditions, including the heart (infective endocarditis), the lungs (carcinoma, cystic fibrosis) and G.I tract (Crohn's, coeliac disease) or liver (cirrhosis). Spoon-shaped nails (koilonychias) suggests iron deficiency.

RADIOLOGICAL ANATOMY

Imaging of the bones and joints

When there are symptoms and/or signs of joint problems or a fracture an X-ray is usually the first imaging investigation to be performed. Two images are taken that are 90° to each other and in some cases the joint above and below the injury, especially if the forearm or lower leg are involved. Information not only about the bones or joints can be gained but also on the tissues surrounding them, e.g. calcification may indicate a tumour or endocrine problem.

Normal radiographic anatomy

Normal bone has a smooth cortex that is thicker along the shaft of a long bone, e.g. humerus, but is thinner in small bones, e.g. carpal. The smooth cortex is interrupted at tendon or ligament insertions and entry points for nutrient arteries to the bone. Medullary trabeculae appear as thin white lines along the planes of weight-bearing forces within that bone.

See Figures 2.36, 2.37 and 2.38 for the osteology and the normal articulation of the shoulder girdle, elbow and wrist joints.

When interpreting an X-ray film assess the overall density of the bone(s). Normal density is seen in Figures 2.36 and 2.40.

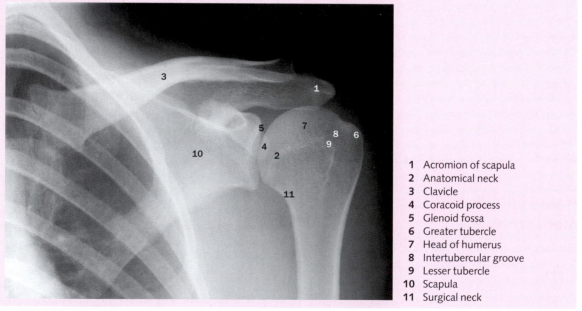

1	Acromion of scapula
2	Anatomical neck
3	Clavicle
4	Coracoid process
5	Glenoid fossa
6	Greater tubercle
7	Head of humerus
8	Intertubercular groove
9	Lesser tubercle
10	Scapula
11	Surgical neck

Fig. 2.36 An anterioposterior (AP) radiograph of the left shoulder joint.

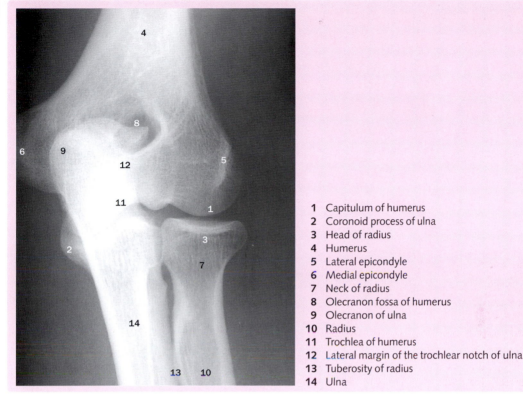

Fig. 2.37 An anterioposterior (AP) radiograph of the left elbow.

1 Capitulum of humerus
2 Coronoid process of ulna
3 Head of radius
4 Humerus
5 Lateral epicondyle
6 Medial epicondyle
7 Neck of radius
8 Olecranon fossa of humerus
9 Olecranon of ulna
10 Radius
11 Trochlea of humerus
12 Lateral margin of the trochlear notch of ulna
13 Tuberosity of radius
14 Ulna

Orthopaedics

In shoulder dislocation the humeral head most commonly lies anterior to the glenoid fossa. On examination there is squaring of the shoulder, i.e. it loses its smooth convex profile and Hamilton's ruler test is positive (a ruler joins the acromion to the lateral epicondyle and the arm appears to bow medially). On X-ray the continuity of the humeral head and the glenoid fossa is lost. In the rare posterior dislocation of the joint a lateral X-ray demonstrates the 'light bulb sign'; this describes the appearance of the humeral head and is diagnostic of the underlying condition.

Orthopaedics

A scaphoid fracture is not always evident on first X-ray. Imaging for a second time 10 days later will reveal the fracture line through the scaphoid bone because the fracture ends undergo calcification (sclerosis) as the fracture begins to heal. A fracture at the base of the first metacarpal that extends into the metacarpophalangeal joint is known as a Bennett's fracture. A fracture of the fifth metacarpal is known as a Boxer's fracture.

How to examine an X-ray methodically

The following is a method of how to examine a film:

- Examine the cortex of each bone. Look at the outline for any breaks in continuity and thickening, thinning or alterations in a normally smooth cortex.

- Examine the medulla of each bone for alterations of texture and areas of whitening (sclerosis – indicating bone thickening) or darkening (rarefaction – indicating bone loss).
- Examine the joint for narrowing of the joint space, loss of the smooth joint surface, formation of bone (osteophytes) and loose bodies.
- Examine the soft tissues for ossification and calcification. If a dense shadow is present, it

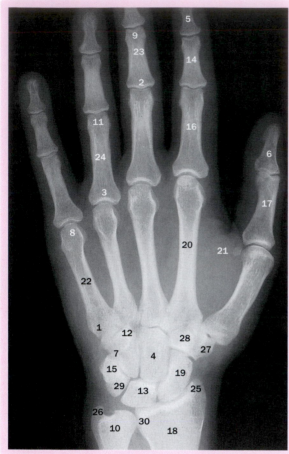

1	Base of fifth metacarpal
2	Base of middle phalanx of middle finger
3	Base of proximal phalanx of ring finger
4	Capitate
5	Distal phalanx of index finger
6	Distal phalanx of thumb
7	Hamate
8	Head of fifth metacarpal
9	Head of middle phalanx of middle finger
10	Head of ulna
11	Head of proximal phalanx of ring finger
12	Hook of hamate
13	Lunate
14	Middle phalanx of index finger
15	Pisiform
16	Proximal phalanx of index finger
17	Proximal phalanx of thumb
18	Radius
19	Scaphoid
20	Second metacarpal
21	Sesamoid bone
22	Shaft of fifth metacarpal
23	Shaft of middle phalanx of middle finger
24	Shaft of proximal phalanx of ring finger
25	Styloid process of radius
26	Styloid process of ulna
27	Trapezium
28	Trapezoid
29	Triquetral
30	Ulnar notch of radius

Fig. 2.38 A dorsalpalmar radiograph of the hand and wrist.

could indicate an abscess, fluid, or solid mass. If there is translucency, it indicates gas or fat.

- Finally, if you have found one abnormality, e.g. a fracture, keep looking because there may be more.

Angiography of the limbs

In Figures 2.39, 2.40, and 2.41 arteriography highlights the arterial supply to the thoracic cage, shoulder girdle, upper arm, forearm and hand.

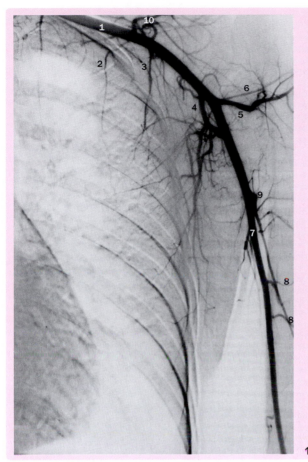

Fig. 2.39 A left axillary arteriogram.

1 Axillary artery
2 Superior thoracic artery
3 Lateral thoracic artery
4 Subscapular artery
5 Posterior circumflex humeral artery
6 Anterior circumflex humeral artery
7 Brachial artery
8 Muscular branches of brachial artery
9 Profunda brachii artery
10 Thoraco-acromial artery

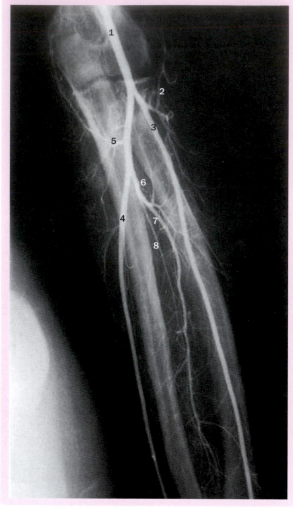

1 Brachial artery
2 Radial recurrent artery
3 Radial artery
4 Ulnar artery
5 Ulnar recurrent artery
6 Common interosseous artery
7 Anterior interosseous artery
8 Posterior interosseous artery

Fig. 2.40 A left brachial arteriogram.

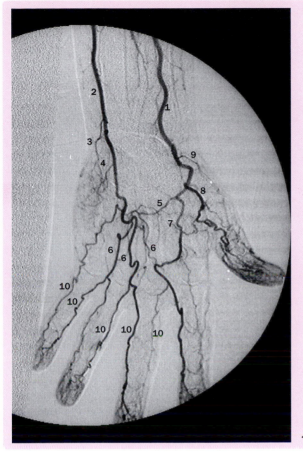

Fig. 2.41 A hand arteriogram.

1 Radial artery
2 Ulnar artery
3 Deep palmar branch of ulnar artery
4 Palmar carpal arch
5 Deep palmar arch
6 Common palmar digital arteries
7 Palmar metacarpal artery
8 Princeps pollicis artery
9 Artery to radial aspect of thumb
10 Proper palmar digital artery

The thorax

Objectives

In this chapter you will learn to:

- Explain the surface markings of the major thoracic viscera (heart, lung, pleurae and great vessels).
- Describe the lymphatic drainage of the breast and be aware of its importance.
- Define the boundaries of the thoracic inlet and state what passes through it.
- Describe the attachments of the diaphragm, and state the structures passing through and peripheral to it.
- Define the divisions of the mediastinum and their contents.
- Describe the major features of each chamber of the heart.
- Explain the blood supply to the heart, including left/right dominance and venous drainage.
- Describe the thoracic sympathetic trunk.
- Describe the lymphatic drainage of the lung.
- Understand the anatomy of the oesophagus, including its course, innervation and blood supply.
- State the structures and their relative positions in the lung root (hilum).
- Describe the divisions of the bronchial tree and explain the concept of a bronchopulmonary segment.
- Outline the blood supply and innervation of the lungs and pleurae.
- Describe the course and distribution of the vagus and phrenic nerves.
- Outline the mechanics of respiration.
- Recognize the bony and soft-tissue features of a normal radiograph of the thorax.
- Have a method for reviewing a chest X-ray (PA and lateral views).

REGIONS AND COMPONENTS OF THE THORAX

The thorax lies between the neck and the abdomen. The thoracic cavity contains the heart, lungs, great vessels, trachea and oesophagus. The lungs lie laterally, and the other structures lie in the mediastinum.

The thoracic cage is formed by the thoracic vertebrae, ribs, costal cartilages and sternum. It protects the contents of the thoracic cavity and some abdominal contents, e.g. the liver and spleen.

Superiorly the thorax communicates with the neck through the thoracic inlet. Inferiorly the diaphragm separates the thorax from the abdominal cavity.

SURFACE ANATOMY AND SUPERFICIAL STRUCTURES

Bony landmarks

The bony landmarks of the thorax are illustrated in Figure 3.1. Clinically, the imaginary vertical lines are used to aid description:

- The midsternal line is the equivalent of the midline of the body.
- The midclavicular line passes halfway between the acromion tip and the midsternal line.
- The anterior axillary line corresponds to the anterior axillary fold.
- The posterior axillary line corresponds to the posterior axillary fold.

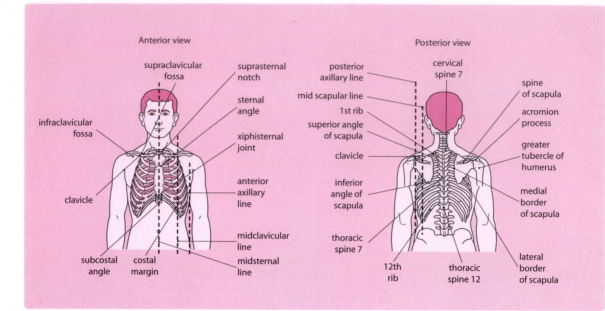

Fig. 3.1 Surface markings of the anterior and posterior thoracic walls.

• The midscapular line passes centrally through the inferior angle of the scapula.

The bony sternum can be palpated in the midline of the thorax anteriorly. However, the pectoralis major muscle overlaps the anterior sternal surface; thus, the width of the sternum is not entirely subcutaneous.

The upper border of the manubrium sterni forms the jugular notch. The manubrium sterni joins the body of the sternum at the manubriosternal joint. The manubriosternal angle is opposite the T4 vertebra and the plane that lies between them marks the level of the aortic arch, the carina of the trachea, entry of azygos vein into the superior vena cava and arbitrary division between the superior and inferior mediastinum. Inferiorly, the body of the sternum articulates with the xiphoid process. The xiphoid process is felt within a triangular depression known as the epigastric fossa.

The costal cartilages of ribs 1–7 articulate with the manubrium and sternum laterally. Anteriorly, the upper six ribs and costal cartilages are covered by pectoralis major. The costal margin begins at the xiphisternum and comprises the costal cartilages of ribs 7–10. This is most evident when the body is hyperextended.

All ribs except the first rib, which lies under the clavicle, can be traced posteriorly.

The second costal cartilage adjoins the sternum at the manubriosternal joint (sternal angle of Louis). The angle can be palpated and is a useful reference point enabling the ribs to be counted (e.g. when attaching the chest ECG electrodes (V1–6)). These are placed as follows: V1 and V2 in the 4th intercostal space (I.C.S) either side of the sternum. V4 in the 5th I.C.S midclavicular line, V3 is equidistant between V2 and V4. Electrode V6 in the 5th I.C.S and V5 is equidistant between V4 and V6.

Posteriorly the spinous processes of the thoracic vertebrae are palpable inferior to the vertebra prominens—the spinous process of C7 vertebra.

Musculature

The muscles covering the thoracic cage are mentioned in Chapter 2.

Posteriorly the triangle of auscultation is formed by the lower border of trapezius, the upper border of latissimus dorsi and laterally by the medial border of the scapula. The rhomboideus major lies in the floor of the triangle (gastric sounds can be heard over this area).

If the trunk is flexed and the scapulae are drawn forwards (protraction) by adduction of the arms (e.g. a patient sitting forwards in bed places arms across thighs), the intercostal spaces normally covered by the scapulae become subcutaneous and is easier to auscultate the lungs (with a stethoscope).

Trachea, lungs and pleurae

The trachea is palpable in the midline, above the jugular notch. It bifurcates behind the manubriosternal angle (at the level of T4) to form the right and left main bronchi.

The dome of the pleura extends about 2.5 cm above the medial end of the clavicle (Fig. 3.29). The anterior border of the right pleura passes down behind the sternal angle to the xiphisternal joint. The anterior border of the left pleura follows a similar course, but at the level of the 4th costal cartilage it deviates laterally to form the cardiac notch. The lower border follows a curved line, being at the level of the 8th rib in the midclavicular line, the 10th rib in the midaxillary line, and the 12th rib adjacent to the vertebral column.

The surface markings of the lungs (Fig. 3.2) during mid-inspiration are similar to those of the pleurae except inferiorly, where they lie at the level of the 6th rib in the midclavicular line, 8th rib in the midaxillary line, and the 10th rib adjacent to the vertebral column, respectively. The oblique fissure corresponds to a line drawn from the third thoracic spinous process to the sixth rib in the midclavicular line (the oblique fissure follows the curve of the fifth rib). The horizontal fissure is drawn from the point of intersection with the right oblique fissure at the midaxillary line to the right fourth costal cartilage anteriorly.

The space between the lower border of the pleura and lung is the costodiaphragmatic recess. In life, it is filled by the lungs in full inspiration.

Heart

The surface markings of the heart are outlined in Figure 3.3. The apex of the heart is taken as lying approximately in the midclavicular line of the fifth intercostal space. This point takes into account differences in adult stature and also applies to children. The surface markings of the heart valves are illustrated in Figure 3.4.

Great vessels

The aortic arch, a continuation of the ascending aorta, begins behind the manubriosternal joint. It arches posteriorly and to the left of the vertebral column, where, again at the level of the manubriosternal joint, the arch ends to become the descending (thoracic) aorta. The aortic arch, brachiocephalic trunk, left common carotid and left subclavian arteries lie behind the manubrium. The brachiocephalic trunk bifurcates into the right common carotid and subclavian arteries behind the right sternoclavicular joint.

The superior vena cava is formed behind the first right costal cartilage by the union of the brachiocephalic veins. The superior vena cava runs inferiorly

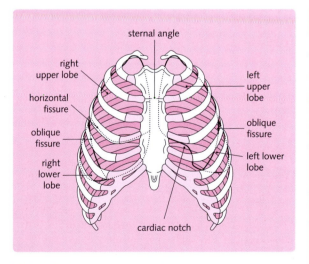

Fig. 3.2 Surface markings of the lungs.

Fig. 3.3 Outline of the surface landmarks of the heart

Border	Area covered
Superior border	From the second left costal cartilage to the third right costal cartilage
Right border	From the third right costal cartilage to the sixth right costal cartilage
Left border	From the second left costal cartilage to the apex of the heart
Inferior border	From the sixth right costal cartilage to the apex
Apex	Lies in the fifth intercostal space, in the midclavicular line

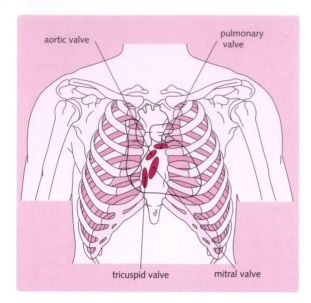

Fig. 3.4 Surface markings of the heart valves.

behind the right sternal border to enter the right atrium behind the third costal cartilage. The azygos vein joins the superior vena cava at the level of the second right costal cartilage.

The internal thoracic artery arising from the subclavian artery run vertically downwards, posterior to the costal cartilages and 1 cm lateral to the sternal edge, as far as the 6th intercostal space. The artery now divides into musculophrenic and superior epigastric arteries.

Diaphragm

The central tendon of the diaphragm lies behind the xiphisternal joint. In mid-respiration the right dome arches upwards to the upper border of the 5th rib in the midclavicular line; the left dome reaches only the lower border of the 5th rib.

Breasts

The breasts lie in the superficial fascia, mainly superficial to the pectoralis major muscle. They contain mammary glandular tissue, which drains through lactiferous ducts into the nipple. The nipple is the greatest prominence of the breast, and it is surrounded by a circular pigmented area called the areola.

The base of the breast usually lies between the 2nd and 6th rib vertically, and from the midaxillary line to the lateral border of the sternum horizontally.

The blood supply to the breast is derived from branches of the internal thoracic artery, the lateral thoracic and the thoracoacromial arteries, and the posterior intercostal arteries. Venous drainage is into the axillary and internal thoracic veins.

Lymph drains into the subareolar plexus and then into either axillary nodes, internal thoracic nodes, or the other breast.

Axillary nodes receive 75% of the lymphatic drainage of the superior and lateral parts of the breast. Lymphatics from the inferior and medial part of the breast drain into lymph nodes along the internal thoracic vessels and then via the bronchomediastinal lymph trunk into the lymphatics at the root of the neck. Lymphatics may communicate with vessels from the opposite breast.

THE THORACIC WALL

The thoracic skeleton is formed by the sternum, the ribs and costal cartilages, and the thoracic vertebrae (Fig. 3.5).

Sternum

The sternum (breast bone) has three components:

- The manubrium is the upper part of the sternum. It articulates with the clavicles and with the 1st and upper part of the 2nd costal cartilages.
- The body of the sternum articulates with the manubrium at the manubriosternal joint superiorly, and with the xiphisternum inferiorly. These are secondary cartilaginous joints. Laterally

Oncology

Breast carcinoma affects 1 in 12 women in the UK. Lymphatic spread dictates the treatment as well as size of lesion. Knowledge of lymphatic drainage is important especially since it can pass to contralateral side. The tumour can cause changes such as dimpling, nipple inversion and erythema (reddening). The dimpling is caused by invasion of the suspensory ligaments that run between the deep fascia and skin. Pulling on and shortening the ligaments causes the overlying skin to have a peau d'orange appearance (like an orange). Nipple inversion occurs by a similar mechanism with the tumour pulling on the nipple/lactiferous ductules.

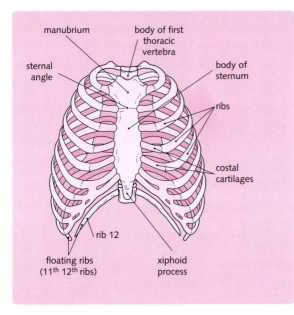

Fig. 3.5 Thoracic skeleton.

- the sternal body articulates with the 2nd to 7th costal cartilages via synovial joints.
- The xiphoid process is the lowest part of the sternum.

Ribs and costal cartilages

There are 12 pairs of ribs. They all articulate with a costal cartilage anteriorly. The upper seven ribs articulate directly with the sternum via their own costal cartilage. The 8th to 10th ribs have costal cartilages that are attached to each other and to the 7th anteriorly, and thence to the sternum.

The floating 11th and 12th ribs have no anterior attachment for their costal cartilages.

Movements of the ribs during respiration are described in Figure 3.35.

Typical ribs

A typical rib has the following features (Fig. 3.6):

- It is a long curved flattened bone with a rounded superior border and a sharp thin inferior border forming the costal groove.
- It has a head with two demifacets for articulation with the numerically similar vertebral body and that of the vertebra immediately above.
- The neck separates the head and the tubercle.
- The tubercle has a facet for articulation with the transverse process of the corresponding vertebra.

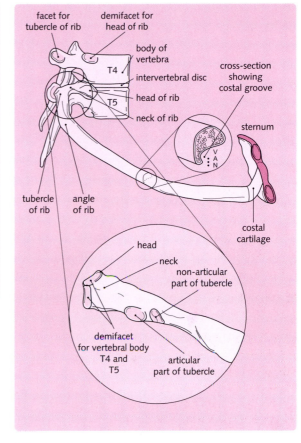

Fig. 3.6 Fifth rib, with the inset showing the posterior surface of the rib.

- The shaft is thin, flat and curved, with an angle at its point of greatest change in curvature.

A&E

Trauma to the root of the neck or a fracture to the angle of a rib (its weakest point) can cause a pneumothorax if the rib fragment punctures the pleura allowing air to enter the pleural cavity. In the medical emergency of tension pneumothorax the hole in the pleura acts as a valve allowing air entry into cavity on inspiration but it closes preventing its escape on expiration. The positive intrathoracic pressure causes the lung to collapse and pushes the mediastinal contents to opposite side (trachea and heart) kinking the superior vena cava and compressing the contralateral lung. Immediate treatment is a chest drain inserted into the 2nd intercostal space in the midclavicular line.

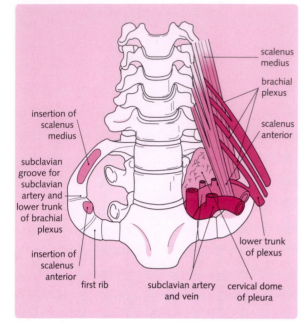

insertion of scalenus medius

subclavian groove for subclavian artery and lower trunk of brachial plexus

insertion of scalenus anterior

first rib

scalenus medius

brachial plexus

scalenus anterior

lower trunk of plexus

subclavian artery and vein

cervical dome of pleura

Fig. 3.7 First rib and its relations to the thoracic inlet.

Atypical ribs

Figure 3.7 shows the 1st rib and its relations in the thoracic inlet. This is the broadest, shortest and most sharply curved rib. The scalene tubercle lies on the inner border for attachment of the scalenus anterior. The subclavian artery and vein pass posterior and anterior to the scalene tubercle, respectively. The subclavian artery forms the subclavian groove on the

rib, and immediately posterior to the artery the lower trunk of the brachial plexus (C8–T1) lies in direct contact with the upper surface of the rib.

The 10th, 11th and 12th ribs have one facet on the head for articulation with their own vertebra.

Thoracic vertebrae

There are 12 thoracic vertebrae with their intervening intervertebral discs (Fig. 3.8).

Openings into the thorax

Thoracic inlet (superior thoracic aperture)

The thoracic cavity communicates with the root of the neck via the thoracic inlet (see Fig. 3.7). The thoracic inlet slopes from behind downwards and forwards and the margins of the inlet include:

- Body of T1 vertebra.
- Medial (inner) border of the 1st rib and its costal cartilage.
- Superior border of the manubrium.

The oesophagus, trachea, and the apices of the lungs, together with important vessels and nerves, pass through the inlet.

Thoracic outlet (inferior thoracic aperture)

The thoracic outlet lies between the thorax and the abdomen. It is bounded posteriorly by the 12th thoracic vertebra and the 12th pair of ribs, anteriorly

Fig. 3.8 Superior (A) and lateral (B) surfaces of a thoracic vertebra.

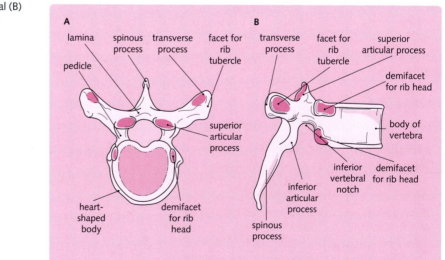

A

lamina

pedicle

spinous process

transverse process

facet for rib tubercle

superior articular process

heart-shaped body

demifacet for rib head

B

transverse process

facet for rib tubercle

superior articular process

demifacet for rib head

body of vertebra

inferior articular process

spinous process

inferior vertebral notch

demifacet for rib head

by the costal margin and xiphoid process and is closed by the diaphragm. Numerous structures pass through the outlet between the thorax and abdomen, which either pierce the diaphragm or pass through a hiatus (hole) in the diaphragm (see Fig. 3.12).

Intercostal spaces

There are eleven intercostal spaces between the ribs.

Each space contains a neurovascular bundle and three layers of intercostal muscles (Fig. 3.9). The innermost muscle layer is lined by endothoracic fascia and parietal pleura. In the intercostal space anteriorly the external intercostal muscle is replaced by the anterior intercostal membrane which runs from the costochondral junction to the sternum. The internal intercostal muscle posteriorly is replaced by the posterior intercostal membrane between the angle of the rib to the superior costotransverse ligament. This ligament is attached between the neck of the rib and the under surface of the transverse process of the vertebral body above.

Intercostal nerves and vessels

The intercostal nerves are the anterior rami of the upper eleven thoracic spinal nerves. The 12th nerve lies below the twelve rib and is known as the subcostal nerve.

Each intercostal nerve runs in a plane between the parietal pleura and the posterior intercostal membrane, and it passes forward in the costal groove of the corresponding rib, between the innermost and internal intercostal muscles. The nerve has a collateral branch that runs along the upper border of the lower rib.

All the intercostal nerves supply the skin and parietal pleura and the intercostal muscles of their respective spaces. The first intercostal nerve (T1) divides into a superior and inferior branch. The larger superior branch passes to the brachial plexus, while the inferior branch passes beneath the first rib to run in the first intercostal space. The 7th to 11th nerves pass from the intercostal space to the anterior abdominal wall to supply the skin, parietal peritoneum and anterior abdominal wall muscles. The subcostal nerve lies entirely in the abdominal wall. Its lateral cutaneous branch pierces the internal and external oblique muscle layers to supply the skin over the hip laterally, between the iliac crest and greater trochanter of femur.

Figure 3.10 shows the arterial supply to the thoracic wall.

The neurovascular bundle structures, from superior to inferior, are VAN (vein, artery, nerve). These run in the costal groove of the rib, with their collateral branches running inferiorly in the intercostal space, above the superior border of the inferior rib. This is important to remember when inserting an intercostal needle (i.e. chest drain) to avoid nerve damage causing paralysis of the intercostal muscle and paradoxical movement on respiration, e.g. inspiration sucks in muscle and expiration causes it to bulge outward.

Fig. 3.9 Muscles of the thorax

Name of muscle (nerve supply)	Origin	Insertion	Action
External intercostal (intercostal)	Inferior border of rib above	Superior border of rib below	All the intercostal muscles assist in both inspiration and expiration during ventilation
Internal intercostal (intercostal)	Costal groove of rib above	Superior border of rib below	
Innermost intercostal (intercostal)	Costal groove of rib above	Adjacent rib below	
Diaphragm (phrenic)	Xiphoid process, lower sixth costal cartilages, L1–L3 vertebrae by crura, and medial and lateral arcuate ligaments	Central tendon	Important muscle of inspiration; increases vertical diameter of thorax by pulling down central tendon

Fig. 3.10 Arterial supply to the thoracic wall

Artery	Origin	Distribution
Anterior intercostal (spaces 1–6)	Internal thoracic artery	Intercostal spaces and parietal pleura
Anterior intercostal (spaces 7–9)	Musculophrenic artery	
Posterior intercostal (spaces 1–2)	Superior intercostal artery (from costocervical trunk of subclavian artery)	
Posterior intercostal (all other spaces)	Thoracic aorta	
Internal thoracic	Subclavian artery	Runs down lateral to the sternum and terminates by dividing into the superior epigastric and musculophrenic arteries
Subcostal	Thoracic aorta	Abdominal wall

Diaphragm

The diaphragm is the primary muscle of respiration. It consists of a peripheral muscular part and a central tendon, and it separates the thoracic and abdominal cavities. As viewed from the front, the diaphragm curves up into two domes, the right dome being higher than the left (Fig. 3.11). When viewed from the side, it assumes an inverted-J shape with a deeper recess behind.

Figure 3.12 lists the openings in the diaphragm and the structures passing through them.

The blood and nerve supply of the diaphragm are shown in Figure 3.13.

To remember the root value of the phrenic nerve (C3, 4, 5) use: C3, 4, 5 keeps the diaphragm alive. But also keep in mind that it has a sensory component that supplies the mediastinal pleura, diaphragmatic pleura and peritoneum.

THE THORACIC CAVITY

The thoracic cavity is filled laterally by the lungs and the pleural cavities. The median partition separating the lungs and pleurae is the mediastinum. This may be divided by a transthoracic plane passing through the sternal angle and T4 vertebra (Fig. 3.14). The superior mediastinum lies above this plane and contains the remnants of the thymus, great vessels, trachea, oesophagus, thoracic duct and sympathetic trunk. The inferior mediastinum lies below the plane, posterior to the body of the sternum and it is further subdivided into:

- The anterior mediastinum, lying between the pericardium and the sternum, which contains lymph nodes and remnants of the thymus (T4–T8).
- The middle mediastinum, which contains the pericardium and heart (T4–T8).
- The posterior mediastinum (T4–T12), lying between the pericardium and the vertebral column, which contains the oesophagus, azygos system of veins thoracic duct, sympathetic trunk, and descending aorta.

Figure 3.15 shows the left and right sides of the mediastinum.

THE MEDIASTINUM

Pericardium

The pericardium is a double-walled fibroserous sac that encloses the heart and the roots of the

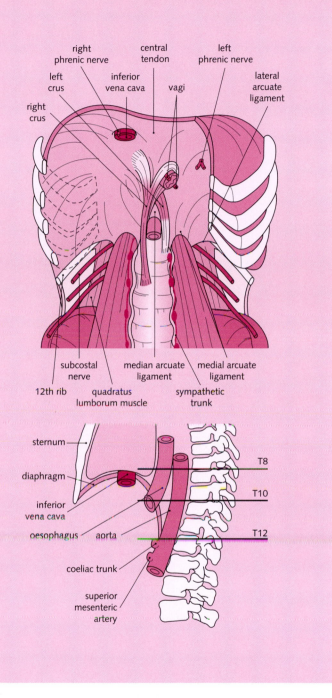

great vessels. It is divided into the fibrous pericardium and the two layers of the serous pericardium (parietal and visceral). The fibrous pericardium is a strong layer that limits the movement of the heart and is attached inferiorly to the central tendon of the diaphragm, anteriorly to the sternum, and superiorly to the tunica adventitia of the great vessels.

The nerve supply to the fibrous and parietal layer of the pericardium is by the phrenic nerve. The

Fig. 3.12 Diaphragmatic apertures and structures passing through them

Opening	Structures
Aortic opening (behind the diaphragm at the level of T12)	Aorta, thoracic duct, azygos and hemiazygos veins
Oesophageal opening (in the muscle of the diaphragm at the level of T10)	Oesophagus, vagus nerves, oesophageal branches of the left gastric vessels and lymphatics
Vena caval opening (in the central tendon at the level of T8)	Inferior vena cava, right phrenic nerve
Structures passing behind the diaphragm	Splanchnic nerves and sympathetic trunk
Structures passing anteriorly to the diaphragm	Superior epigastric vessels and lymphatics
Structures passing laterally to the diaphragm	Lower six intercostal vessels and nerves.

Cardiology

The pericardium can become inflamed e.g. by bacteria, viruses, iatrogenic (post-operation) and is known as pericarditis. It causes central chest pain worse on inspiration and relieved by sitting forwards. The phrenic nerve supply can cause referred pain to the skin above the shoulder (C3 and 4). More important is bleeding into the pericardium from trauma or an aortic dissection (a tear in the endothelium allows blood to track between tunica intima and media layers). As the blood collects it causes compression of the heart (cardiac tamponade) due to its indistensible fibrous component. Untreated cardiac output decreases and causes death. This medical emergency requires drainage (pericardiocentesis) with a needle inserted to left of xiphoid process towards the inferior angle of the left scapula.

Fig. 3.13 Nerves and vessels of the diaphragm

Innervation	Motor supply: phrenic nerves (C3–C5);
	Sensory supply: centrally by phrenic nerves (C3–C5), peripherally by intercostal nerves (T5–T11) and subcostal nerve (T12)
Arterial supply	Superior phrenic arteries; musculophrenic arteries; inferior phrenic arteries; pericardiacophrenic arteries
Venous drainage	Musculophrenic and pericardiacophrenic veins drain into internal thoracic vein; inferior phrenic veins
Lymphatic drainage	Diaphragmatic lymph nodes drain to posterior mediastinal nodes eventually; superior lumbar lymph nodes; lymphatic plexuses on superior and inferior surfaces communicate freely

visceral layer has no somatic innervation, and so it is insensitive to pain.

Pericardial sinuses

The reflection of the serous pericardium around the large veins forms a recess posterior to the left atrium called the oblique sinus. The oesophagus is a posterior relation to the oblique sinus. The reflection around the aorta and the pulmonary trunk anteriorly and around the great veins posteriorly, forms the transverse sinus. The transverse space separates the arterial outflow and venous inflow of the heart (Fig. 3.16).

Heart

This is the muscular organ responsible for pumping blood throughout the body (Fig. 3.17). It lies free in the pericardium, connected only to the great vessels.

The walls of the heart consist mainly of heart muscle (myocardium), lined internally by the endocardium and externally by the epicardium (visceral serous pericardium).

The heart has four chambers, two atria and two ventricles. The right side of the heart pumps blood to the lungs while the left side propels blood throughout the remainder of the body.

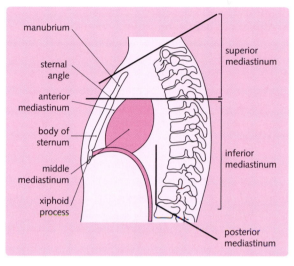

Fig. 3.14 Subdivisions of the mediastinum.

Chambers of the heart

Right atrium

This chamber consists of the right atrium proper and an atrial appendage, the right auricle (Fig. 3.18). The atrium has a smooth and rigded parts are separated externally by a groove, the sulcus terminalis, and internally by a ridge, the crista terminalis. The area posterior to the crista terminalis is smooth walled, while the region anterior to it is ridged by muscle fibres – the musculi pectinati. Three veins enter the atrium, the superior vena cava, inferior vena cava and coronary sinus.

Interatrial septum

This forms the posterior wall of the right atrium. In the lower part of the septum is a depression, called the fossa ovalis. This represents the foramen ovale of the fetal heart. The anulus ovalis (limbus fossa ovalis) forms the crescentic upper margin of the fossa and is formed from the lower edge of the septum secundum of the fetal heart.

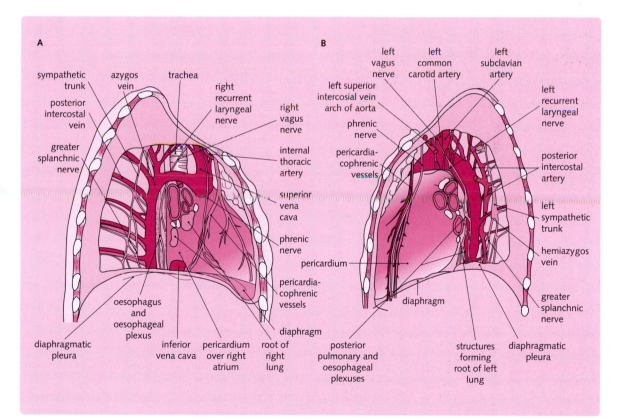

Fig. 3.15 (A) Right surface of the mediastinum and the right posterior thoracic wall. (B) Left surface of the mediastinum and the left posterior thoracic wall. Mediastinal pleura has been removed.

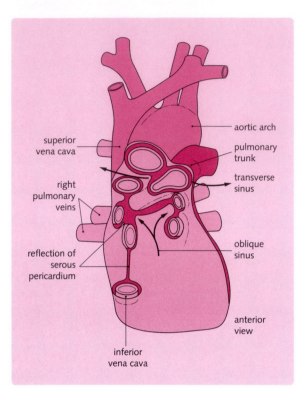

superior
vena cava

aortic arch

pulmonary
trunk

transverse
sinus

right
pulmonary
veins

reflection of
serous
pericardium

oblique
sinus

anterior
view

inferior
vena cava

Fig. 3.16 Pericardial sinuses and reflections (the heart has been removed). Anterior view. (Adapted from *Gray's Anatomy*, 38th edn, edited by L H Bannister et al. Pearson Professional Ltd.)

Failure of the foramen ovale to close after birth to form the fossa ovalis forms an atrial septal defect (ASD). This allows oxygenated blood to pass from the left atrium into the right atrium and causes the right atrium to become dilated. The increased blood volume in the right side of the heart causes pulmonary hypertension.

Right ventricle

This chamber communicates with the right atrium via the tricuspid valve (Fig. 3.18), and with the pulmonary artery through the pulmonary valve. The ventricle becomes funnel shaped as it approaches the pulmonary orifice—this region is known as the infundibulum.

The tricuspid valve has three cusps (anterior, posterior, and septal), the bases of which are attached to the fibrous ring of the skeleton of the heart.

The bases of the three cusps of the pulmonary valve are attached to the arterial wall at the site of three dilations or pulmonary sinuses.

The ventricular wall has irregular muscular elevations:

- Prominent muscular ridges called trabeculae carneae.
- Moderator band—transmits part of the conducting system of the heart and runs from the septal wall to the anterior wall.
- Papillary muscles—attached to the ventricular wall and to the cusps of the tricuspid valve via fibrous cords, the chordae tendineae.

Left atrium

This consists of a main cavity and an atrial appendage, the left auricle. The interior is smooth, but the auricle is ridged. The left atrium forms most of the base of the heart. The four pulmonary veins open into the posterior wall. The left atrioventricular orifice is protected by the bicuspid mitral valve.

Left ventricle

The left ventricle is responsible for pumping blood throughout the entire body except the lungs. Consequently, its wall is three times thicker than that of the right ventricle, and pressures in this chamber are up to six times greater.

There are well-developed trabeculae carneae and two large papillary muscles.

The outflow tract of the ventricle is the aortic vestibule.

The mitral valve guards the left atrioventricular orifice. It is bicuspid (anterior and posterior cusps), with attached chordae tendineae similar to the tricuspid valve.

The three-cusped aortic valve is similar to the pulmonary valve. Above each cusp the aortic wall bulges to form the aortic sinuses. The right aortic sinus gives rise to the right coronary artery; the left sinus gives rise to the left coronary artery.

The interventricular septum is of equal thickness to the rest of the left ventricle, and consequently it bulges into the right ventricle. Where it attaches to the fibrous ring, it is thinner and more fibrous—this is the membranous part of the septum. It transmits the atrioventricular bundle of the conducting system.

A defect in the interventricular septum (in either its muscular or membranous part) is called a ventricular septal defect (VSD). The majority of VSDs in the muscular part of the septum close spontaneously unless large. Failure to close requires surgery because the high pressure in the left ventricle forces blood to cross the defect into the right ventricle, dilating it.

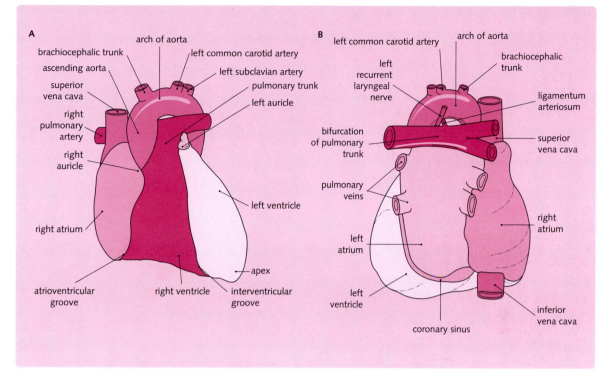

A

brachiocephalic trunk
arch of aorta
ascending aorta
left common carotid artery
superior vena cava
left subclavian artery
pulmonary trunk
right pulmonary artery
left auricle
right auricle
left ventricle
right atrium
right ventricle
left ventricle
atrioventricular groove
right ventricle
interventricular groove
apex

B

left common carotid artery
arch of aorta
left recurrent laryngeal nerve
brachiocephalic trunk
ligamentum arteriosum
bifurcation of pulmonary trunk
superior vena cava
pulmonary veins
right atrium
left atrium
left ventricle
inferior vena cava
coronary sinus

Fig. 3.17 Anterior (A) and posterior (B) surfaces of the heart.

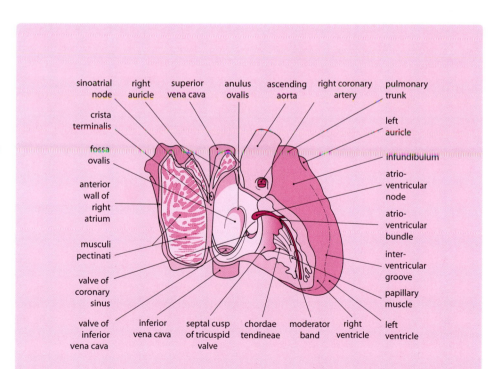

Fig. 3.18 Interior of right atrium and right ventricle.

sinoatrial node
right auricle
superior vena cava
anulus ovalis
ascending aorta
right coronary artery
pulmonary trunk
crista terminalis
left auricle
fossa ovalis
infundibulum
anterior wall of right atrium
atrio-ventricular node
musculi pectinati
atrio-ventricular bundle
inter-ventricular groove
valve of coronary sinus
papillary muscle
valve of inferior vena cava
inferior vena cava
septal cusp of tricuspid valve
chordae tendineae
moderator band
right ventricle
left ventricle

Skeleton of the heart

The atria and ventricles are attached to a pair of fibrous rings around the atrioventricular orifices. The fibrous rings separate the muscle fibres of the atria and ventricles, with the atrioventricular bundle of the conducting system forming the only physiological connection between the atria and ventricles.

The bases of the cusps of the atrioventricular valves and the membranous part of the atrioventricular septum are also attached to the fibrous skeleton.

There are fibrous rings that support the aortic and pulmonary valves.

Blood supply of the heart

Figure 3.19 illustrates the blood supply of the heart. The ascending aorta has two branches, which arise from the aortic sinuses. These branches are the right and left coronary arteries. Both run in the coronary groove and supply the myocardium through a series of important branches (Fig. 3.19).

Left and right dominance of the heart is a reference to the coronary artery from which the posterior interventricular branch arises. Right dominance is more common: where the posterior interventricular branch arises from the right coronary artery.

The left coronary artery (LCA) is short and divides into circumflex and anterior interventricular (or left anterior descending) branches. The circumflex branch runs in the coronary groove supplying the left atrium and left ventricle. The anterior interventricular branch runs in the anterior interventricular groove supplying both ventricles and interventricular septum before anastomosing at the apex with the posterior interventricular artery.

The right coronary artery (RCA) gives off branches to the right atrium and right ventricle as it descends in the coronary groove (Fig 3.19). It has a right marginal branch that runs along the inferior border of the heart and supplies the right ventricle. On the inferior surface of the heart, the RCA anastomoses with the circumflex artery of the LCA as well as giving off a posterior interventricular (or right posterior descending) branch that runs in the posterior interventricular groove and supplies both ventricles and the interventricular septum.

The RCA in 60% of individuals supplies the sinoatrial node and in 90% of individuals also supplies the atrioventricular node. The atrioventricular bundle and its right terminal branch are supplied by the RCA. The left terminal branch is supplied by both the RCA and LCA.

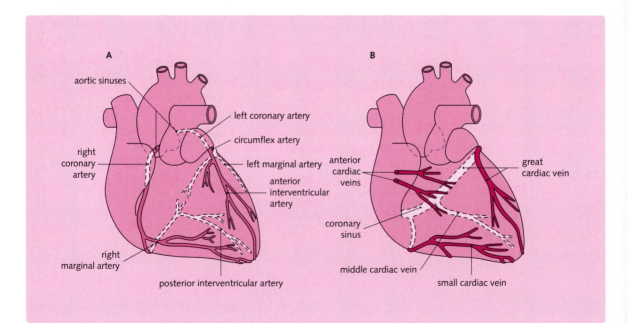

Fig. 3.19 Blood supply of the heart. (A) coronary arteries; (B) cardiac veins.

Venous drainage of the heart

Most of the venous blood in the heart drains into the coronary sinus, which lies in the posterior atrioventricular groove. It is a continuation of the great cardiac vein, and it opens into the right atrium.

The middle and small cardiac veins empty directly into the coronary sinus.

The remaining blood is returned to the heart via the anterior cardiac veins which drain into the right atrium and other small veins (venae cordis minimae) that open directly into the heart chambers.

Conducting system of the heart

The heart contracts rhythmically at about 70 beats per minute.

The sinoatrial node (pacemaker) lies in the upper part of the sulcus terminalis of the right atrium. Impulses generated here are transmitted across the atria, causing them to contract. The atrioventricular node which lies in the atrial septum just above the attachment of the septal cusp of the tricuspid valve conducts the impulses to the atrioventricular bundle.

The atrioventricular bundle lies in the membranous part of the interventricular septum. At this point, the bundle divides into two branches, one for each ventricle:

- The right branch conducts the impulse to the apex of the right ventricle and, via the moderator band, to its anterior wall. The impulses are then distributed throughout the muscle through purkinje fibres.
- The left branch pierces the septum and passes down on the left side beneath the endocardium. It divides into an anterior and a posterior branch.

The heart is innervated by the left and right vagus nerves and by branches of the sympathetic trunk. Figure 3.20 gives details of the nerve supply.

Great vessels of the thorax

Figure 3.21 outlines the thoracic aorta and its branches. The aortic arch and its three branches that supply the head, neck and upper limb are posterior to the manubrium. The descending thoracic aorta begins at the level of the sternal angle to the left of the midline and passes posterior to the diaphragm (in the midline) through the aortic hiatus opposite vertebra T12.

Referred pain from a myocardial infarction is transmitted through the cardiac branches of the cervical sympathetic trunk. Afferent fibres enter the spinal cord of the upper five thoracic nerves, and pain is referred to dermatomes that these spinal nerves supply, e.g. the medial surface of the left upper limb.

Fig. 3.20 Outline of the nerve supply of the heart

Nerve type	Origin	Action
Sympathetic nerves	Cervical and upper thoracic part of the sympathetic trunk via the cardiac plexuses	Increase the rate and force of contraction
Parasympathetic nerves	Vagus nerves via the cardiac plexuses	Reduce the rate and force of contraction

Fig. 3.21 Aorta and its branches in the thorax

Artery	Course and origin	Branches
Ascending aorta	Originates from the left ventricle, ascends and becomes the aortic arch at the level of the sternal angle	Right and left coronary arteries
Aortic arch	Arches posteriorly to the left of the trachea and the oesophagus, and continues as the descending aorta	Brachiocephalic trunk, left common carotid artery, left subclavian artery
Descending aorta	Descends to the left of the vertebral column, moves anterior to reach the midline, and leaves the thorax by passing behind the diaphragm at T12	Posterior intercostal arteries, subcostal arteries and visceral branches
Bronchial	Arises from the descending aorta	To bronchi and visceral pleura
Oesophageal	Arises from the descending aorta	To oesophagus
Superior phrenic	Arises from the descending aorta	To diaphragm
Posterior intercostal	Arises from the descending aorta	To intercostal muscles and thoracic wall

Figure 3.22 shows an anterior view of the aortic arch and pulmonary trunk.

Pulmonary trunk

This vessel divides inferior to the arch of the aorta to form the right and left pulmonary arteries which transport deoxygenated blood to the lungs.

The ligamentum arteriosum (Fig. 3.22) is a fibrous band that connects the bifurcation of the pulmonary trunk to the aortic arch. It is the remnant of the ductus arteriosus, which in the fetus conducts blood from the pulmonary trunk to the aorta, bypassing the lungs.

Superior vena cava

The superior vena cava is formed by the union of the right and left brachiocephalic veins. It carries blood from the upper limbs and head and neck (before entering the pericardium). It receives the azygos vein which receives pericardial, bronchial, mediastinal, oesophageal, vertebral venous plexus, posterior and superior intercostal venous tributaries. Thus, the

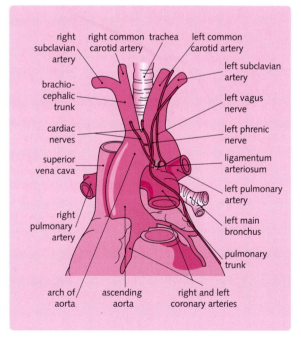

Fig. 3.22 Aorta and pulmonary trunk.

superior vena cava also drains thoracic structures indirectly. The superior vena cava drains into the right atrium.

Inferior vena cava

The vein pierces the central tendon of the diaphragm opposite T8 vertebra and almost immediately it enters the right atrium.

Figure 3.23 shows the superior and inferior venae cavae and their main tributaries.

Pulmonary veins

Two pulmonary veins leave each lung, carrying oxygenated blood to the left atrium of the heart. The veins branch and four pulmonary veins enter the left atrium.

Azygos system of veins

Figure 3.24 shows the azygos system of veins and the thoracic duct. These pass through the aortic hiatus.

Nerves of the thorax

The right phrenic nerve descends on the cervical pleura posterior to the right brachiocephalic vein into the thorax. Within the thorax, the right phrenic nerve is lateral to the right brachiocephalic vein then the superior vena cava before it passes over the fibrous pericardium overlying the right atrium (Fig. 3.15A). It passes through the diaphragm with the inferior vena cava (Fig. 3.11).

The left phrenic nerve descends on the cervical pleura behind the left brachiocephalic vein then it is

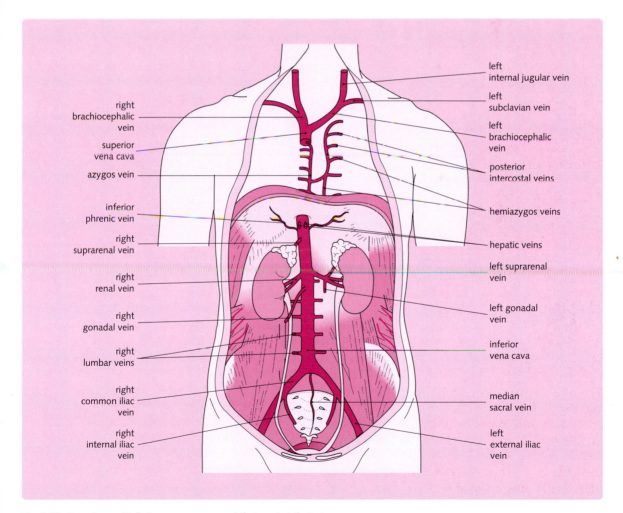

Fig. 3.23 Superior and inferior venae cavae and their main tributaries.

Fig. 3.24 Azygos system of veins and the thoracic duct.

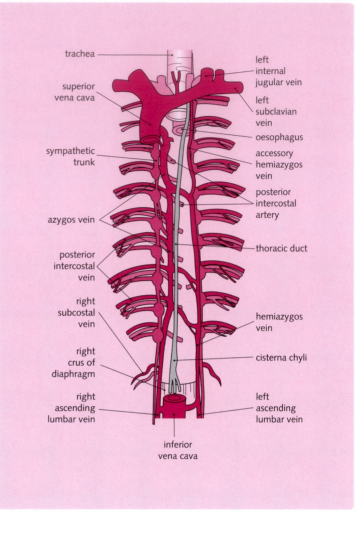

posterior to this vein and anterior to the left subclavian artery as the nerve passes into the thorax. In the thorax, the left phrenic nerve lies in the interval between the left common carotid and left subclavian arteries and it crosses the left vagus nerve superficially. The nerve then crosses the aortic arch and over the left superior intercostal vein (Fig. 3.15B) before it passes over the fibrous pericardium overlying the left ventricle to pierce the left hemi diaphragm (Fig. 3.11).

The vagus nerves descend in the carotid sheath posterior to the common carotid artery and internal jugular vein in the carotid sheath towards the thoracic inlet. The thoracic structures innervated by these nerves are summarized in Figure 3.25.

The right vagus nerve descends over the right subclavian artery then between the brachiocephalic trunk and right brachiocephalic vein into the thorax. Within the thorax, the nerve passes behind the brachiocephalic trunk to cross the trachea antero-posteriorly (Fig. 3.15). It gives off cardiac branches in the root of the neck to supply the heart. The nerve passes deep to the azygos vein and then posterior to the lung hilum to form plexuses that supply the lungs and oesophagus. The nerve trunk is then reformed and descends along the oesophagus before leaving the thorax with it through the diaphragm (Fig. 3.11).

The left vagus nerve descends over the right subclavian artery posterior to the left brachiocephalic vein into the thorax. It pass between the left common carotid and left subclavian arteries and is crossed superficially by the left phrenic nerve. As it descends over the aortic arch, the left superior intercostal vein crosses it superficially. The nerve gives off cardiac

Fig. 3.25 Nerves of the thorax

Nerve (origin)	Course and distribution
Vagus, cranial nerve X (medulla oblongata)	Enters superior mediastinum posterior to the sternoclavicular joint and brachiocephalic vein to supply the pulmonary plexus, oesophageal plexus, and cardiac plexus
Phrenic (anterior rami of C3–C5)	Enters thorax and runs between mediastinal pleura and pericardium to supply motor and sensory innervation to the diaphragm. It also has a sensory supply mediastinal pleura, pericardium and diaphragmatic peritoneum (in abdominal cavity)
Intercostal nerves (anterior rami of T1–T11)	Run between internal and innermost layers of intercostals muscles and supply skin, intercostal muscles and parietal pleura. The lower six intercostal nerve also supply the skin, musculature and parietal peritoneum of the abdominal wall
Subcostal nerve (T12)	Follows inferior border of 12th rib and passes into the abdominal wall. Its lateral cutaneous branch pierces the internal and external oblique muscle layers to supply the skin over the hip laterally, inferior between the iliac crest and greater trochanter of femur
Recurrent laryngeal nerve (cranial nerve X)	Loops around subclavian artery on right and arch of aorta on left, and ascends in the tracheoesophageal groove; supplies intrinsic muscles of larynx (except cricothyroid) and sensation below level of vocal folds
Cardiac plexus (cranial nerve X and sympathetic trunks)	Fibres pass along coronary arteries to sinoatrial node; parasympathetic fibres (from vagus nerve) reduce heart rate and force of contraction. Sympathetic nerve (from spinal cord levels T1–T5) increase heart rate and force of contraction
Pulmonary plexus (cranial nerve X and sympathetic trunks)	Plexus forms in hilum (root) of lung and extends along branches of bronchi; parasympathetic fibres (from vagus nerve) constrict bronchioles, sympathetic fibres (from spinal cord segments T2–T6) dilate bronchioles
Oesophageal plexus (cranial nerve X and sympathetic trunks)	Vagus nerve and sympathetic nerves form a plexus around oesophagus to supply muscle and glands.

branches in the root of the neck to supply the heart and its left recurrent laryngeal branch that hooks under the aortic arch (Fig. 3.15) to ascend between the trachea and oesophagus. The left vagus nerve passes posterior to the lung hilum to form plexuses that supply the lungs and oesophagus before reforming to exit the thorax with the oesophagus through the diaphragm (Fig. 3.11).

Figure 3.25 summarizes the other main nerves of the thorax.

Thoracic sympathetic trunk

The sympathetic trunks follow a paravertebral course and run on either side of the entire vertebral column. Superiorly the trunks lie over the heads of the ribs, but inferiorly they lie over the body of the vertebrae. They pass into the abdomen from the thorax behind the medial arcuate ligaments of the diaphragm.

There is usually a ganglion for each thoracic spinal nerve, but the first ganglion usually merges with the inferior cervical ganglion to form the stellate ganglion.

White and grey rami communicantes from the sympathetic ganglia communicate with the thoracic spinal nerves.

Medial branches from the thoracic sympathetic ganglia innervate thoracic viscera. The branches from the upper five to six ganglia form a plexus on the thoracic aorta and supply the heart, lung, oesophagus and trachea. The branches from the lower ganglia form the splanchnic nerves.

The sympathetic trunk gives rise to the greater, lesser, and least splanchnic nerves. The greater nerve is formed by branches from the 5th to 9th ganglia. The lesser nerve is formed by branches from the 10th to 11th ganglia, and the least nerve is a branch of the 12th ganglion. These pass into the abdomen behind the diaphragm to relay in the coeliac ganglion and supply abdominal structures.

Lymphatic drainage of the thorax

Figure 3.26 shows the lymphatic drainage of the thoracic cavity.

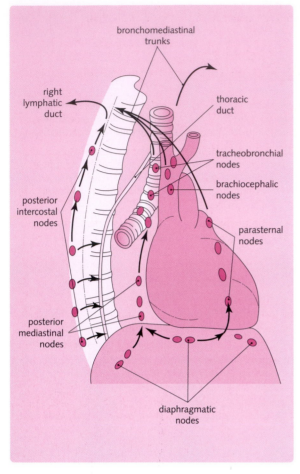

Fig. 3.26 Lymphatic drainage of the thoracic cavity (right hemithorax).

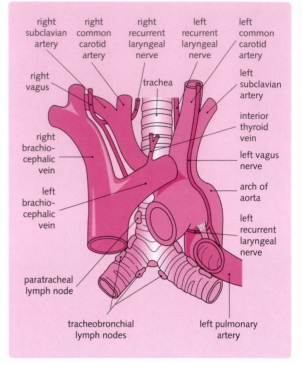

Fig. 3.27 Trachea and its main relations anteriorly and laterally.

The thoracic duct (Fig. 3.24) receives lymph from:

- The lower half of the body.
- The left posterior intercostal nodes.
- The left side of the head and neck, and the left upper limb, via the left jugular and subclavian lymph trunks, respectively.

The right lymph duct receives lymph from the posterior right thoracic wall. The right side of the head and neck, and the right upper limb drain into the right jugular and subclavian trunks, respectively. These vessels open into the great veins either independently or as a single trunk, the right lymph trunk.

Thymus

This is the major organ responsible for the maturation of T lymphocytes. It is a large bilobed organ at birth, lying in the superior and anterior divisions of the mediastinum, anterior to the great vessels. The gland involutes after puberty.

Trachea

The trachea (Fig. 3.27) commences in the neck, at the lower border of the cricoid cartilage (level of C6 vertebral body). It passes into the superior mediastinum, anterior to the oesophagus and close to the midline. At the level of T4 vertebra, the trachea bifurcates into the right and left main bronchi. The right main bronchus is shorter, wider, and more vertical than the left—foreign bodies are therefore more likely to lodge in this bronchus or one of its branches.

Oesophagus

This organ commences as a continuation of the laryngopharynx at the level of C6 vertebra. In the thorax the oesophagus lies between the trachea and the vertebral column. It then passes through the diaphragm at the level of T10 vertebra and after 1–2 cm enters the stomach. Fibres from the right crus of the diaphragm form a sling around the oesophagus.

Fig. 3.28 Blood and nerve supply, and lymphatic drainage of the oesophagus. (Adapted from *Anatomy as a Basis for Clinical Medicine*, by E C B Hall-Craggs, Williams & Wilkins.)

	Upper oesophagus	Middle oesophagus	Lower oesophagus
Arterial supply	Inferior thyroid artery	Oesophageal branches of the aorta	Left gastric artery
Venous drainage	Brachiocephalic vein	Azygos vein	Oesophageal tributaries of the left gastric veins which drain finally into the portal vein
Nerve supply	Recurrent laryngeal nerves and sympathetic fibres from cell bodies in the middle cervical ganglion running on the inferior thyroid artery	Fibres from the anterior and posterior oesophageal plexus from the vagus nerves; sympathetic fibres from the sympathetic trunks and greater splanchnic nerves	
Lymphatic drainage	Deep cervical nodes near the origin of the inferior thyroid artery	Tracheobronchial and posterior mediastinal nodes	Preaortic nodes of the coeliac group

The upper oesophageal sphincter lies at the level of cricopharyngeus. This is the narrowest part of the oesophagus. Other normal constrictions in the oesophagus are found where it is crossed by the aortic arch and left main bronchus, and where it pierces the diaphragm. The left atrium is an anterior relation to the oesophagus and causes constriction when the atrium become dilated in mitral valve incompetence (during left ventricular contraction blood regurgitates back into the left atrium).

Figure 3.28 outlines the blood supply, lymphatic drainage, and nerve supply of the oesophagus.

PLEURAE AND LUNGS

Pleurae

The pleurae surround the lungs. The pleura is divided into two layers: the parietal and visceral pleurae (Fig. 3.29).

Blood from the inferior third of the oesophagus drains into the oesophageal tribuatries of the left gastric vein through the oesophageal hiatus of the diaphragm. As a result the venous blood enters the portal venous system and then the liver before re-entering the systemic venous circulation. Oesophageal varices (dilated tortuous veins) can develop if there is portal system hypertension due to cirrhosis of the liver.

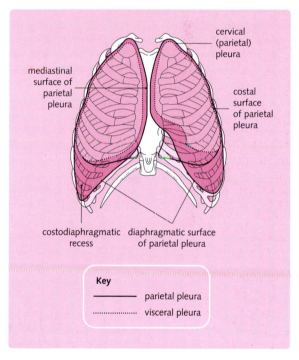

Fig. 3.29 Pleurae.

The parietal pleura lines the thoracic wall (costal pleura), the thoracic surface of the diaphragm (diaphragmatic pleura), and the lateral aspect of the mediastinum (mediastinal pleura). At the thoracic inlet, it arches over the lungs as the cervical pleura. It lies 2.5 cm above the medial end of the clavicle at this point.

The visceral pleura completely invests the outer surface of the lung and invaginates into the fissures of the lungs. Consequently, it is firmly adherent to the lungs.

The two layers become continuous with each other at the root of the lung. Here, there is a double layer of pleura that hangs down as the pulmonary ligament.

The pleural cavity lies between the two pleural layers. It is a potential space and, in health, contains a small quantity of clear pleural fluid.

Where the parietal pleura is reflected off the diaphragm onto the thoracic wall, a recess is formed that is not filled with lung except in deep inspiration. This is the costodiaphragmatic recess. A similar recess is formed between the thoracic wall and mediastinum (costomediastinal recess).

The nerve supply of the pleura is described in Figure 3.30. The visceral pleura has no somatic innervation, and it is, therefore, insensitive to pain.

Blood supply of the pleurae

The parietal pleura is supplied by the intercostal arteries and branches of the internal thoracic artery. Venous drainage and lymphatic drainage are similarly shared.

The visceral pleura is supplied by the bronchial arteries. It shares venous and lymphatic drainage with the lung.

Endothoracic fascia

This layer of loose connective tissue separates the parietal pleura from the thoracic wall. It includes the suprapleural membrane, which covers the dome of the parietal pleura where it projects into the root of the neck.

Lungs

The lungs in life are light, spongy, and elastic. The surface changes from a pink colour at birth to a mottled darker colour in later life because of deposition of carbon particles from atmospheric pollution. This is more pronounced in city-dwellers and smokers.

Each lung lies free in the pleural cavity except at its root, where it is attached to the mediastinum.

Surfaces and borders of the lungs

These are indicated in Figures 3.31 and 3.32. Each lung has an apex that projects into the neck about 2.5 cm above the medial end of the clavicle, a base that lies on the diaphragm, a costal surface, and a mediastinal surface.

The hilum (root) of the lung (Fig. 3.32) lies on the mediastinal surface where the bronchi and neurovascular bundles enter the lungs.

Bronchi and bronchopulmonary segments

The trachea divides into the right and left main bronchi. These are fibromuscular tubes reinforced by incomplete rings of cartilage. They are lined by respiratory epithelium.

In the lung, the main bronchus divides into secondary (lobar) bronchi, which in turn divide into tertiary (segmental) bronchi. The latter supply the bronchopulmonary segments, which are the functional units of the lungs (Fig. 3.33).

Bronchopulmonary segments are wedge shaped, with the base lying peripherally and the apex lying

Fig. 3.30 Nerve supply of the pleura	
Pleura	**Nerve supply**
Costal	Segmentally by the intercostal nerves
Mediastinal	The phrenic nerve
Diaphragmatic	The phrenic nerve centrally, the lower five intercostal nerves peripherally
Visceral	Autonomic nerve supply from the pulmonary plexus

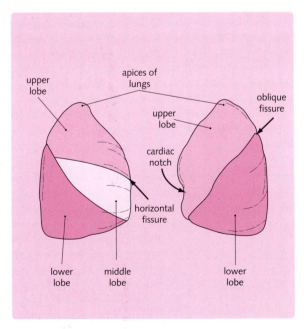

Fig. 3.31 Surface of the lungs.

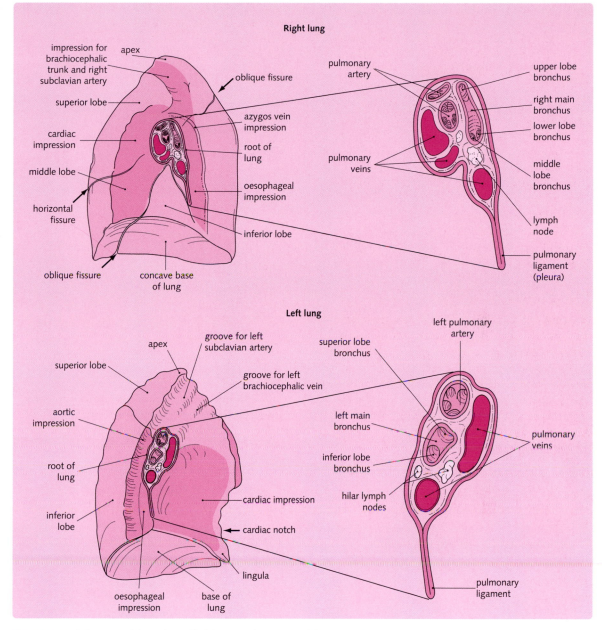

Right lung

impression for brachiocephalic trunk and right subclavian artery

apex

oblique fissure

superior lobe

azygos vein impression

cardiac impression

root of lung

middle lobe

oesophageal impression

horizontal fissure

inferior lobe

oblique fissure

concave base of lung

pulmonary artery

upper lobe bronchus

right main bronchus

lower lobe bronchus

pulmonary veins

middle lobe bronchus

lymph node

pulmonary ligament (pleura)

Left lung

apex

groove for left subclavian artery

superior lobe bronchus

left pulmonary artery

superior lobe

groove for left brachiocephalic vein

aortic impression

left main bronchus

pulmonary veins

root of lung

inferior lobe bronchus

inferior lobe

cardiac impression

hilar lymph nodes

cardiac notch

lingula

oesophageal impression

base of lung

pulmonary ligament

Fig. 3.32 Medial aspect of the right and left lungs and contents of their roots. Impressions are only seen in fixed lungs.

towards the root of the lung. There are 10 segments in each lung. Each segment has its own segmental bronchus, segmental artery, lymphatic vessels, and autonomic nerves. The veins are between segments. Within each segment, the segmental bronchus repeatedly subdivides and reduces in diameter with each division. The airway that is no longer supported by cartilage is now called a bronchiole. These subdivide further and they eventually give rise to millions of

The right principle bronchus is wider and more vertical than the left and thus is prone to have inhaled foreign objects lodged within it. The basal superior bronchopulmonary segment is at 90° to the bronchial tree. In supine patients, bronchial secretions drain into this segment and cause pneumonia.

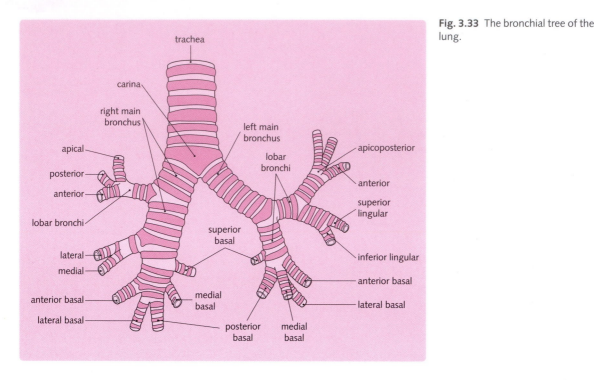

Fig. 3.33 The bronchial tree of the lung.

alveoli. Alveoli are thin-walled sacs of epithelium surrounded by capillaries that bring blood into close contact with air which is within each alveolus.

Blood supply of the lungs

The lungs have a dual blood supply:

• Bronchial arteries from the thoracic aorta supply the walls of the bronchi, the connective tissue of the lung and the visceral pleura. Bronchial veins drain into the azygos system of veins.

• Pulmonary arteries transport deoxygenated blood to the alveolar capillaries. The pulmonary veins return oxygenated blood to the lungs.

There are anastomoses between the pulmonary and bronchial circulations.

Nerve supply of the lungs

Sympathetic and parasympathetic nerves from the pulmonary plexuses, which lie anterior and posterior to the lung roots, supply the smooth muscle of the bronchial tree, the vessels, and the mucous membrane.

Lymphatic drainage of the lungs

Figure 3.34 illustrates the lymphatic drainage of the lungs. Lung carcinoma is very common and it is important to have an understanding of where it may spread.

Mechanics of respiration

Respiration consists of an inspiratory and an expiratory phase as the thoracic cavity diameters increase and decrease respectively (Fig. 3.35). These diameters are the:

• Anteroposterior diameter: lies between the sternum and costal cartilages anteriorly and the

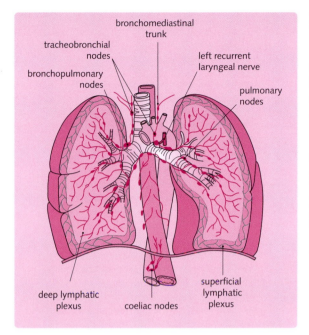

tracheobronchial
nodes

bronchomediastinal
trunk

bronchopulmonary
nodes

left recurrent
laryngeal nerve

pulmonary
nodes

deep lymphatic
plexus

coeliac nodes

superficial
lymphatic
plexus

Fig. 3.34 Lymphatic drainage of the lungs.

Oncology

Bronchial carcinoma accounts for 27% of cancer deaths and has a poor prognosis. It spreads via the lymphatic vessels and the tracheobronchial nodes around the carina (tracheal bifurcation) are commonly involved, causing the carina to widen. The left recurrent laryngeal nerve may become involved as it hooks under the aortic arch (around the ligamentum arteriosum) and superior to the left principal bronchus. This causes paralysis of the left laryngeal musculature (except cricothyroid muscle), causing the vocal cords to adopt a mid-abducted position. The patient complains of a hoarse, weakened voice and has a bovine cough.

Clinical examination

In patients with severe obstructive airway disease, e.g. asthma, chronic obstructive pulmonary disease (COPD) make use of their accessory respiratory muscles e.g. sternocleidomastoid, pectoralis major, scalene, latissimus dorsi, and anterior abdominal muscles. The patient may lean against a table top with their arm to fix the insertion of latissimus dorsi. The muscle is now used to move the rib cage. Other signs include contraction of sternocleidomastoid and scalene muscles, intercostal recession (indrawing of the spaces), suprasternal recession, Harrison's sulcus (intercostal recession – seen in paediatrics) and pursing of lips (this creates positive air pressure to keep smaller airways open that normally collapse and ease work of breathing).

- Vertical diameter: lies between the apex of the pleural cavity superiorly and the diaphragm inferiorly. Its diameter is increased by the diaphragm flattening during contraction.

Types of respiration

In adult males, diaphragmatic movement is greater than thoracic movement and, therefore, males are said to have an abdominal type of respiration. Adult females have a greater thoracic movement and, therefore, use a thoracic type of respiration. Infants under the age of two depend on diaphragmatic movements because their ribs are horizontal. In adults the normal rate of respiration is 14 breaths per minute; however, children have a higher rate.

RADIOLOGICAL ANATOMY

Imaging of the thorax

The chest X-ray is a common imaging tool to assess the lungs, heart and great vessels.

The traditional views taken are named after the direction the X-ray beam is projected, i.e. posteroanterior (PA) and lateral. The films are taken with the patient in maximal inspiration to prevent the artificial appearance of an enlarged heart (cardiomegaly) or pulmonary oedema.

Before any attempt to interpret the X-ray, its quality should be evaluated because poor quality can cause difficulties. Check the:

vertebral column and ribs posteriorly. Its diameter is increased by forward movement of the sternum and the upper ribs are raised superiorly (resembles the movement of a pump handle). The axis of movement passes through the neck of the rib.
- Transverse diameter: lies between corresponding right and left ribs. Its diameter is increased by the lower ribs being raised superiorly and outwards (resembles the movement of a bucket handle). The axis of movement passes through the costochondral junction (anteriorly) and the head of the rib (posteriorly).

Fig. 3.35 Movements and muscles involved in respiration

Movements	Effect	Muscles involved
Quiet inspiration	Increased vertical diameter	Diaphragm contracts causing flattening of the domes
Quiet inspiration	Increased anteroposterior diameter	Scalenus muscles contract and fix the first rib. The upper intercostal muscles contract to elevate the upper ribs at their sternal ends towards the first rib, and this pushes the sternum forwards—known as the pump handle movement
Quiet inspiration	Increased transverse diameter	Scalenus muscles contract fixing the first rib. The intercostal muscles contract raising the lower ribs along an anteroposterior axis that runs through the costochondral joint (anteriorly) and costovertebral joint (posteriorly). The lower ribs are raised upward and outward in a bucket handle movement
Forced inspiration	Increase of all three diameters	In addition to the diaphragm contracting, the scalenus and sternocleidomastoid muscles elevate the ribs and manubrium. The intercostal muscles forcefully contract elevating the ribs. Quadratus lumborum lowers and fixes the twelfth rib. This allows a forceful diaphragmatic contraction. The erector spinae muscles arch the back and increase the thoracic volume. With the humerus and scapula fixed the pectoral and serratus anterior muscles raise the ribs
Quiet expiration	Decrease of all three diameters	Elastic recoil of the lungs and controlled relaxation of the intercostal and diaphragmatic muscles causes this passive movement
Forced expiration	Decrease of all three diameters	Contraction of the anterior abdominal wall muscles depresses the ribs and reinforces the elastic recoil of the lungs. The abdominal contents are pushed up forcing the diaphragm upwards. The intercostal muscles contract and prevent bulging of their intercostal spaces

- Projection of the film i.e. posteroanterior (PA), anteroposterior (AP) or lateral. An AP film will artificially enlarge the heart.
- Orientation. The heart is not always on the left (dextrocardia).
- Rotation. The medial ends of the clavicle should be the same distance from an intervening thoracic vertebral spinous process. If not rotation is present.
- Penetration of tissue. The thoracic vertebral bodies should only be slightly visible through the cardiac shadow. If the vertebral bodies cannot be seen through the cardiac shadow the film is under-penetrated.
- Degree of inspiration. If between five to seven ribs can be counted anteriorly (i.e. adjacent to the costochondral joints) or ten ribs posteriorly (i.e. adjacent to the costovertebral joints) then it is adequate.

Normal radiographic anatomy of a PA chest X-ray

In a normal PA chest radiograph (Fig. 3.36) the right superior mediastinum, lateral to the thoracic spine has a curved shadow, the superior vena cava (20). This merges with the right atrium (18) or right cardiac border, inferiorly. The inferior border of the heart is formed by the right ventricle with the left ventricle contributing to formation of the apex and left heart border.

The pulmonary arteries (8, 19) can be seen arising from the mediastinum, especially on the right where a V-shape is formed by the upper and lower branches of the pulmonary artery. The left pulmonary artery (8) is not as prominent as it lies above the auricle of the left atrium (9). The aorta arch or knuckle (6) is seen superior to the pulmonary trunk (7). The descending aorta (11) runs inferiorly to the aortic hiatus at T12 to pass posterior to the diaphragm.

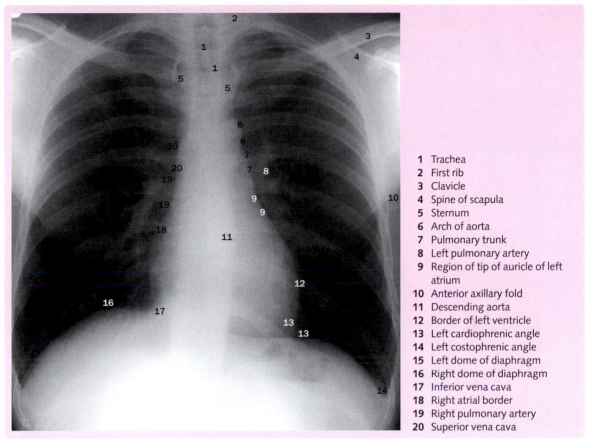

Fig. 3.36 An adult male chest posteroanterior radiograph.

1	Trachea
2	First rib
3	Clavicle
4	Spine of scapula
5	Sternum
6	Arch of aorta
7	Pulmonary trunk
8	Left pulmonary artery
9	Region of tip of auricle of left atrium
10	Anterior axillary fold
11	Descending aorta
12	Border of left ventricle
13	Left cardiophrenic angle
14	Left costophrenic angle
15	Left dome of diaphragm
16	Right dome of diaphragm
17	Inferior vena cava
18	Right atrial border
19	Right pulmonary artery
20	Superior vena cava

The right hemi diaphragm (16) is higher due to the position of the liver and because the heart 'pushes' down the left hemi diaphragm (15).

The trachea (1), if followed inferiorly, is seen faintly as it bifurcates at T4 (sternal angle) with the aortic knuckle to the left and inferiorly.

The scapulae do not overlie the lungs and the anterior axillary fold (10) formed by the pectoralis major muscle is seen.

Radiology

The carina (point of tracheal bifurcation) can be seen on a PA chest X-ray. The angle it forms can widen in bronchial carcinoma due to tracheobronchial node enlargement. These nodes are positioned around the carina and enlarge due to metastatic spread.

How to examine a PA chest X-ray methodically

The following is a method of how to examine a PA film:

- Lungs: Each should be of an equal lucency. Normally the horizontal fissure run between the right hilum and right sixth rib in the mid-axillary line.
- Costophrenic angles: Normally they are well defined.
- Diaphragm: The right diaphragm is normally higher than the left due to the position of the liver.
- Heart: Its diameter should be less than half the transthoracic diameter.
- Hilum: Normally they are concave.
- Mediastinum: Its edge should be well defined. However, the angle between the heart and diaphragm (cardiophrenic angle) may not be but this is normal.

- Trachea: Is a central structure but at the aortic knuckle is slightly to the right.
- Bones: Follow edges of clavicle, scapulae, ribs and vertebrae for continuity of the cortical bone.

Areas of darkness indicate a fracture. Compare one side with the other.

- Soft tissue: Are there any enlargements?

Normal radiographic anatomy of a lateral chest X-ray

In a normal lateral chest radiograph (Fig. 3.37) a retrosternal space posterior to the sternum (6) and anterior to the ascending aorta contains lung. Any change in lucency indicates an anterior mediastinal mass i.e. thymoma.

The right ventricle (8), if enlarged, may also distend into this space. The left atrium (15) forms the posterior border of the cardiac shadow.

The left hemi diaphragm (14) is seen with the gas bubble of the fundus of the stomach underneath it.

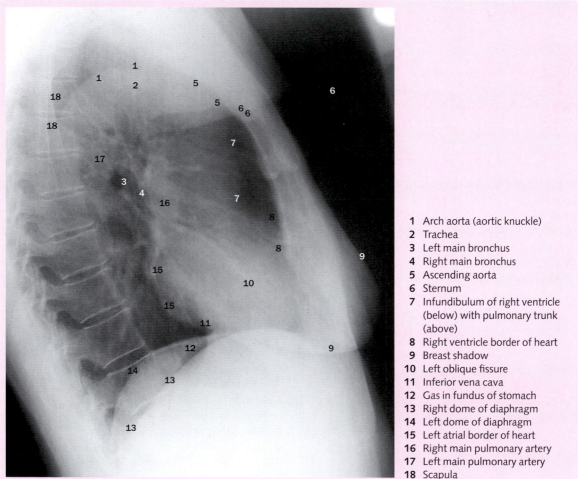

1. Arch aorta (aortic knuckle)
2. Trachea
3. Left main bronchus
4. Right main bronchus
5. Ascending aorta
6. Sternum
7. Infundibulum of right ventricle (below) with pulmonary trunk (above)
8. Right ventricle border of heart
9. Breast shadow
10. Left oblique fissure
11. Inferior vena cava
12. Gas in fundus of stomach
13. Right dome of diaphragm
14. Left dome of diaphragm
15. Left atrial border of heart
16. Right main pulmonary artery
17. Left main pulmonary artery
18. Scapula

Fig. 3.37 An adult female chest lateral radiograph.

The shadow of the inferior vena cava (11) is seen running between the diaphragm and the inferior border of the heart.

The trachea (2), if followed inferiorly, divides into a steeper inclined right main bronchus (4) accompanied by the right pulmonary artery (16) and a shallower left main bronchus (3) with left pulmonary artery.

The ascending aorta (5) forms a smooth curved shadow as it becomes the aortic arch (1) then the descending aorta which is superimposed upon the thoracic vertebrae.

How to examine a lateral chest X-ray methodically

The following is a method of how to examine a lateral film:

- Diaphragm: The right hemi diaphragm passes through the heart across the width of the thorax.

The left hemi diaphragm appears to stop at the posterior border of the heart and has the gas bubble of the gastric fundus beneath it. Is the costophrenic angle clearly defined?

- Lungs: The lung anterior to the heart should be of an equal lucency to that posterior to the heart. Is the retrosternal space clear?
- Check the hila and position of the lung fissures.
- The lower thoracic vertebral bodies become darker. Note any change in shape, or size.

Angiography of the great vessels

Figure 3.38 shows the branches of the aortic arch and their subsequent divisions to form the arterial supply of the head, neck, and thoracic cage.

1	Ascending aorta
2	Brachiocephalic trunk
3	Left common carotid artery
4	Left subclavian artery
5	Right subclavian artery
6	Right common carotid artery
7	Vertebral artery
8	Internal thoracic artery
9	Inferior thyroid artery
10	Ascending cervical artery
11	Thyrocervical trunk
12	Suprascapular artery
13	Costocervical trunk
14	Superior thoracic artery
15	Lateral thoracic artery
16	Deltoid branch of the thoraco-acromial artery

Fig. 3.38 Aortic arch arteriogram.

The abdomen

Objectives

In this chapter you will learn to:

- Understand the boundaries of the abdominal cavity, both skeletal and muscular.
- Outline the surface anatomy of the abdomen, including surface markings of organs.
- Know the boundaries and contents of the inguinal canal.
- Describe the structure and nerve supply of the peritoneum, including its recesses/pouches.
- List the relations of the stomach.
- Know the morphological differences between different gut sections.
- Describe the anatomy of the colon.
- Describe the anatomy of the liver, including its peritoneal reflections and the biliary tree.
- Discuss the blood and nerve supply of the gastrointestinal tract, with its lymphatic drainage.
- Describe the anatomy of the kidneys and suprarenal glands.
- Recognize the bony and soft-tissue features of a normal radiograph of the abdomen.
- Have a method for reviewing an abdominal X-ray.

REGIONS AND COMPONENTS OF THE ABDOMEN

The abdominal cavity is separated from the thoracic cavity by the diaphragm. Because the domes of the diaphragm arch high above the costal margin, the upper part of the abdomen—including the liver, the spleen, the upper poles of the kidneys, and the suprarenal glands—is protected by the bony thoracic cage. The bony pelvis surrounds the lower part.

Posteriorly, the vertebral column protects the abdominal contents, but anteriorly and laterally the abdomen is more vulnerable to injury, with only a muscular wall for protection.

Over the anterior abdominal wall, a part of the superficial fascia condenses into a strong but thin membranous layer under the fat. This allows the fatty layer of the superficial fascia to move freely, allowing the abdomen to expand. This membranous superficial fascia (Scarpa's fascia) fades over the thoracic wall superiorly, and it fuses with the fascia lata of the thigh inferiorly. In males it continues into the scrotum and penis as the superficial perineal fascia (of Colles) and the superficial fascia of the penis respectively. In the female the superficial perineal fascia lines the labia majora, and is perforated by the vagina.

The anterolateral abdominal wall is composed of three muscle layers which fuse anteriorly to surround the rectus abdominis.

The abdominal cavity contains most of the alimentary tract (stomach, duodenum, and small and large intestines) together with its derivatives (liver and pancreas). Some viscera (e.g. small intestines and transverse colon) are intraperitoneal: suspended by mesenteries (sheets formed from double folds of peritoneum), while others (e.g. duodenum, pancreas) are retroperitoneal: bound down to the posterior abdominal wall behind peritoneum.

Abdominal pain is a very common presentation—knowledge of embryology and anatomy will help diagnosis (Fig. 4.1).

SURFACE ANATOMY AND SUPERFICIAL STRUCTURES

To facilitate description, the abdomen is divided into regions. The simplest method is to divide the abdomen into four quadrants by a vertical and a

Fig. 4.1 Origin and blood supply of the abdominal viscera

Part of fetal gut	Organs	Blood supply	Usual site of presentation of abdominal pain
Foregut	Oesophagus, stomach, first and second part of duodenum, liver, spleen, pancreas	Coeliac artery	Epigastric region
Midgut	Remainder of duodenum, jejunum, ileum, caecum, appendix, ascending colon, right two-thirds of transverse colon	Superior mesenteric artery	Umbilical region
Hindgut	Remainder of transverse colon, descending colon, rectum	Inferior mesenteric artery	Suprapubic region

horizontal line through the umbilicus; however, for more accurate description, it is divided into nine regions (Fig. 4.2):

- Two vertical midclavicular lines, each extending down to the midinguinal point.
- A lower transverse line running between the two tubercles of the iliac crest (intertubercular plane).
- An upper transverse line lying midway between the pubic symphysis and jugular notch (transpyloric plane) – although some clinicians use the subcostal plane (level of L2 – beneath the ribcage).

The linea alba is a midline depression running from the xiphisternum to the pubis. The linea semilunaris is a slightly curved line marking the lateral margin of rectus abdominis.

The inguinal ligament lies between the anterior superior iliac spine and the pubic tubercle. The deep inguinal ring lies at the midinguinal point (halfway between the anterior superior iliac spine and the midline).

The umbilicus lies at the level of L3.

Liver

The inferior border extends from the right 10th costal cartilage in the midclavicular line to the left 5th rib in

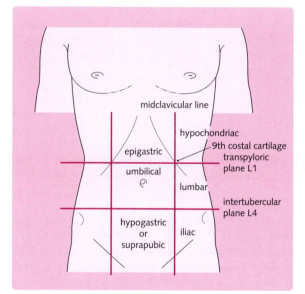

Fig. 4.2 Regions of the abdomen.

the midclavicular line. The upper border runs between the left and right 5th ribs; both points are in the midclavicular line. The right border runs from the 5th right rib to the 10th costal cartilage.

Fundus of the gall bladder

The fundus of the gall bladder lies behind the 9th right costal cartilage at the intersection of the linea semilunaris with the costal margin in the transpyloric plane.

Spleen

The spleen lies deep to the left 9th, 10th and 11th ribs behind the midaxillary line. It is not palpable unless

The body wall has three muscle layers in the abdomen. These layers fuse centrally to form the rectus sheath that surrounds the rectus abdominus.

enlarged, at which point the spleen extends inferiorly and anteriorly below the costal margin.

Pancreas

The head lies in the 'C' shaped concavity of the duodenum at the level of L2. The neck lies in the transpyloric plane (L1). The pancreas continues left, curving upwards towards the hilum of the spleen.

Kidneys

The hilum lies in the transpyloric plane, 5 cm from the midline. The upper pole of the kidneys lie deep to the 12th rib posteriorly. The right kidney is lower than the left due to the liver, but they both lie roughly opposite the first three lumbar vertebrae.

Ureters

Each ureter begins at the hilum of the kidney in the transpyloric plane. They run inferiorly over psoas major anterior to the tips of transverse processes of lumbar vertebrae (as seen on a urogram) to the sacroiliac joint before entering the pelvis.

THE ABDOMINAL WALL

Skeleton

Figure 4.3 shows the skeleton of the abdominal and pelvic cavities (see Chapter 5).

The costal margin and floating ribs have been described previously (see Chapter 3). The characteristics of a lumbar vertebra are outlined in Figure 4.4.

The hip bones articulate with the sacrum at the sacroiliac joint (a synovial joint) and with each other at the pubic symphysis (a secondary cartilaginous joint). Each pelvic bone is formed by ilium, ischium and pubis.

The iliac bones protect the underlying structures, providing a site for muscle attachment. The upper border—the iliac crest—runs from anterior superior iliac spine (ASIS) to the posterior superior iliac spine (PSIS). The iliac tubercle is the highest point of the crest. The three muscle layers of the anterolateral abdominal wall arise from the iliac crest, along with latissimus dorsi, quadratus lumborum, and thoracolumbar fascia.

The pectineal line lies on the superior surface of the superior ramus of the pubic bone, and medial to it lie

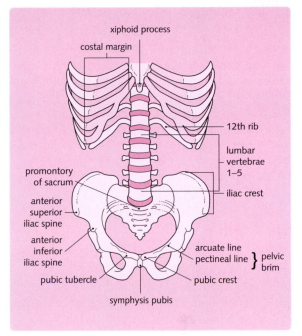

Fig. 4.3 Skeleton of the abdomen and pelvis.

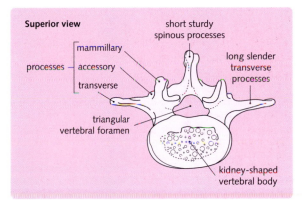

Fig. 4.4 A typical lumbar vertebra.

the pubic tubercle and pubic crest. It continues posteriorly as the arcuate line, which forms part of the pelvic brim.

Thoracolumbar fascia

The lumbar part of this fascia arises from vertebrae in three sheets:

- Tips of the lumbar spinous processes (posterior sheet).
- Tips of the lumbar transverse processes (middle sheet).

- The anterior aspect of the lumbar transverse processes (anterior sheet).

The anterior and middle sheets enclose quadratus lumborum; the middle and posterior sheets enclose erector spinae. The three sheets fuse laterally and provide attachment for the internal oblique and transversus abdominis muscles. The thoracic part is formed only by the posterior sheet. This attaches to the thoracic spines and angles of the ribs as far as the first rib. Its superior edge forms the lateral arcuate ligament (**see p. 105**).

Muscles of the anterolateral abdominal wall

Figure 4.5 outlines these muscles. The conjoint tendon is formed by the lowest fibres of internal oblique and transversus abdominis, inserting into the pubic crest and most medial part of the pectineal line, with the conjoint tendon.

Rectus sheath

Each rectus abdominis muscle is enclosed in a fibrous sheath formed by the aponeurotic tendons of the three lateral muscles (Fig. 4.6).

The external oblique muscle contributes to the anterior layer of the sheath over its entire extent. Below the costal margin, the internal oblique aponeurosis splits around the rectus muscle, forming the anterior and posterior layers, the aponeurosis of transversus abdominis contributing to the posterior layer.

Midway between the symphysis pubis and the umbilicus, all three aponeuroses pass anterior to the rectus muscle, leaving an inferior free margin to the posterior layer of the sheath – the arcuate line. Below the arcuate line, the posterior surface of rectus abdominis is in direct contact with transversalis fascia. The inferior epigastric artery enters the sheath at this level, passing superiorly on the deep surface of rectus abdominis. The posterior wall of the sheath is also deficient above the costal margin, where the rectus muscle lies directly on the underlying costal cartilages.

Nerve and blood supply to the anterolateral abdominal wall

The principal nerves and arteries of the anterolateral abdominal wall are shown in Figure 4.7. Nerves run in a 'neurovascular plane' between transversus abdominis and internal oblique. All the nerves except the ilioinguinal give lateral cutaneous branches.

Fig. 4.5 Muscles of the anterolateral abdominal wall			
Name of muscle (nerve supply)	**Origin**	**Insertion**	**Action**
External oblique (outermost layer) (T6–T12 spinal nerves)	Lower 8 ribs	Becomes aponeurotic and attaches to the xiphoid process, linea alba, pubic crest, pubic tubercle, and iliac crest	Flexes and rotates trunk; pulls down ribs in forced expiration
Internal oblique (spinal nerves T6–T12, iliohypogastric and ilioinguinal nerves)	**Thoracolumbar** Fascia, iliac crest, lateral two-thirds of inguinal ligament	Lower three ribs and costal cartilages, xiphoid process, linea alba, symphysis pubis; forms conjoint tendon with transversus	Assists in flexing and rotating trunk; pulls down ribs in forced expiration
Transversus abdominis (innermost layer) (spinal nerves T6–T12, iliohypogastric and ilioinguinal nerves)	Lower six costal cartilages, Thoracolumbar fascia, iliac crest, lateral third of inguinal ligament	Xiphoid process, linea alba, symphysis pubis, forms conjoint tendon with internal oblique	Compresses abdominal contents with external and internal oblique
Rectus abdominis (spinal nerves T6–T12)	Symphysis pubis and pubic crest	Costal cartilages 5–7 and xiphoid process	Compresses abdominal contents and flexes vertebral column

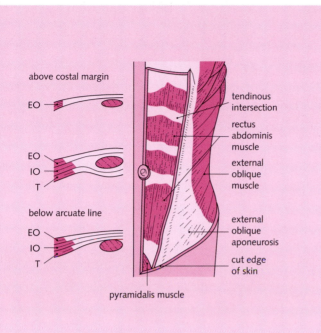

Fig. 4.6 Rectus sheath and rectus abdominis muscle. (EO, external oblique; IO, internal oblique; T, transversus abdominis).

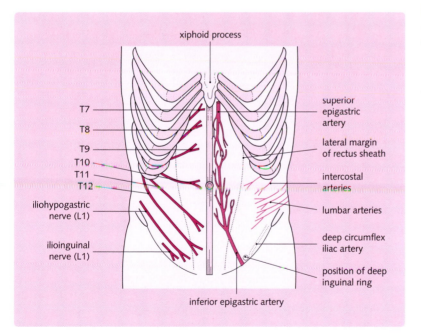

Fig. 4.7 Innervation (left) and arterial supply (right) of the anterolateral abdominal wall.

Venous drainage of the anterolateral abdominal wall

The superficial veins include the superficial epigastric and thoracoepigastric veins. These drain ultimately into the femoral vein and axillary veins, respectively.

The superior and inferior epigastric veins and the deep circumflex iliac veins follow the arteries and drain into the internal thoracic and external iliac veins.

The lower two posterior intercostal veins drain into the azygos veins. Of the four lumbar veins, the lower

Abdominal incisions

- A midline incision passes through the linea alba: allows rapid and bloodless access.
- A paramedial incision passes through the anterior wall of the rectus sheath, the rectus muscle is displaced laterally and the posterior sheath is then divided. Postoperatively the rectus muscle covers and strengthens the scar.
- A subcostal incision is made 2.5 cm below and parallel to the costal margin (on the right for biliary surgery and on the left to expose the spleen).
- A gridiron incision is made centred at McBurney's point. Each muscle layer is incised individually in line with its fibres, so the strength of the wall is virtually unaffected, although there is a risk of damaging the iliohypogastric and ilioinguinal nerves.
- Transverse incisions are made across the rectus abdominis muscle—it is supplied segmentally, so there is no danger of denervation.

The fibres of oblique muscles run diagonally. The fibres of transversus abdominis run horizontally.

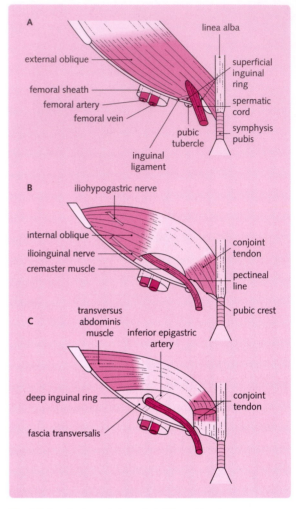

Fig. 4.8 Inguinal canal viewed at different levels.
(A)   Superficial inguinal ring in external oblique muscle.
(B, C) Internal oblique and transversus muscles and the conjoint tendon.
(C)   Deep inguinal ring in fascia transversalis.

two drain into the inferior vena cava. The upper two join to form the ascending lumbar vein, and, with the subcostal vein, drain into the azygos vein on the right and hemiazygos vein on the left.

Inguinal region

Inguinal ligament

This is the lower edge of the external oblique aponeurosis, extending from ASIS to the pubic tubercle. It gives origin to internal oblique and transverse abdominis and the fascia lata of the thigh.

Inguinal canal

This is a narrow tunnel, about 6 cm long, lying above the medial half of the inguinal ligament from deep inguinal ring to superficial ring (Figs 4.8 and 4.9). It contains the spermatic cord and ilioinguinal nerve in males, and the round ligament and ilioinguinal nerve in females.

The superficial inguinal ring is a triangular slit in the external oblique aponeurosis, just above and lateral to the pubic tubercle. The contents of the inguinal canal exit through this ring.

The deep inguinal ring is an opening in the transversalis fascia lying just above the midinguinal point. The contents of the spermatic cord pass through the deep inguinal ring.

The ilioinguinal nerve enters the canal by running between the external oblique aponeurosis and the internal oblique muscle – not via the deep ring.

Region	Components
Fig. 4.9 Composition of the inguinal canal	
Anterior wall	External oblique aponeurosis; reinforced laterally by internal oblique
Floor	Lower edge of the inguinal ligament; reinforced medially by the lacunar ligament, which lies between the inguinal ligament and the pectineal line
Roof	Lower edges of the internal oblique and transversus muscles: these muscles arch over the front of the cord laterally, to behind the cord medially, where their joint tendon—the conjoint tendon—is inserted into the pubic crest and pectineal line of the pubic bone
Posterior wall	The strong conjoint tendon medially and the weak transversalis fascia laterally

---

Inguinal hernias

An inguinal hernia occurs when abdominal viscera (usually intestine) protrudes along the inguinal canal. There are two types based on whether the sac lies outside or inside an inguinal triangle formed by inferior epigastric artery (laterally), the linea albea (medially) and the inguinal ligament (inferiorly).

- An indirect hernia is where the herniation tracks through the inguinal canal, passing through the deep inguinal ring, within the spermatic cord. If large enough it passes through the superficial ring into the scrotum (sometimes within a persistent processus vaginalis). The neck of the sac lies lateral to the inferior epigastric artery (lateral to the inguinal triangle). These are most common in children due to a patent processus vaginalis.
- A direct hernia is where a weakness in the abdominal wall between the deep inguinal ring and the midline allows a hernia to enter the canal posteriorly, lying outside the spermatic cord with the neck medial to the inferior epigastric artery (inside the inguinal triangle). These are most common in older men.

Spermatic cord

The structures entering the deep inguinal ring pick up a covering from each layer of the abdominal wall as they pass through the canal to form the spermatic cord (Fig. 4.10). The spermatic cord is not complete until it emerges from the superficial inguinal ring with all of its coverings.

Contents:

- The ductus deferens.
- Arteries—testicular artery (from the abdominal aorta) and the artery to the ductus deferens (from superior and inferior vesical arteries).
- Veins—the pampiniform plexus of veins.
- Lymphatics—accompany the veins from the testis to the para-aortic nodes.
- Nerves—the genital branch of the genitofemoral nerve supplies the cremaster muscle and sympathetic nerves go to arteries and smooth muscle of the vas.
- The processus vaginalis—the obliterated remains of the peritoneal connection with the tunica vaginalis of the testis.

Scrotum

This structure contains the testis, epididymis, and lower end of the spermatic cord. Beneath the thin skin is the superficial fascia, which contains the dartos muscle but no fat. This smooth muscle has sympathetic innervation and contracts in response to cold, pulling the testes closer to the body and wrinkling the skin. The fascia also forms a median partition, separating the testes. Beneath the dartos muscle is a layer of membranous fascia: the superficial perineal fascia (of Colles). This is continuous with the membranous layer of the superficial fascia of the anterior abdominal wall (Scarpa's fascia).

Blood supply, lymphatic drainage and nerve supply of the scrotum

The superficial and deep external pudendal arteries (branches of the femoral artery of the thigh) supply

---

Cremasteric reflex

In the male, the genital branch of the genitofemoral nerve supplies the cremaster muscle. Its femoral branch supplies a small area of skin on the thigh. Stimulation of this skin causes the cremaster muscle to contract, raising the testis towards the inguinal canal – testing L1. This reflex is very active in children, often leading to a misdiagnosis of undescended testes.

Fig. 4.10 Left testis, epididymis, coverings and contents of the spermatic cord (DIR – Deep Inguinal Ring; SIR – Superficial Inguinal Ring).

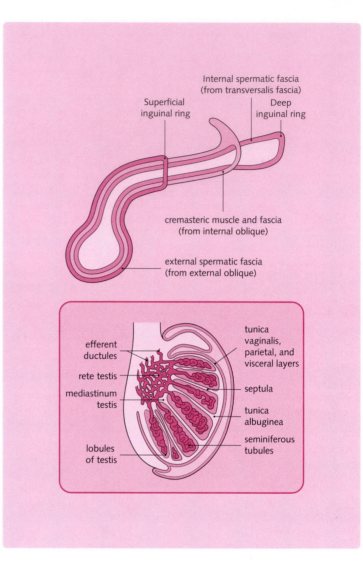

the scrotum. The venous drainage is to the great saphenous vein via venous tributaries. The lymphatic drainage is the medial superficial inguinal lymph nodes of the thigh.

The ilioinguinal nerve supplies the anterior one third of the scrotum. The posterior two thirds is innervated by the posterior scrotal branch of the perineal nerve (medially) and the perineal branch of the posterior femoral cutaneous nerve (laterally).

Testis

This oval organ lies at the lower end of the spermatic cord (Fig. 4.10). It has the epididymis attached to its posterolateral surface. The anterior and posterior surfaces lie free in a serous space formed by the tunica vaginalis.

The testis is surrounded by a tough fibrous capsule, the tunica albuginea. It gives rise to numerous septa that divide the testis into lobules containing the seminiferous tubules. Posteriorly the tubules form the

It is important to remember that the scrotum is part of the body wall and receives a local arterial and nerve supply, while the testis is an abdominal structure that is supplied by an abdominal artery and drains to abdominal lymphatics

rete testis and the efferent ducts, which open into the head of the epididymis.

Epididymis

This is a long coiled tube attached to the posterior border of the testis. Its head lies at the upper pole of the testis, and is joined by the efferent ductules before giving rise to the body and tail.

It stores and matures sperm.

Ductus deferens

Muscular contractions of the ductus transmit sperm from the epididymis to the prostatic urethra during ejaculation (sympathetic innervation). It receives its blood supply from a small branch of the superior vesical artery.

Blood supply of the testis

The testicular artery enters the spermatic cord and supplies the testis and the epididymis.

The pampiniform plexus provides venous drainage. In the inguinal canal it merges into four veins, which join to form two veins that leave the deep inguinal ring. The left testicular vein drains into the left renal vein, and the right into the inferior vena cava. The pampiniform venous plexus surrounds the testicular artery, acting as a countercurrent heat exchanger,

cooling the arterial blood to maintain a testicular temperature of 35°.

Lymphatics drain into the para-aortic nodes (not local inguinal nodes).

Descent of the testis

The testis develops in the posterior abdominal wall of the embryo, but then migrates preceded by the gubernaculum through the inguinal canal into the scrotum: it reaches the deep inguinal ring by 4 months, and it is inside the canal at 7 months, then progresses through the superficial ring to reach the scrotum at around birth.

A diverticulum of peritoneum—the processus vaginalis—precedes the testis as it passes through the inguinal canal into the scrotum. All but the part at the lower end is obliterated – this becomes the tunica vaginalis.

THE PERITONEUM

The peritoneum is the serous membrane lining the abdominal cavity. It consists of two continuous layers, separated by serous fluid.

The parietal layer lines the anterior and posterior abdominal walls, the diaphragm's inferior surface and the pelvic cavity.

The visceral layer leaves the abdominal wall and covers viscera.

Embryology

During development, the foregut, midgut and hindgut are suspended from the posterior abdominal wall by the dorsal mesentery (a mesentery is the double layer of peritoneum that connects an organ to the body wall. Between the two layers of peritoneum are blood vessels, lymphatics and nerves—Fig. 4.11). These organs are known as intraperitoneal.

Retroperitoneal organs lie against the posterior abdominal wall and are covered only by peritoneum on their anterior surface (e.g. the kidneys).

Undescended testis

The testis may not descend completely, stopping at any point along its descent. The testis may undergo malignant change if it remains undescended.

Testicular swellings

- Hydrocele is an accumulation of serous fluid within the tunica vaginalis, usually due to a persistent processus vaginalis.
- Haematocele is an accumulation of blood within the tunica vaginalis, usually due to rupture of branches of the testicular artery as a result of trauma.
- Varicocele is due to varicose veins of the pampiniform plexus, caused by failures of valves in the testicular vein or problems in the kidneys or renal veins.
- Spermatocele is retention cyst within the epididymis containing spermatozoa.

An incision through the anterior abdominal wall will enter the greater sac. Note that, technically, all viscera are covered by peritoneum and do not lie within the greater sac.

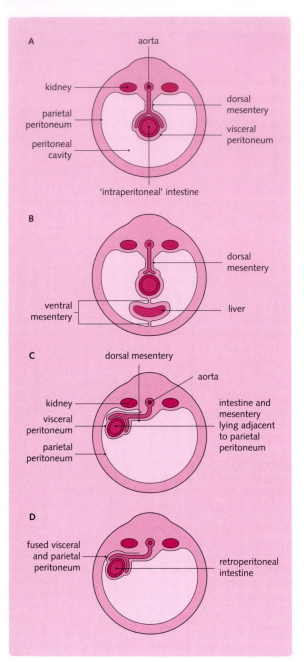

Fig. 4.11 The embryonic

(A)	Dorsal and
(B)	ventral mesenteries
(C and D)	and the formation of the retroperitoneal part of the intestines. (Adapted from *Anatomy as a Basis for Clinical Medicine*, by E C B Hall-Craggs. Courtesy of Williams & Wilkins.)

A ventral mesentery is present only in the terminal parts of the oesophagus and stomach and the upper

part of the duodenum (foregut). Growth of the liver divides the mesentery into the falciform ligament and the lesser omentum (Fig. 4.12).

Nerve supply of the peritoneum

The parietal peritoneum is supplied segmentally by the nerves supplying the overlying muscles and skin. The peritoneum covering the inferior surface of the diaphragm is supplied by the intercostal nerves peripherally and by the phrenic nerve (C3, 4, 5) centrally. The parietal peritoneum in the pelvis is supplied by the obturator nerve. The visceral peritoneum does not have a somatic innervation, so is insensitive to pain.

Peritoneal folds of the anterolateral abdominal wall

Peritoneal folds may sometimes be referred to as ligaments, e.g. phrenicocolic ligament is a transverse peritoneal fold between the splenic flexure of the colon and the diaphragm.

Anterolateral peritoneal folds are shown in Figure 4.13 and include:

- Median umbilical fold—contains the remnant of urachus (median umbilical ligament).
- Medial umbilical fold—contains remnants of the umbilical arteries (medial umbilical ligaments).
- Lateral umbilical fold—contains the inferior epigastric vessels.

The falciform ligament (an anterior peritoneal fold between the diaphragm and the umbilicus) contains the ligamentum teres hepatis (the remnant of the umbilical vein) in its free margin.

Greater and lesser sacs

Between the parietal and visceral peritoneum is a potential space containing a small quantity of peritoneal fluid to allow free movement of viscera. This space is the general peritoneal cavity. In males it is

Diaphragm

The diaphragm and its innervation originate in the neck. Irritation of the diaphragm by thoracic or abdominal pathology (e.g. infection in the subphrenic recess) may cause pain in the shoulder due to shared C3 and C4 root values – an example of 'referred pain'.

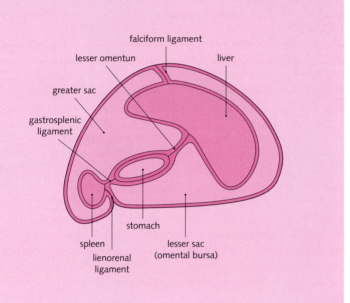

Fig. 4.12 Transverse section of abdomen (looking downwards)

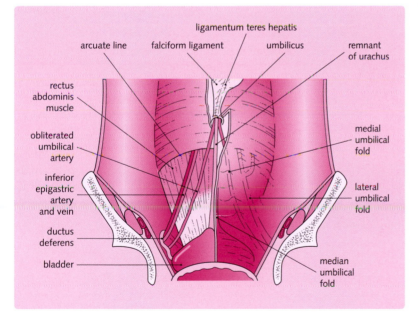

Fig. 4.13 Peritoneal folds of the anterior abdominal wall, viewed from the posterior aspect.

completely closed; however, in females the cavity communicates with the exterior via the reproductive tract.

The peritoneal cavity is divided into greater and lesser sacs. The lesser sac (omental bursa) is a diverticulum of peritoneum behind the stomach, formed by changes in position of viscera during development. The lesser sac communicates with the greater sac through the epiploic (omental) foramen. The epiploic (omental) foramen is bounded by:

- Superiorly—caudate process of liver.
- Anteriorly—portal vein in the free edge of the lesser omentum.
- Inferiorly—first part of the duodenum.
- Posteriorly—inferior vena cava.

The greater sac (the remainder of the cavity) can be divided descriptively into compartments by the transverse mesocolon: the supracolic is above and the infracolic and pelvic compartments below (Fig. 4.14).

The infracolic compartment is subdivided further by the root of the mesentery (of the small intestine) into upper right and lower left. The compartment is bounded laterally by the paracolic gutters lying lateral to ascending and descending colons.

The supracolic compartment is divided into left and right parts by the falciform ligament. Between the upper surface of the liver and the diaphragm on either side of the falciform ligament are two spaces: subphrenic recesses. Under the liver on the right of the falciform ligament, but above the right kidney, is the right subhepatic recess, also known as the hepatorenal or Morrison's pouch – it communicates with the right paracolic gutter. The left subhepatic

Fig. 4.14 (A) Sagittal section of the upper abdomen to show the recesses of the right supracolic compartment. (B) Posterior abdominal wall showing lines of peritoneal reflection and how the greater sac compartments are divided (liver, stomach, small intestine, caecum, transverse and sigmoid colons have been removed). (B) is adapted from *Gray's Anatomy*, 38th edn. by L H Bannister et al. Pearson Professional Ltd.

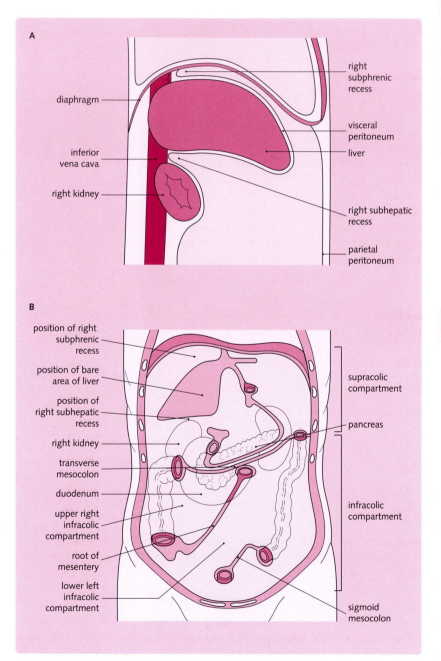

recess has similar boundaries, but forms part of the lesser sac.

In the pelvic compartment the peritoneum lies over and between pelvic viscera. The pouches formed differ between genders. Males have a rectovesical pouch. Females have vesicouterine and rectouterine pouches (see Chapter 5).

These recesses and pouches are important because they determine the spread and accumulation of fluids in the peritoneal cavity: in a supine patient, the hepatorenal pouch is the lowest part; when prone the rectouterine or rectovesical pouch is the lowest part (where fluid will accumulate).

Greater and lesser omenta

The greater omentum is the largest peritoneal fold, arising from the greater curvature of the stomach and the superior duodenum to hang down over the intestines. It is filled with fat. The transverse colon and its mesentery are fused to the posterior aspect of the omentum.

The lesser omentum connects the lesser curvature of the stomach and the proximal part of the duodenum to the liver. It can be subdivided into two parts: a hepatogastric ligament between liver and stomach and a hepatoduodenal ligament between liver and duodenum.

THE ABDOMINAL ORGANS

Oesophagus

After passing through the diaphragm, accompanied by vagal trunks, the oesophagus turns forward and to the left to enter the cardiac part of the stomach. Blood and nerve supply are shown in Figure 3.28.

Stomach

This is a dilated muscular bag lying between the oesophagus and the duodenum (Fig. 4.15). It is a relatively mobile organ, being fixed at its ends. The gastro-oesophageal junction lies at the level of T10,

Gastro-oesophageal reflux disease (GORD)

Gastro-oesophageal reflux is a very common problem in young children and in adults, causing epigastric discomfort and regurgitation of acidic stomach contents. Ulceration of the oesophagus may occur. A number of factors normally prevent reflux of stomach contents into the oesophagus. These include:

- The sphincteric action of the lower oesophageal muscle.
- The sling of the right crus of the diaphragm. This compresses the oesophagus when the diaphragm contracts.
- A mucosal flap projecting from the stomach lining.
- Positive intra-abdominal pressure acting on the abdominal oesophagus.

Hiatus hernia – If the sling action of the right crus is weakened (typically in middle-aged patients), the abdominal oesophagus, cardia and fundus of the stomach can slide superiorly through the diaphragmatic opening.

and the pyloric sphincter (gastroduodenal sphincter) lies at the level of L1. The stomach is intraperitoneal, with peritoneum forming the lesser and greater omenta and the lesser and greater curvatures.

The mucosal lining of the stomach is thrown into folds or rugae which allow considerable dilation. The wall is muscular and comprises outer longitudinal, middle circular and inner oblique muscle layers.

The relations of the stomach comprise:

- Anterior—the anterolateral abdominal wall, left costal margin, and diaphragm.
- Posterior (stomach bed)—the left suprarenal gland, upper pole of the left kidney, pancreas, spleen, splenic artery, and left colic flexure.

The stomach and oesophagus are foregut derivatives, and, therefore, they receive their blood supply from the coeliac trunk: a branch of the abdominal aorta (Fig. 4.15).

The greater omentum is the 'policeman' of the abdomen—it moves to a site of infection and adheres to it, preventing spread.

The right and left gastric arteries supply the lesser curvature while the right and left gastroepiploics supply the greater curvature.

Fig. 4.15 Blood supply of the stomach.

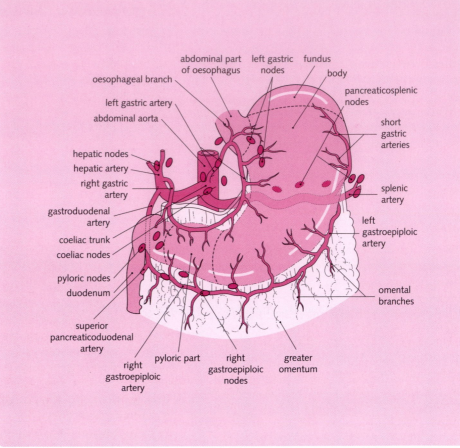

Lymphatic drainage is to the coeliac nodes, lymphatic vessels being distributed with arteries.

Duodenum

The duodenum is C-shaped. It is mostly retroperitoneal and firmly attached to the posterior abdominal wall, although the first 2.5 cm are intraperitoneal. It is divided into four parts:

- The first part passes posteriorly to the right side of the vertebral column, along the transpyloric plane at the level of L1.
- The second part passes downwards and receives the major duodenal papilla – the opening of the bile and main pancreatic ducts at the level of L2.
- The third part crosses the vertebral column at the level of L3.
- The fourth part ascends to the level of L2 and opens into the jejunum.

Figure 4.16 shows the relations of the duodenum.

The duodenum receives its blood supply from:

- Superior pancreaticoduodenal arteries from the gastroduodenal branch of the hepatic artery, a branch of the coeliac trunk.
- Inferior pancreaticoduodenal arteries from the superior mesenteric artery.

Duodenal lymph drains into channels that accompany the superior and inferior pancreaticoduodenal vessels to the coeliac and superior mesenteric nodes.

Jejunum and ileum

The jejunum and ileum are intraperitoneal – attached to the posterior abdominal wall by the mesentery,

Gastric ulcer

A perforated gastric ulcer in the posterior stomach wall may erode the splenic artery, causing haemorrhage. It may also erode the pancreas, giving pain referred to the back.

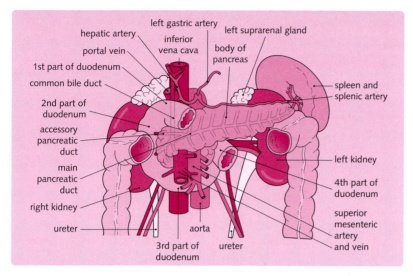

Fig. 4.16 Relations of the duodenum. Note the splenic vein is hidden behind the pancreas and, therefore, not drawn, and the inferior mesenteric vein has been omitted for clarity.

giving them great freedom to move. Their total length is approximately 6–7 m.

Figure 4.17 outlines the differences between the jejunum and ileum.

The blood supply to the jejunum and ileum isfrom the jejunal and ileal branches of the superior mesenteric artery. These form a series of anastomotic loops to make arterial arcades from which straight arteries (vasa recta) pass to the mesenteric border of the gut. The straight arteries (vasa recta) are end arteries—occlusion may result in infarction.

Lymphatic drainage is to superior mesenteric nodes.

Parasympathetic fibres from the vagus nerve increase peristalsis and secretion, whereas sympathetic fibres from T9 and T10 inhibit peristalsis.

Large intestine

This consists of the caecum, appendix, colon, rectum, and upper part of the anal canal.

Caecum and appendix

The caecum and the vermiform appendix lie in the right iliac fossa. The caecum lies free in the abdominal cavity, invested by peritoneum. The ileum enters the caecum obliquely, invaginating into it to form the ileocaecal orifice. The blood supply to the caecum is from the ileocolic artery.

The appendix is a blind-ending tube, usually 6–9 cm long, with lymphoid tissue in its wall (which may inflame). It opens into the posteromedial wall of the caecum, 2 cm below the ileocaecal orifice. The vermiform appendix has its own mesentery (the mesoappendix) and the colon's taeniae coli merge to form a complete longitudinal muscle layer (their convergence marks the base of the appendix).

Blood supply is from the appendicular artery, a branch of the posterior caecal artery from the superior mesenteric artery. It is an end artery, and any swelling of the appendix may obstruct the artery, causing necrosis and perforation.

Duodenal ulcer

95% of duodenal ulcers occur in the posterior wall of the 1st part of the duodenum. Should an ulcer perforate, duodenal contents will enter the abdominal cavity, causing peritonitis. A posterior ulcer may also erode the gastroduodenal artery, causing severe haemorrhage. An anterior ulcer may be sealed off by the greater omentum.

Meckel's diverticulum

This is a remnant of the connection between the gut tube and the embryonic yolk sac, projecting from the ileum approximately 60 cm from the ileocaecal junction in roughly 2% of people. It may contain pancreatic as well as acid-secreting gastric mucosa, which can erode intestinal mucosa and cause bleeding. It presents a pain distribution similar to that of appendicitis.

Fig. 4.17 Distinguishing characteristics of the jejunum and ileum

Characteristic	Jejunum	Ileum
Colour	Deep red	Paler pink
Wall	Thick and heavy	Thin and light
Vascularity	Greater	Less
Vasa recta	Long	Short
Arcades	A few large loops	Many short loops
Peyer's patches (aggregated lymphoid follicles)	No	Yes—towards the terminal part of the ileum
Plicae circulares (mucosal folds increasing surface area)	More and larger	Less and smaller/absent
Fat	Less—stops at the mesenteric border with the jejunum	More—encroaches onto the ileum

The base of the appendix is usually identified externally at McBurney's point, one third of the way along a line joining the anterior superior iliac spine and the umbilicus.

The position of the appendix can vary:

- In 65% of cases it lies retrocaecal.
- In 30% it is in a pelvic position (passing down over the pelvic brim).
- The remaining 5% occupy a variety of positions.

Colon

Most of the colon has an incomplete longitudinal muscle layer in three bands: the taeniae coli. In the sigmoid (pelvic) colon the taeniae coli are wider, and in the terminal part they coalesce to form a complete longitudinal muscle layer. Haustrations (sacculations) are pouches along the length of the colon, formed by taeniae coli which 'bunch together' the colonic wall.

Bulbous pouches of peritoneum distended with fat project from the surface – appendices epiploicae. They become larger and more developed along the length of the colon. The blood supply reaches these appendices from the colonic mucosa by perforating the muscular wall.

Ascending colon

This extends from the ileocolic junction to the right colic (hepatic) flexure. On the medial and lateral sides of the ascending colon the peritoneum runs posteriorly forming the paracolic gutters. The

The ascending and descending colons are held onto the posterior abdominal wall, i.e. they are retroperitoneal. The transverse and sigmoid colons are suspended by mesenteries and are mobile.

Appendicitis

This occurs when the appendix is obstructed by swelling of lymphoid tissue. As the organ swells it causes periumbilical colicky pain which localizes in the right iliac fossa (due to irritation of the parietal peritoneum).

Acute infection can cause thrombus formation in the appendicular artery – resulting in gangrene and rupture, causing peritonitis (with increased pain, nausea/vomiting and abdominal rigidity).

Treatment is surgical removal (appendectomy).

Diverticulae

Mucous membrane may herniate through the perforations in the muscle layer of the colon made by the blood vessels supplying the appendices epiploicae. Such a hernia is called a diverticulum. These may become inflamed (diverticulitis) – causing abdominal pain.

colon lies retroperitoneal, fixed to lumbar and iliac fascia.

Transverse colon

This extends from the right colic (hepatic) flexure to the left colic (splenic) flexure, the former being lower due to the right lobe of the liver. It is intraperitoneal, suspended by the transverse mesocolon, so can move around.

Descending colon

This extends from the left colic (splenic) flexure to the pelvic brim. There are paracolic gutters on its medial and lateral sides formed by the peritoneum posteriorly. It lies retroperitoneal, fixed to lumbar and iliac fascia.

Sigmoid (pelvic) colon

This extends from the descending colon to the pelvic brim. It hangs free from the sigmoid mesocolon. The mesocolon is an inverted V-shape, the base of which lies over the sacroiliac joint. From here, one part runs to the midinguinal point along the external iliac vessels, and the other runs to the level of the S3 where the rectum begins.

The colon is supplied by the superior mesenteric artery up to the proximal two thirds of the transverse colon, and the inferior mesenteric artery thereafter (Fig. 4.18).

The branches anastomose near the medial margin of the entire colon, forming an arterial circle, the marginal artery, from which short vessels pass to the gut wall. The venous drainage follows the arterial supply to the portal venous system.

Spleen

The spleen is a large lymphoid organ. It filters the blood and helps in mounting immunological responses against blood-borne pathogens.

Blood supply and innervation

The poorest part of the marginal artery's supply to the colon is between the middle colic and left colic arteries at the splenic flexure. This site is thus most prone to ischaemia and infarction.

In Hirschsprung's disease nerve plexuses are absent from the wall of a section of hindgut and constricts, leading to bowel obstruction, constipation and vomiting. It is confirmed by biopsy – the affected section must be surgically removed.

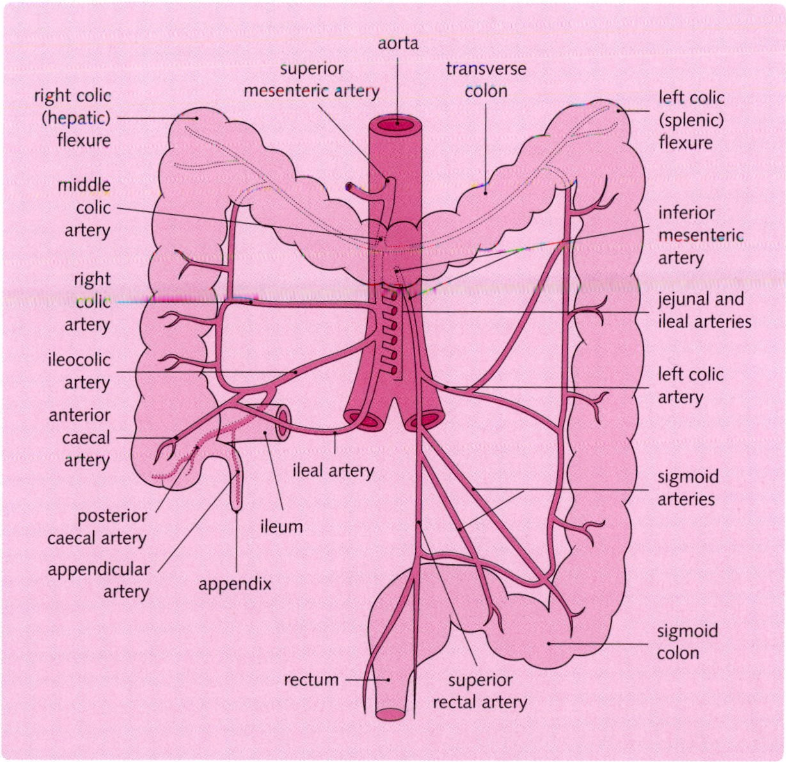

Fig. 4.18 Colon and its blood supply.

The spleen has a convex diaphragmatic surface fitting into the concavity of the diaphragm. The anterior and superior borders are notched and sharp, but the posterior and inferior borders are rounded.

The spleen has a visceral surface with four impressions: the gastric impression for the stomach, the renal impression for the kidney, the colic impression for the splenic flexure of the colon and a pancreatic flexure within the hilus of the spleen itself. It is connected to the greater curvature of the stomach by the gastrosplenic ligament and to the posterior abdominal wall at the left kidney by the splenorenal ligament. It is completely enclosed by peritoneum except at the hilum.

The splenic artery from the coeliac trunk is a tortuous vessel that passes along the superior border of the pancreas and anterior to the left kidney. Between the layers of the splenorenal ligament, the splenic artery divides into five or more branches, which enter the hilum (and the short gastric and left gastroepiploic arteries to the stomach).

The splenic vein joins the inferior mesenteric vein, and this runs posterior to the body of the pancreas to unite with the superior mesenteric vein to form the hepatic portal vein.

Lymphatic drainage is to the pancreaticosplenic and coeliac nodes.

Liver

The liver is a wedge-shaped organ lying in the right hypochondrium. It is largely under cover of the costal margin, and it is invested by peritoneum except over its bare area.

The liver has four lobes, although this is a purely anatomical description and does not reflect functional subdivisions (Fig. 4.19). The falciform ligament divides the liver into right and left lobes. Posteriorly, there is a caudate lobe lying between the inferior vena cava and the fissure for the ligamentum venosum, and a quadrate lobe lying between the gall bladder fossa and the ligamentum teres. Functionally, the quadrate and caudate lobes are part of the left lobe as they are supplied by the left hepatic artery, left branch of the portal vein, and deliver bile to the left bile duct.

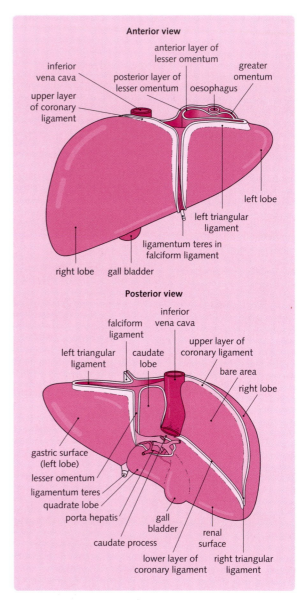

Fig. 4.19 Anterior and posterior views of the liver.

Ruptured spleen and splenectomy

The spleen is very susceptible to trauma on the left side, particularly involving fracture of the 9th to 11th ribs. If ruptured, it may bleed profusely, resulting in collapse of the patient and shock. Emergency splenectomy may be life saving in these cases; however, these patients are vulnerable to infection and often require life-long antibiotics. Partial removal of the spleen is preferable, as it is followed by rapid regeneration.

If the entire spleen must be removed (e.g. in splenic anaemia), then the surgeon must be aware of small accessory spleens that occur near the hilum in around 10% of people.

The falciform ligament runs up the anterior surface of the liver. At the superior surface of the liver the left layer of peritoneum passes to the left and returns to form the left triangular ligament. The right layer forms the upper layer of the coronary ligament, the right triangular ligament, and the lower layer of the coronary ligament (Fig. 4.19).

The area between the upper and lower parts of the coronary ligament is the bare area of the liver. This area is devoid of peritoneum and lies in contact with the diaphragm.

The right and left layers of peritoneum meet on the visceral surface of the liver to form the hepatogastric and hepatoduodenal ligaments, part of the lesser omentum.

Between the caudate and quadrate lobes, the two layers surround the porta hepatis. The porta hepatis, the inferior vena cava, the gall bladder, and the fissures of the ligamentum venosum and ligamentum teres, form an H-shaped pattern. The ligamentum venosum is the remnant of the fetal ductus venosus, which transported blood from the portal and umbilical veins to the hepatic veins.

The porta hepatis contains the right and left branches of the hepatic artery, the hepatic ducts, and the hepatic portal vein (Fig. 4.19):

- The hepatic artery (a coeliac trunk branch) supplies oxygenated blood to the liver and branches to form the cystic artery supplying the gall bladder.
- The hepatic portal vein carries the products of digestion from the gut to the liver.
- The right and left hepatic ducts drain bile into the common hepatic duct. The latter joins the cystic duct to form the bile duct.

These three structures form the portal triad that lies in the right free margin of the lesser omentum.

There are also three hepatic veins that drain the liver which pass directly from the posterior surface of the liver into the inferior vena cava.

Lymphatics drain into the hepatic nodes lying around the porta hepatis. They also drain the gall bladder. The hepatic nodes drain into the coeliac nodes. Lymphatics of the bare area drain into the posterior mediastinal nodes.

Nerve supply is from the vagal trunks and the coeliac plexus.

Gall bladder and biliary tract

The gall bladder lies in a fossa on the visceral surface of the liver. It has a fundus, a body, and a neck (Fig. 4.20).

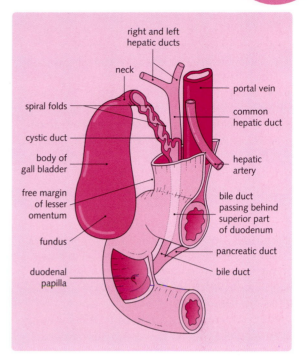

Fig. 4.20 Gall bladder and biliary tract. (Adapted from *Anatomy as a Basis for Clinical Medicine*, by E C B Hall-Craggs. Courtesy of Williams & Wilkins.)

Bile secreted by the liver is stored and concentrated by the gall bladder which releases it into the duodenum after a meal.

The cystic duct drains the gall bladder and joins the common hepatic duct to form the common bile duct. This passes through the free margin of the lesser omentum behind the first part of the duodenum to enter the second part of the duodenum with the pancreatic duct at the hepatopancreatic ampulla (of Vater) which opens at the major duodenal papilla. The sphincter of Oddi is a layer of circular muscle surrounding the ampulla, controlling the flow of bile and pancreatic secretions. The mucosa lining the neck of the gall bladder and cystic duct is thrown into folds, forming a spiral valve.

Blood supply is from the cystic artery, usually a branch of the right hepatic artery.

Pancreas

The pancreas has both exocrine and endocrine functions. It lies behind the peritoneum on the posterior abdominal wall, roughly at the level of the transpyloric plane (see Fig. 4.16). It has a head, neck, body, and tail:

- The head lies in the concavity of the duodenum, anterior to the inferior vena cava and left renal vein. The bile duct travels through it.
- The uncinate process is an extension of the head; the superior mesenteric artery and vein pass behind it.
- The neck overlies the superior mesenteric vessels and the portal vein.
- The body crosses the left renal vein and the aorta. The splenic vessels run close to this part of the pancreas.
- The tail is accompanied by the splenic vessels and lymphatics in the lienorenal (splenorenal) ligament, to touch the hilum of the spleen.

The main pancreatic duct opens into the duodenum with the bile duct at the major duodenal papilla. The accessory duct opens into the duodenum 2 cm proximal at the minor duodenal papilla.

The splenic artery (a coeliac trunk branch) supplies the neck, body, and tail of the pancreas. The superior and inferior pancreaticoduodenal arteries supply the head. The splenic vein drains the pancreas. Lymphatics drain into the coeliac and superior mesenteric nodes.

Vessels of the gut

The foregut, midgut and hindgut are supplied by the branches of the coeliac trunk, the superior mesenteric artery and the inferior mesenteric artery, respectively.

The coeliac trunk arises from the abdominal aorta at the level of T12. It gives off the left gastric, common hepatic and splenic arteries (see Fig. 4.15).

The superior mesenteric artery arises from the abdominal aorta at the level of L1 (transpyloric plane). It gives off the inferior pancreaticoduodenal, jejunal and ileal, ileocolic, right colic and middle colic arteries (Fig. 4.18).

The inferior mesenteric artery arises from the abdominal aorta, opposite L3. It gives off the left colic, sigmoid and superior rectal arteries (Fig. 4.18).

Venous drainage of the gut

Venous blood rich in nutrients from the intestines travels in the hepatic portal system of veins to the liver (Fig. 4.21). The portal vein is formed by the union of the superior mesenteric vein with the splenic vein posterior to the neck of the pancreas. The inferior mesenteric vein usually joins the splenic vein.

The portal vein passes posterior to the first part of the duodenum to run in the lesser omentum's free edge. On reaching the porta hepatis the vein divides into left and right branches supplying left and right lobes of the liver. Within the sinusoids of the liver the hepatic portal blood comes into contact with hepatocytes where metabolic exchanges take place. From the sinusoids, blood passes via the hepatic veins to the inferior vena cava and then the heart.

Nerve supply of the gastrointestinal tract

The gut receives sympathetic and parasympathetic nerves that travel with the gut arteries. See the section on nerves of the posterior abdominal wall for more detail.

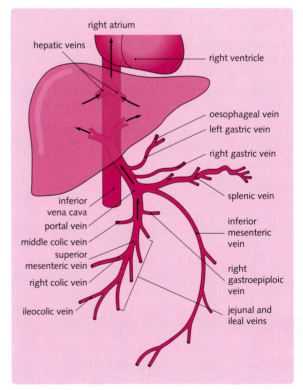

Fig. 4.21 Hepatic portal venous system.

Obstruction of the hepatic portal system (e.g. due to liver cirrhosis or tumour), causes portal hypertension and increased flow through veins which connect portal and systemic veins, causing these veins to enlarge.

- Lower end of the oesophagus between left gastric vein and azygos tributaries – enlargement results in oesophageal varices, which may rupture, causing haematemesis
- Superficial para-umbilical veins – enlargement causes caput medusae: enlarged systemic veins radiating out from the umbilicus.
- Anal canal between superior and inferior rectal veins – enlargement results in haemorrhoids (although it is important to note that portal hypertension is not the major cause of haemorrhoids).
- There are also anastomoses where gut viscera lie retroperitoneal (e.g. the ascending and descending colon or the bare area of the liver); however, these do not give rise to significant clinical symptoms.

Lymphatic drainage of the gut

Lymph from the mucosa of the gut passes through a number of filters including:

- Lymphoid follicles, e.g. Peyer's patches.
- The epicolic nodes, which lie in the gut margin of the mesentery.
- The paracolic nodes, which lie in the mesentery between the gut margin and the root of the mesentery.

Lymphatics run with the arteries, following the same pattern of supply, ultimately to lymph nodes anterior to the aorta (preaortic nodes) at the roots of the three gut arteries.

All the lymph eventually enters the coeliac nodes and from here passes into the cisterna chyli—the origin of the thoracic duct.

THE POSTERIOR ABDOMINAL WALL

The posterior abdominal wall offers protection to the abdominal contents. It is composed of the bodies of the five lumbar vertebrae and their intervertebral discs, and the psoas, iliacus, and quadratus lumborum muscles.

The lumbar vertebrae project forwards into the abdominal cavity with a forward convexity (lumbar lordosis). The inferior vena cava and the aorta lie in front of the bodies of the vertebrae.

On either side of the vertebral bodies lie the paravertebral gutters. The kidneys and suprarenal glands lie in these gutters (Fig. 4.22).

Muscles of the posterior abdominal wall

These are outlined in Figure 4.23. The iliolumbar ligament is a ligament passing from the transverse process of L5 vertebra to the posterior part of the iliac crest.

Fascia of the posterior abdominal wall

Fascia covers the muscles of the posterior abdominal wall: psoas fascia covering psoas major and thoracolumbar fascia already mentioned.

The superior edge of the thoracolumbar fascia forms the lateral arcuate ligament slung between the middle of the 12th rib and the transverse process of L1 vertebra. From here, the medial arcuate ligament (the superior edge of psoas fascia) extends to the side of L1 or L2 vertebra. Tendinous fibres of the diaphragm pass in front of the aorta in the midline to form the median arcuate ligament.

Vessels of the posterior abdominal wall

Abdominal aorta

The abdominal aorta passes through the diaphragm at the level of T12. It passes inferiorly on the bodies of the lumbar vertebrae. In front of L4 it divides into the common iliac arteries (Fig. 4.24).

Pus from a tuberculous infection of a lumbar vertebra may track laterally into the fascial sheath around psoas major. It then tracks down under the inguinal ligament into the femoral triangle, where it produces a soft swelling, close to the insertion of psoas on the lesser trochanter of the femur.

Fig. 4.22 Structures of the posterior abdominal wall.

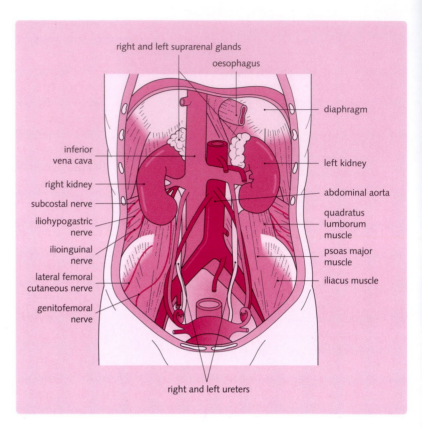

right and left suprarenal glands

oesophagus

diaphragm

inferior vena cava

left kidney

right kidney

abdominal aorta

subcostal nerve

quadratus lumborum muscle

iliohypogastric nerve

psoas major muscle

ilioinguinal nerve

iliacus muscle

lateral femoral cutaneous nerve

genitofemoral nerve

right and left ureters

Fig. 4.23 Muscles of the posterior abdominal wall. (Adapted from *Clinical Anatomy. An Illustrated Review with Questions and Explanations*, 2nd edn, by R S Snell, Little Brown & Co.)

Name of muscle (nerve supply)	Origin	Insertion	Action
Psoas major (L1–L3)	Transverse process, bodies, and intervertebral discs of T12 and L1–L5 vertebrae	Lesser trochanter of femur	Flexes thigh on trunk
Quadratus lumborum (T12–L3)	Iliolumbar ligament, iliac crest, transverse processes of lower lumbar vertebrae	12th rib	Depresses 12th rib during respiration; laterally flexes vertebral column
Iliacus (femoral nerve)	Iliac fossa	Lesser trochanter of femur	Flexes thigh on trunk

Aortic aneurysm

An abdominal aortic aneurysm usually occurs below the renal arteries and may be detected on deep palpation as a pulsatile mass just to the left of the midline that may be moved from side to side. Should it rupture, rapid haemorrhage ensues – usually fatal. Aortic aneurysms may be repaired using a prosthetic graft.

Inferior vena cava

This vessel is formed on the right side of the aortic bifurcation at the level of L5, by the union of the two common iliac veins (see Fig. 3.23). It ascends to the right of the aorta and passes behind the liver to pierce the diaphragm at the level of T8 and almost immediately enters the heart.

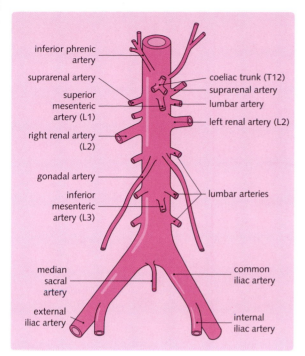

inferior phrenic artery
suprarenal artery
superior mesenteric artery (L1)
right renal artery (L2)
gonadal artery
inferior mesenteric artery (L3)
median sacral artery
external iliac artery

coeliac trunk (T12)
suprarenal artery
lumbar artery
left renal artery (L2)
lumbar arteries
common iliac artery
internal iliac artery

Fig. 4.24 Branches of the abdominal aorta.

Nerves of the posterior abdominal wall

Somatic nerves

The upper four lumbar spinal nerves emerge from their intervertebral foramina into psoas major, which they supply. Their anterior rami divide and unite to form the lumbar plexus (Fig. 4.25), which is mostly concerned with sensory and motor innervation to the lower limb. However, some branches are motor and sensory to the anterior abdominal wall, e.g. iliohypogastric nerve, and sensory to the parietal peritoneum, e.g. obturator nerve. The lumbosacral trunk joins the first three sacral nerves to contribute to the sacral plexus.

Autonomic nerves

Also **see p.132**. The autonomic nerve supply of the abdomen is composed of the following:

- Parasympathetic supply from the vagal trunks and pelvic splanchnic nerves (S2,3,4).
- Sympathetic supply from the lumbar sympathetic trunks and the thoracic and lumbar splanchnic nerves.
- Prevertebral autonomic plexuses surrounding the aorta (coeliac, aortic and superior hypogastric), which distribute the nerve fibres.

Sympathetic nerves

The lumbar sympathetic trunk comprises preganglionic fibres from the lower thoracic trunk and from L1 and L2 nerves (via white rami). This trunk enters the abdomen posterior to the medial arcuate ligament of the diaphragm. It runs down on the medial border of psoas major.

There are usually four lumbar ganglia. These give somatic branches (grey rami communicantes) to all five lumbar nerves, supplying the body wall and lower limb, and visceral branches (lumbar splanchnic nerves) that join the prevertebral plexuses. Fibres from the third and fourth lumbar ganglia join with fibres from the aortic plexus in front of L5 vertebra to form the superior hypogastric plexus. The superior hypogastric plexus divides into the right and left hypogastric nerves, which run into the pelvis to join the inferior hypogastric plexus. The sympathetic trunks do not give branches to the abdominal viscera.

The greater and lesser splanchnic nerves are preganglionic – they pierce the crura of the diaphragm to synapse in the coeliac ganglion. The least splanchnic nerves relay in a small renal ganglion close to the renal artery.

From the coeliac ganglion, postganglionic fibres form the coeliac plexus around the origin of the coeliac trunk. Fibres either pass directly or via superior and inferior mesenteric plexuses along branches of the aorta to supply all abdominal viscera.

The suprarenal gland also receives preganglionic fibres directly from the lesser splanchnic nerve – stimulation causes the release of adrenaline.

Functions of the sympathetic nerves include vasomotor, motor to the sphincters, inhibition of peristalsis, and carries sensory fibres from all of the abdominal viscera.

Parasympathetic nerves

The vagal trunks supply foregut and hindgut: they enter the abdomen on the surface of the oesophagus, directly supplying the stomach. Branches to the coeliac plexus then supply the remainder of the gut as far as the distal two-thirds of the transverse colon. Branches to the renal plexus pass to the kidneys.

The pelvic splanchnic nerves (from S2 to S4) join the inferior hypogastric plexus. Some fibres pass up into prevertebral plexuses to be distributed to the distal part of the transverse colon and descending and sigmoid colons (hindgut).

Parasympathetic activation of the gut causes stimulation of peristalsis and secretomotor activity of glands (remember 'rest and digest').

Fig. 4.25 Lumbar plexus and the relationship of the branches to the psoas muscle. The spinal root values of the branches are shown in parentheses. Note that the sciatic nerve is not part of the lumbar plexus and is shown only for completeness.

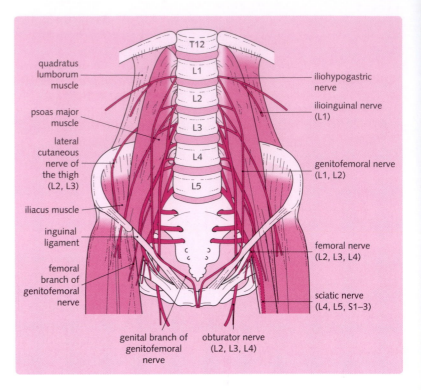

Kidneys

The kidneys are retroperitoneal organs lying mostly under cover of the costal margin in the paravertebral gutters of the posterior abdominal wall. Their position varies with respiration, but they lie approximately opposite the first three lumbar vertebrae. The right kidney is slightly lower than the left kidney, as it lies below the liver (Fig. 4.26).

Each kidney is surrounded by perinephric fat. The renal fascia encloses both structures and separates the kidney from the suprarenal gland. The fascia is firmly attached to the renal vessels and the ureter at the hilum of the kidney.

The renal arteries supply the kidneys (Fig. 4.27), which divide at the hilum into anterior and posterior branches. These are further subdivided into segmental and interlobular arteries (end arteries). Venous drainage is via segmental veins, which join together to form the renal vein – this joins the inferior vena cava at the level of L2. The left renal vein is longer because it passes in front of the aorta to reach the inferior vena cava.

The sympathetic nerve supply arises from the coeliac, renal, and superior hypogastric plexuses – it is vasomotor and accompanied by afferent pain fibres. The parasympathetic nerve supply is from the vagus.

Ureters

The ureters form at the renal pelvis. They descend on the psoas muscle retroperitoneally and cross the common iliac artery at its bifurcation at the pelvic brim. They turn towards the bladder at the level of the ischial spine.

The ureter narrows in three places:

- At the pelvoureteric junction.
- Where it crosses the pelvic brim.
- As it passes through the bladder wall.

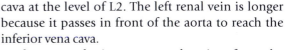

In the hilum of the kidney, the structures from anterior to posterior are vein, artery, ureter.

Kidney transplant

A transplanted kidney is placed in the iliac fossa. The renal vessels are sutured to the external iliac vessels and the ureter is sutured to the bladder.

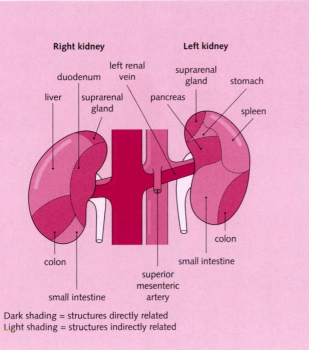

Fig. 4.26 Kidneys and their main anterior relations.

Right kidney
Left kidney

left renal
vein

duodenum

suprarenal
gland

stomach

liver

suprarenal
gland

pancreas

spleen

colon

small intestine

superior
mesenteric
artery

colon

small intestine

Dark shading = structures directly related
Light shading = structures indirectly related

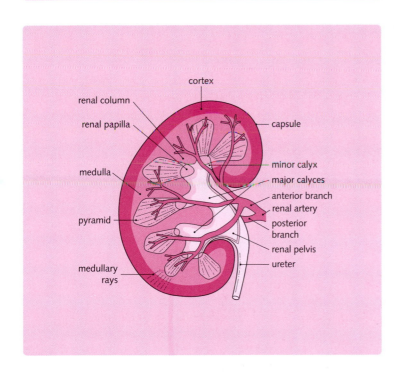

Fig. 4.27 Macroscopic structure and arterial supply of the kidney.

cortex

renal column

renal papilla

capsule

minor calyx

major calyces

medulla

anterior branch
renal artery

posterior
branch

pyramid

renal pelvis

ureter

medullary
rays

Blood supply is segmental and arises from the renal artery, abdominal aorta, gonadal and vesical arteries, common and internal iliac arteries, and the middle rectal artery. The ureter has a sympathetic nerve supply from the coeliac and hypogastric plexuses. Parasympathetic fibres come from the pelvic splanchnic nerves. The pain afferents accompany the sympathetic nerves.

Suprarenal gland

The suprarenal gland lies on the medial aspect of the superior pole of each kidney, and it is separated from it by renal fascia. The pyramidal left suprarenal lies posterior to the stomach (lesser sac intervening) and the comma-shaped right suprarenal lies posterior to the inferior vena cava, liver and hepatorenal pouch. The suprarenal glands consist of a central medulla that secretes adrenalin and a peripheral cortex that secretes several essential hormones.

Each suprarenal gland is supplied by three main vessels:

- The superior suprarenal artery – a branch of the inferior phrenic artery.
- The middle suprarenal – a branch of the renal artery.
- The inferior suprarenal – a direct branch of the aorta.

On the right a single suprarenal vein drains into the inferior vena cava directly. On the left a single suprarenal vein drains into the left renal vein.

Lymph from the kidneys and the suprarenal glands drains into the para-aortic lymph nodes.

RADIOLOGICAL ANATOMY

Imaging of the abdomen

An abdominal plain X-ray is also known as a KUB or kidneys, ureters and bladder film. It is most commonly taken in an anteroposterior (AP) view with the patient in a supine position.

Normal radiographic anatomy of an AP abdominal X-ray

In a normal AP abdominal radiograph (Fig. 4.28) the differences between soft-tissue structures and fluid are difficult to distinguish. The liver (11) is a homogeneous structure situated in the upper right quadrant. The abdomen contains fat, which surrounds the organs and outlines these structures. The spleen (8) is seen in the upper left quadrant with the gas in the stomach (2) adjacent. Other structures that are outlined are the bladder (9), the left obturator internus muscle (10), left kidney (3) and right kidney (1).

Retroperitoneal muscles that are outlined by fat are the left (5) and right (6) psoas muscles as well as the obturator internus muscle. The quadratus lumborum muscle can also be seen outlined by fat, which is lateral to the psoas muscle shadow. Gas on a normal plain X-ray is seen in the stomach (2) and (descending) colon (4, 7) as a radiolucent or dark area.

The bone structures visible are the 11th and 12th ribs, lumbar spine, sacrum and pelvis. If solid matter is seen as a mottled appearance with small bubbles, it suggests it is faecal matter (12).

Normal radiographic anatomy of an abdominal contrast study

Contrast medium is used to highlight the anatomy of the intestines; barium sulphate is most commonly used. In Figure 4.29 the anatomy of the foregut and midgut is illustrated. The stomach (1) empties into the duodenum (2) through the narrow pyloric sphincter. The C-shaped duodenum comprises the superior, descending (2a), horizontal (2b) and ascending (2c) parts. The jejunum (3) begins at the duodenojejunal flexure (attached to the ligament of Treitz) and the ileum (4) is its continuation. The jejunum and ileum can be distinguished on an X-ray because the jejenum has more mucous folds (plicae circulares).

A double-contrast image is shown in Figure 4.30. In this technique barium has been refluxed from the rectum (10) to the caecum (2) and terminal ileum (1) and air introduced. The parts of the large intestine e.g. transverse colon, can be visualized along with the smooth mucosal surface, which is interrupted by haustra (sacculations).

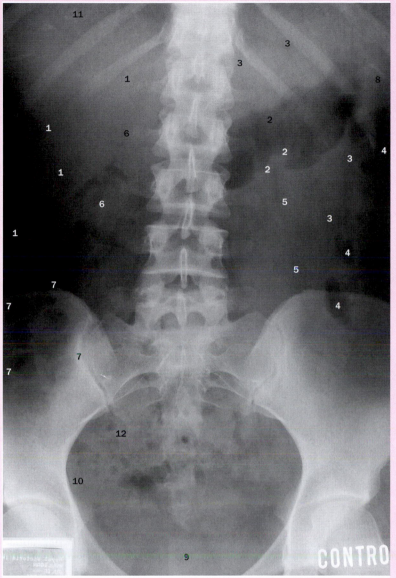

Fig. 4.28 Abdominal radiograph in a supine projection.

1 Outline of right kidney
2 Gas in stomach
3 Outline of left kidney
4 Outline of gas in descending
5 Outline of left psoas muscle
6 Outline of right psoas muscle
7 Outline of gas in caecum and
   ascending colon
8 Spleen
9 Bladder
10 Obturator internus muscle
11 Liver
12 Faeces in sigmoid colon

How to examine an AP abdominal X-ray methodically

Examine the following features in sequence:

- Check the patient details and the technical quality of the X-ray, i.e. the projection (is it AP?) and orientation (left from right).
- Bones: Look at the lower ribs, lumbar vertebrae and pelvis for continuity of the cortex areas of darkness (i.e. fracture) or white lesions (i.e. metastatic deposits). Costal cartilages may be calcified.

On a plain abdominal X-ray, the portions of the bowel can be distinguished by the mucosal folds and their position. The jejunum has numerous folds crossing the lumen, more so than the ileum, which has fewer folds. Both jejenum and ileum are seen centrally on the X-ray. The colon is characterized by folds (haustra) that do not cross the lumen and the colon is seen peripherally on the X-ray as an inverted U-shape surrounding the centrally positioned small intestine.

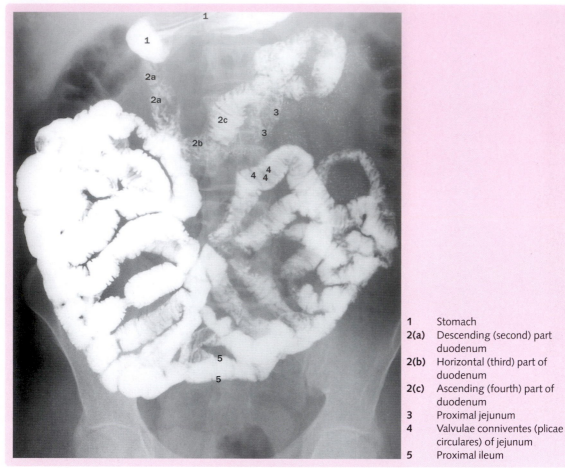

1	Stomach
2(a)	Descending (second) part duodenum
2(b)	Horizontal (third) part of duodenum
2(c)	Ascending (fourth) part of duodenum
3	Proximal jejunum
4	Valvulae conniventes (plicae circulares) of jejunum
5	Proximal ileum

Fig. 4.29 Abdomen barium follow-through showing duodenum and small intestine.

Radiology

Organ displacement particularly of the intestines may occur due to enlargement of the spleen or liver (typically). Hepatomegaly causes the hepatic flexure and proximal transverse colon to become compressed inferior to the right kidney. Splenomegaly causes an inferior displacement of the splenic flexure.

Examine the hip joint for narrowing of the joint space, loss of the smooth joint surface, formation of bone (osteophytes) and loose bodies.

- Viscera and muscles
  - Liver: Its shadow is seen in the upper right quadrant; enlargement will move the intestines inferiorly.
  - Spleen: In the upper left quadrant it should be the size of the patient's fist.
  - Kidneys: Have a smooth outline, but their position varies with inspiration.
  - Bladder (and uterus): Is the bladder distended?
  - Psoas major muscle: Its outline can be followed inferiorly into the pelvis to its insertion into the lesser trochanter of the femur. If this outline is lost or not visible it can indicate that fluid, e.g. blood, is present within the abdomen or that an abnormal mass is present.
  - Quadratus lumborum: The outline of this muscle can be seen lateral to the psoas muscle. Similarly, if its outline is lost or not visible it can indicate that fluid or an abnormal mass is present.
- Gastrointestinal tract
  - Stomach: On an erect AP film a gas bubble should be seen in the fundus. However, if the film is supine, gastric fluid accumulates in the fundus.

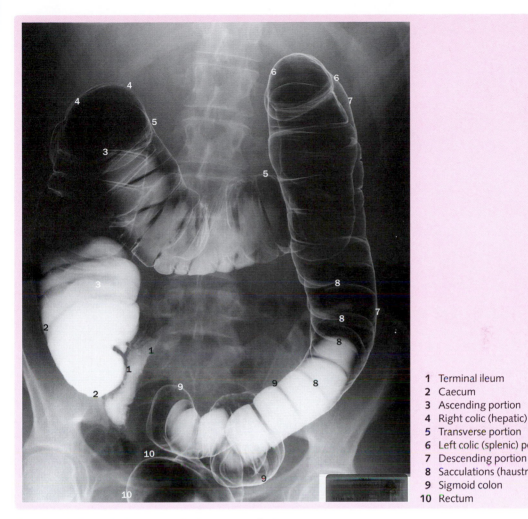

Fig. 4.30 Abdomen double-contrast barium enema of colon.

1 Terminal ileum
2 Caecum
3 Ascending portion
4 Right colic (hepatic) flexure
5 Transverse portion
6 Left colic (splenic) portion
7 Descending portion
8 Sacculations (haustrations)
9 Sigmoid colon
10 Rectum

- Small intestine: Is visualized centrally on the X-ray film.
- Large intestine: Begins in the right iliac fossa. The appendix may not be visible unless appendoliths (calcified faecal matter) are present. Identify the flexures and note their position. Faecal matter may be seen distally in the colon.
- Abdominal aorta and branches: These can be visualized if they are calcified, a process that occurs with age (atherosclerosis). Note the position of the aorta, its bifurcation at L4 and the common iliac artery bifurcation at the sacro-iliac joint.

Angiography of the abdominal aortic branches

In Figures 4.31, 4.32 and 4.33 the branches of the abdominal aorta and their subsequent divisions to form the arterial supply of the foregut (coeliac trunk), midgut (superior mesenteric artery) and hindgut (inferior mesenteric artery) can be seen.

When looking at the aorta, check that the walls of the vessel are parallel to one another. If they are not it suggests that an abdominal aortic aneurysm is present.

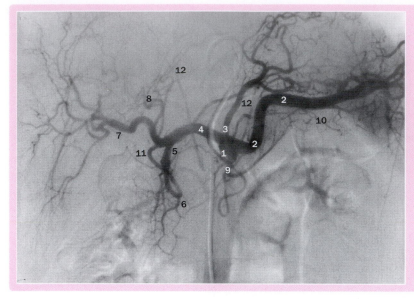

1   Tip of catheter in coeliac trunk
2   Splenic artery
3   Left gastric artery
4   Hepatic artery
5   Gastroduodenal artery
6   Superior pancreaticoduodenal
    artery
7   Right hepatic artery
8   Left hepatic artery
9   Dorsal pancreatic artery
10 Left gastro-epiploic artery
11 Right gastro-epiploic artery
12 Phrenic artery

Fig. 4.31 Coeliac trunk arteriogram.

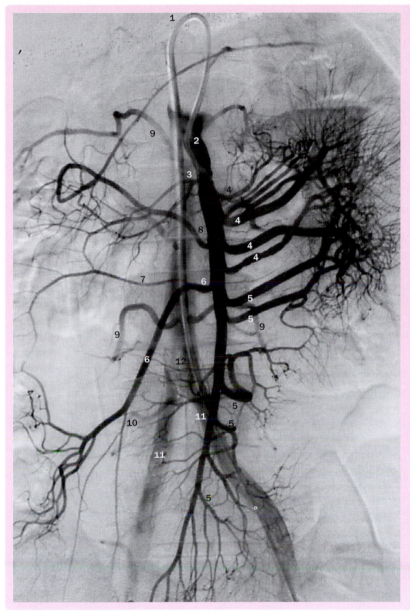

Fig. 4.32 Superior mesenteric arteriogram.

1 Tip of catheter in superior mesenteric artery
2 Superior mesenteric artery
3 Inferior pancreaticoduodenal artery
4 Jejunal branches of superior mesenteric artery
5 Ileal branches of superior mesenteric artery
6 Ileocolic artery
7 Right colic artery
8 Middle colic artery
9 Lumbar arteries arising from abdominal aorta
10 Appendicular artery
11 Common iliac artery
12 Aorta

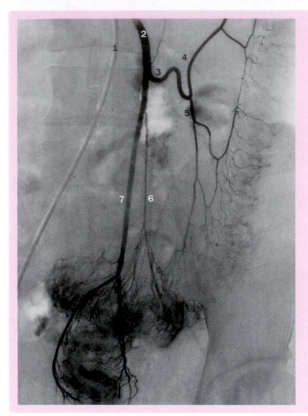

1   Catheter in the abdominal aorta
2   Inferior mesenteric artery
3   Left colic artery
4   Ascending left colic artery
5   Descending left colic artery
6   Sigmoid arteries
7   Superior rectal artery

Fig. 4.33 Inferior mesenteric arteriogram.

The pelvis and perineum

Objectives

In this chapter you will learn to:

- Describe the main features of the pelvic bones, including surface landmarks and sex differences.
- Discuss the anatomy of the pelvic floor and wall muscles and understand the function of the perineal body.
- Describe the peritoneum in the pelvis.
- Describe the anatomy of the rectum and anal canal.
- Describe the anatomy of the bladder and the course of the ureters in the pelvis.
- Describe the anatomy of the male and female reproductive tracts.
- Outline the vessels, nerves and lymphatic drainage of the pelvis.
- Describe how the perineum is divided into triangles. What are their contents?
- Describe how the superficial perineal space is formed and its contents in male and female.
- Describe the male and female external genitalia.

REGIONS AND COMPONENTS OF THE PELVIS

The pelvis lies below the abdomen, enclosed by bony, muscular, and ligamentous walls.

The bony pelvis is formed by the two hip bones, the sacrum and coccyx and is open superiorly (at the pelvic inlet) and inferiorly (the pelvic outlet). It has an upper part, the greater pelvis, flanked by the iliac bones, and a lower part, the lesser pelvis. The greater and lesser pelves meet at the pelvic brim (Figs 5.1 and 4.3).

The pelvic cavity is continuous with the abdominal cavity and is lined by peritoneum of the greater peritoneal sac. It is limited inferiorly by the pelvic diaphragm, beneath which lies the perineum.

The contents of the pelvis include:

- The coils of the small intestine.
- The rectum and sigmoid colon.
- The ureters and bladder.
- The ovaries, uterine tubes, uterus and vagina in females.
- The ductus deferens, seminal vesicles and prostate in males.
- The lumbosacral trunk, obturator nerve, sympathetic trunks and sacral plexus.

- The common iliac arteries, gonadal arteries and superior rectal arteries.

SURFACE ANATOMY AND SUPERFICIAL STRUCTURES

Bony landmarks

The iliac crest can be felt along its entire length. The anterior superior iliac spine is at the anterior border of the iliac crest and lies in the fold of the groin superiorly. The posterior superior iliac spine is at the posterior end of the iliac crest, lying under a skin dimple at the level of S2 vertebra.

The pubic tubercle can be felt on the upper border of the pubis. The symphysis pubis joins the two pubic bones and is palpable. The pubic crest is a ridge of bone on the superior surface of the pubic bone, medial to the pubic tubercle. The pubic arch runs from the pubic symphysis to the ischial tuberosity.

The spinous processes of the sacrum fuse to form the median sacral crest. The crest can be felt beneath the skin in the buttock cleft. The sacral hiatus is found at the lower end of the sacrum, about 5 cm above the coccyx. The coccyx may be palpated about 2.5 cm behind the anus in the natal cleft.

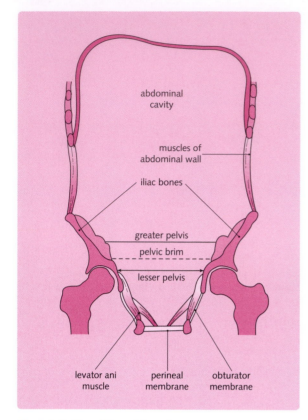

Fig. 5.1 Outline of the pelvic cavity.

Viscera

The adult bladder is a pelvic organ, but when full it may be palpated through the anterior abdominal wall.

The non-pregnant uterus is not usually palpable. In pregnancy its fundus may be palpated from about week 12. At term, the fundus is usually at the level of the xiphisternum.

THE BONY PELVIS AND PELVIC WALL

Bony pelvis

The bony pelvis is formed by the two hip bones, sacrum and coccyx (Fig. 5.2). The hip bones meet anteriorly at the pubic symphysis; posteriorly they articulate with the sacrum at the sacroiliac joints, thus forming a ring that protects the pelvic contents.

The pelvis is divided into greater pelvis (false pelvis) above the pelvic brim (pelvic inlet) and lesser

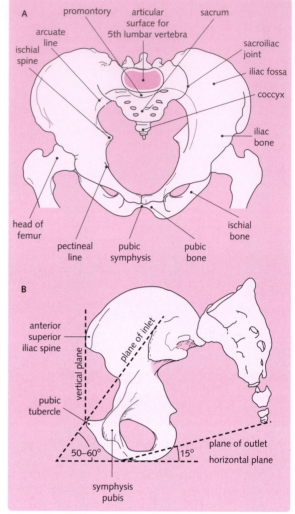

Fig. 5.2 (A) Pelvic girdle. (B) Pelvic inlet and outlet.

pelvis (true pelvis) between the pelvic inlet and pelvic outlet (Fig. 5.3). The pelvic inlet lies at about 45° to the pelvic outlet.

Sacrum

The sacrum consists of the fused five sacral vertebrae (Fig. 5.4). There are four anterior and four posterior sacral foramina for passage of the anterior and posterior rami of the sacral spinal nerves. The median sacral crest represents the fused spinal processes of the sacral vertebrae.

The sacrum articulates with the ilium on either side via its alar surface at the sacroiliac joints.

Fig. 5.3 Boundaries of pelvic apertures

Pelvic inlet	Pelvic outlet
Superior border of the pubic symphysis	Inferior margin of the pubic symphysis
Posterior border of the pubic crest	Inferior ramus of the pubis and the ischial tuberosity
Pectineal line	Sacrotuberous ligaments
Arcuate line of the ilium	Tip of the coccyx
Anterior border of the ala of the sacrum	
Sacral promontory	

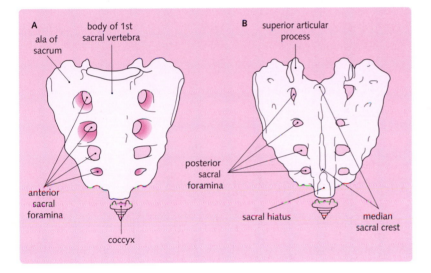

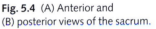

Fig. 5.4 (A) Anterior and (B) posterior views of the sacrum.

Hip bone

This is formed by the fusion of the ilium, the ischium, and the pubic bone shortly after puberty (Fig. 5.5).

Ilium

The iliac fossa gives rise to the iliacus muscle, and the articular surface forms the sacroiliac joint. The iliac crest, and the anterior superior and posterior superior iliac spines lie superiorly, with corresponding anterior inferior and posterior inferior iliac spines (Fig. 5.5).

The ilium contributes to forming the acetabulum and the bony margin of the greater sciatic notch.

Pubis and ischium

The pubic bones articulate in the midline at the pubic symphysis (see Fig. 5.5). On the upper surface of the body are the pubic crest and pubic tubercle. Each pubic bone has a superior and inferior ramus. The pectineal line runs along the superior ramus and joins with the arcuate line of the ischium to form the pelvic brim. The superior ramus forms the superior border of the obturator foramen. The inferior ramus unites the pubis with the ischial bone to form the ischiopubic ramus. This leads to the body of the ischium and the ischial tuberosity, which bears the weight in a sitting position.

The posterior border of the ischium contributes to the formation of the greater and lesser sciatic notches. The two notches are separated by the ischial spine. The sacrotuberous and sacrospinous ligaments transform the notches into the greater and lesser sciatic foramina.

Fig. 5.5 Medial view of the hip bone.

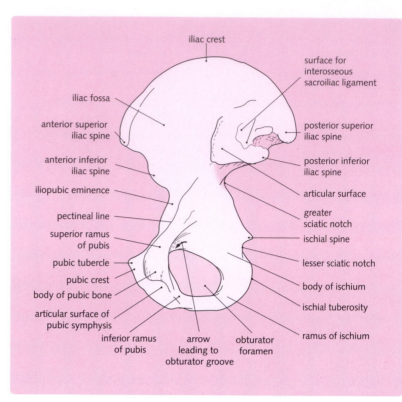

The three bones of the hip all contribute to the formation of the acetabulum.

Fig. 5.6 Differences between the male and female pelves

	Male	Female
Acetabulum	Large	Small
Build	Robust	Light
Inferior pelvic aperture	Relatively small	Relatively large
Obturator foramen	Round	Oval
Pubic arch	Narrow	Wide
Superior pelvic aperture	Usually heart-shaped	Usually oval or rounded

The position of the pelvis

The pelvis in a standing individual is tilted, such that the anterior superior iliac spine and the superior border of the pubic symphysis lie in the same vertical plane. A horizontal plane runs through the superior border of the pubic symphysis, ischial spine and coccyx.

Male and female pelves

The male and female pelves may show a great deal of sexual dimorphism (Fig. 5.6).

The largest diameter of the pelvic inlet is the transverse diameter (Fig. 5.7), while the largest diameter of the pelvic outlet is the anteroposterior diameter.

Pelvic joints

Pubic symphysis

This is a secondary cartilaginous joint between the two pubic bones (see Fig. 5.5). It is usually immobile,

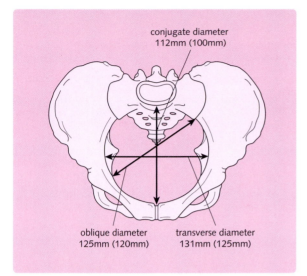

Fig. 5.7 Female pelvic inlet and its average diameters (male average diameters).

conjugate diameter
112mm (100mm)

oblique diameter
125mm (120mm)

transverse diameter
131mm (125mm)

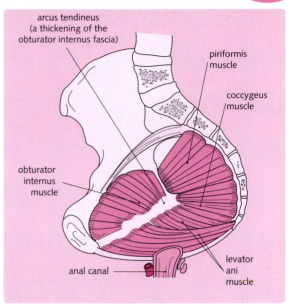

Fig. 5.8 Pelvic wall and its muscles.

arcus tendineus
(a thickening of the
obturator internus fascia)

piriformis
muscle

coccygeus
muscle

obturator
internus
muscle

anal canal

levator
ani
muscle

Birth

As the fetal head enters the pelvic inlet its maximum diameter lies across the pelvis, but as it descends through the birth canal the head rotates through 90 degrees, so that its maximum diameter lies anteroposteriorly at the pelvic outlet. Failure of this rotation leads to arrest in the delivery, and instrumental assistance or a caesarean section may be required.

reinforced by the superior pubic ligament and the inferior arcuate pubic ligament.

Sacroiliac joint

This is a synovial joint, but allows only minimal movement – strengthened by strong interosseous and anterior and posterior sacroiliac ligaments. The sacrospinous and sacrotuberous ligaments prevent rotation at the joint. The joint transmits all the body weight to the hip bones.

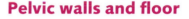

During pregnancy an ovarian hormone (relaxin) causes the pelvic joints and ligaments to relax. As a result greater movements occur in the pelvis and vertebral column.

Pelvic walls and floor

The side walls of the pelvis are formed by the hip bone with obturator internus (Fig. 5.8). The posterior wall is formed by the sacrum and piriformis as it passes into the greater sciatic foramen.

Figure 5.9 outlines the muscles of the pelvic wall and floor. Levator ani takes origin from the tendinous arch (a thickening of the fascia over obturator internus running from the body of the pubis to the ischial spine). Levator ani and coccygeus form a continuous section of muscle known as the pelvic diaphragm, inserting into a series of midline structures. This forms a bowl of muscle around the terminal parts of the rectum, prostate and urethra in the male, and the vagina and urethra in the female (Fig. 5.10).

Perineal body

The perineal body is a midline knot of fibromuscular tissue lying posterior to the prostate or vagina and is an important point of insertion for many muscles, giving it an essential supporting role for pelvic and perineal structures. Parts of levator ani, bulbospongiosus, the external sphincter of the anal canal, and the superficial and deep transverse perineal muscles are fused with it.

Anococcygeal body

The anococcygeal body is a midline raphe running from the anorectal junction to the tip of the coccyx,

121

Fig. 5.9 Muscles of the pelvic wall and floor

Name of muscle (nerve supply)	Origin	Insertion	Action
Coccygeus (4th and 5th sacral nerves)	Ischial spine	Inferior aspect of sacrum and coccyx	Supports pelvic viscera, flexes coccyx
Levator ani (pudendal nerve, 4th sacral nerve)	Ischial spine Body of pubis Fascia of obturator internus	Perineal body Anococcygeal body Walls of prostate, vagina, rectum, and anal canal	Supports pelvic viscera; sphincter to anorectal junction and vagina Counteracts increased abdominal pressure, e.g. defaecation, parturition
Piriformis (first and second sacral nerves)	Anterior aspect of sacrum	Greater trochanter of femur	Rotates femur laterally at hip and stabilizes hip joint
Obturator internus (nerve to obturator internus; L5, S1, S2)	Obturator membrane and adjacent hip bone	Greater trochanter of femur	Rotates femur laterally at hip and stabilizes hip joint

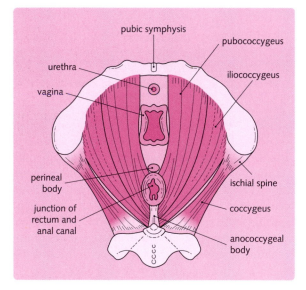

Fig. 5.10 Pelvic floor viewed from below.

Perineal tear, episiotomy

During childbirth, the tension on the perineal body can damage or tear it – as this is an important site of muscle attachment this can result in urinary and faecal incontinence and even pelvic organ prolapse. To prevent this, an incision can be made obliquely and posteriorly from the vagina, protecting the perineal body from harm and leaving a clean incision that can be easily sutured. This is an episiotomy.

into which levator ani inserts. It also separates the two ischioanal fossae behind the anal canal.

Pelvic fascia

Over the pelvic wall the fascia forms a strong covering over obturator internus and piriformis, continuous with that of the abdomen. The spinal nerves lie external to the fascia and vessels lie internal to it. The sacral plexus lies between the fascia and piriformis.

Over the pelvic floor, the fascia consists of loose areolar tissue. This condenses around neurovascular bundles to form ligaments, and also gives rise to the puboprostatic and pubovesical ligaments in the male and female, respectively. These fibromuscular bands, on either side of the median plane, run from the pubic bone to the bladder neck – immobilizing it and supporting the bladder. The deep dorsal vein of the penis (or clitoris) passes between the ligaments.

The fascia varies in thickness over the pelvic viscera.

Pelvic peritoneum

In the male, the peritoneum lines the pelvic wall and cavity inferiorly. From the anterior abdominal wall the peritoneum is reflected onto and attaches to the superior surface of the bladder, meaning that as the bladder fills and enlarges it peels the peritoneum away from the anterior abdominal wall. Behind the bladder, the peritoneum descends before ascending

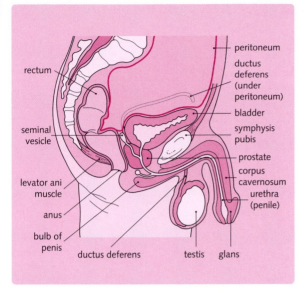

Fig. 5.11 A section through the male pelvis, illustrating the rectum and rectovesical pouch.

onto the rectum then sacrum, forming the rectovesical pouch (Fig. 5.11).

In the female the peritoneum turns superiorly to adhere to the uterus from the bladder, and it forms the vesicouterine pouch. The fold of peritoneum containing the uterus runs from side to side of the pelvic cavity and is known as the broad ligament of the uterus. From the superior aspect of the uterus and upper vagina the peritoneum ascends to cover the rectum then sacrum. This reflection forms the rectouterine pouch (or Pouch of Douglas) (Fig. 5.15).

THE PELVIC CONTENTS

Pelvic organs

Rectum

The rectum commences as a continuation of the sigmoid colon (where the sigmoid mesocolon ends) at

The rectovesical (in males) and rectouterine (in females) pouches are the lowest part of the peritoneal cavity in the sitting position and can be a site for collection of pus.

the level of S3 vertebra. It ends at the anorectal junction by piercing the pelvic floor at the border of puborectalis to become the anal canal. The rectum lacks appendices epiplociae, distinguishing it from the colon. Taeniae coli and therefore haustrations are also absent.

The rectum is concave anteriorly, following the sacrum – it also has three lateral curves (right, left and right), a transverse fold containing mucous membrane and circular muscle projecting into the lumen of the rectum from the convexity of each curve. These may provide support for faecal material. Its lowest part dilates as the rectal ampulla.

The rectum has no mesentery. Peritoneum covers the upper third of the rectum at the front and sides, and the middle third of the rectum at the front. The lower third lies below the level of the peritoneum, with the peritoneum reflected onto the bladder or vagina to form the rectovesical or rectouterine pouch (Fig. 5.11).

Posteriorly the rectum is related to the sacrum, coccyx and pelvic floor.

Vessels and nerves of the rectum

Blood supply is from the superior, middle and inferior rectal arteries. The superior rectal artery is a continuation of the inferior mesenteric artery. The others are discussed in the section describing the blood supply to the pelvis.

The rectal plexus of veins drains into the inferior mesenteric vein (draining to the portal system) and the middle and inferior rectal veins. These are systemic veins, so the rectum is a site of portosystemic anastomosis.

The nerve supply of the rectum consists of:

- Sympathetic—hypogastric plexus.
- Parasympathetic—pelvic splanchnic nerves, which are motor to the rectal muscles.

Lymphatics accompany branches of the superior and middle rectal arteries and eventually drain to the preaortic nodes at the origin of the inferior mesenteric vessels.

Ureters in the pelvis

The ureters (arising in the abdomen) cross the pelvic brim at the bifurcation of the common iliac vessels (Fig. 5.12). They continue into the lesser pelvis posteriorly towards the ischial spines (internal to the obturator nerve and vessels), then turn forward to enter the base of the bladder near its superior angle obliquely to prevent reflux. Here, in males, the ductus

Fig. 5.12 Course of the ureter in the pelvis of the male.

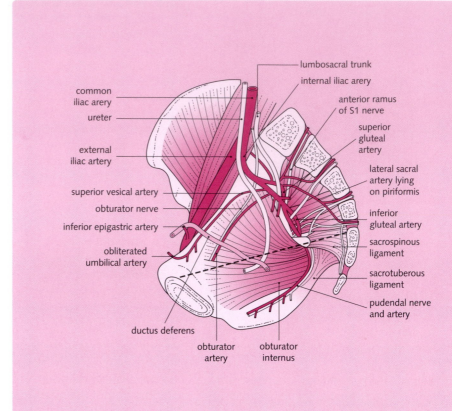

Rectal exam

This is made by asking the patient to lie on their left side, in the fetal position with their knees drawn up to their chest. A gloved, lubricated finger is inserted facing posteriorly and a sweep made clockwise.
In the male the following structures can be palpated:

- Anteriorly: the bulb of the penis, the membranous urethra, the prostate (allowing detection of prostate cancer).
- Posteriorly: The sacrum, the coccyx.
- Posterolaterally: The ischial spines.

In the female the structures palpated are:

- Anteriorly: The body of the uterus, the cervix.
- Posteriorly: same as in the male.

The rectum is distinguished from the sigmoid colon by the lack of a mesentery.

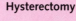

Hysterectomy

The ureter may be damaged in hysterectomy (removal of the uterus) when it may be tied while attempting to tie off the uterine artery.

To recall that the female ureter is crossed by the uterine artery superiorly, remember 'bridge over troubled water'.

deferens crosses the ureter superiorly; in females, the uterine artery crosses the ureter (near the lateral fornices of the vagina).

Bladder

The undistended bladder is a pyramid-shaped organ (Fig. 5.13). The apex points towards the pubic symphysis and attaches the median umbilical ligament.

Fig. 5.13 Base of the bladder and related structures in the male.

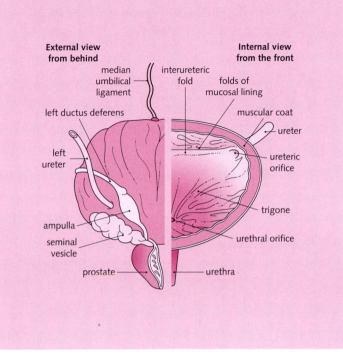

External view from behind

median umbilical ligament

left ductus deferens

left ureter

ampulla

seminal vesicle

prostate

Internal view from the front

interureteric fold

folds of mucosal lining

muscular coat

ureter

ureteric orifice

trigone

urethral orifice

urethra

The base is triangular and faces posteriorly. In males, most of the base lies below the rectovesical pouch. The ductus deferens and the seminal vesicles are attached to the surface, and the ureter enters the base of the bladder at its superolateral angle. In females, the base is firmly attached to the vaginal wall and the upper part of the cervix by connective tissue.

Two inferolateral surfaces become continuous with each other at the retropubic space.

The bladder wall is composed of three layers. An outer serous (peritoneal) layer lines the superior surface of the bladder. A smooth muscle layer, the detrusor muscle, is an interlacing network of fibres, giving the bladder's internal surface a trabeculated appearance. The detrusor muscle has a parasympathetic nerve supply. However, a second superficial layer of smooth muscle (with sympathetic innervation) exists in the trigone, extending into the proximal urethra. An inner mucosal layer of urothelium (transitional epithelium) lines the bladder.

The urethra leaves the neck of the bladder. Here, in males, the muscle is circularly arranged – forming the internal urethral sphincter, which prevents retrograde ejaculation (sperm entering the bladder) and has sympathetic supply. In females this sphincter is lacking.

Suprapubic cystostomy

In males and females a distended bladder rises above the symphysis pubis and lifts the peritoneum away from the anterior abdominal wall. A needle can be inserted above the symphysis pubis to drain the bladder (suprapubic cystostomy).

Internal surface of the bladder

When the bladder is empty, the mucosa is thick and folded. As it fills, the mucosa becomes thinner and smoother. Note that it is mainly the superior part of the bladder that distends – it is imbedded in loose fat while the inferior part is fixed by ligaments – this is reflected in the domains of arterial supply.

The trigone is a triangular area lying between the urethral orifice and the two ureteric orifices (Fig 5.13). It is the least mobile part of the bladder, with mucosa that is always smooth. The interureteric fold (formed by the continuous longitudinal muscle of the ureters) connects the two ureteric orifices.

The ureters pierce the mucosa obliquely, and the valve-like flap of mucosa produced is important in preventing reflux of urine when intravesical pressure

Abnormal insertion of ureters

Abnormal insertion of the ureters in the bladder (where they do not take an oblique course) may lead to reflux of urine up the ureters and even to the kidneys. This is a common problem in children and it may result in hypertension and renal failure due to backpressure of urine.

increases. The ureteric orifices are closed by this pressure and opened by peristaltic activity.

Vessels and nerves of the bladder

Blood supply is from the superior and inferior vesical arteries, with minor contributions from the obturator, uterine, inferior gluteal and vaginal arteries.

In males, veins form the vesicoprostatic plexus lying in pelvic fascia, which drains into the internal iliac veins. A similar plexus is formed in females.

The nerve supply comprises:

- Parasympathetic (motor)—pelvic splanchnic nerves – contract detrusor, relax sphincters.
- Sympathetic—the superior hypogastric and pelvic plexuses – relax detrusor, contract sphincters.

The male urethra

The male urethra is 20 cm long, commencing at the bladder neck and terminating at the external urethral orifice (Fig. 5.14). It has three parts:

The prostatic urethra has an elevated central ridge on its posterior wall, the urethral crest. The crest expands to form the seminal colliculus on which lies the orifice of prostatic utricle and the orifices of the ejaculatory ducts.

The membranous urethra lies between the apex of the prostate and the bulb of the penis. It is

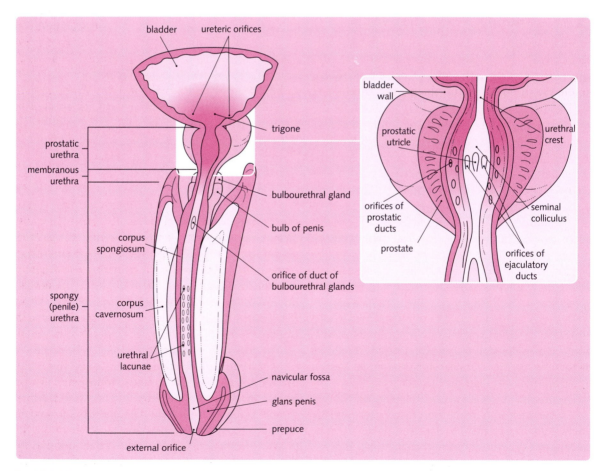

Fig. 5.14 Male urethra (showing details of the prostatic urethra).

surrounded by the sphincter urethrae and the perineal membrane. The bulbourethral glands lie on either side of it.

The spongy urethra passes through the bulb, corpus spongiosum and glans of the penis. Immediately before the external urethral orifice, the urethra expands to form the navicular fossa.

Numerous urethral glands open throughout the course of the urethra.

The female urethra

The female urethra is only 4 cm long. It runs from the bladder neck, through the pelvic floor and the perineal membrane, to open into the vestibule, anterior to the vaginal opening.

Male reproductive organs in the pelvis

Ductus (vas) deferens

The ductus deferens passes from the epididymis to the pelvic cavity via the inguinal canal. At the deep inguinal ring it hooks around the inferior epigastric artery, crossing the external iliac vessels to enter the pelvic cavity. It crosses the obturator neurovascular bundle and the ureter to reach the base of the bladder (see Fig. 5.13). The terminal part dilates, forming the ampulla, and it joins the duct of the seminal vesicle to form the ejaculatory duct, which opens into the prostatic urethra on the colliculus.

Seminal vesicles

The seminal vesicles are two elongated lobular sacs lying lateral to the ampulla of the ductus deferens (see Fig. 5.13). They produce seminal fluid.

Prostate

The prostate is a chestnut-shaped organ that lies below the bladder and above the perineal membrane with the prostatic urethra running through it (see Fig. 5.14). It has a base that is attached to the bladder neck, and an apex that points inferiorly.

The female urethra, being shorter than that of the male, is more prone to urinary tract infections by ascending organisms.

Prostatic hypertrophy

This is almost inevitable in men over 45 years old as a result of normal ageing. Usually the lateral lobes are affected; however, hypertrophy of the median lobe by itself can obstruct the prostatic urethra, reducing urinary outflow. Enlargement can be detected on rectal examination. If an enlarged smooth prostate is palpated it is benign; however, in malignant disease (e.g. prostatic carcinoma, usually affecting the median lobe) the prostate is hard with irregular craggy nodules. Prostate cancer has a very high mortality rate and the connection of prostatic veins to the internal vertebral venous plexus allows metastasis to lumbar vertebral bodies.

The prostate has right and left lobes united by an isthmus. The median lobe lies above and behind the lateral lobes and it receives the ejaculatory ducts.

The fibrous true capsule of the prostate completely surrounds the gland, in turn surrounded by a thick sheath of pelvic fascia – the false capsule. The two are separated by the prostatic plexus of veins.

Blood supply is from the inferior vesical artery. Veins drain to the prostatic plexus, which eventually drains into the internal iliac veins.

The female reproductive tract

Vagina

The vagina opens into the vestibule at the vaginal orifice and passes upwards and backwards to be continuous with the cervix at the external os (see Fig. 5.15). The vaginal fornix surrounds the part of the cervix that projects into the vagina: the posterior part is deepest and related to the rectouterine pouch of Douglas; the lateral parts are related to the ureters. Anteriorly, the vagina is separated from the bladder and urethra by loose connective tissue. The anal canal and rectum lie posteriorly.

The upper part of the vagina is supplied by the uterine artery, the middle and inferior parts by the vaginal branches of the internal iliac and internal pudendal arteries. Veins drain into the uterine and vaginal plexuses. The internal vagina has lymphatic drainage to the iliac nodes and the external vagina to the superficial inguinal nodes. It is lined by stratified squamous epithelium.

Uterus

This is a muscular organ that accommodates the developing embryo. The wall consists of serosa, the myometrium (a thick smooth muscle layer) and a lining of endometrium.

The uterus has three parts (Fig. 5.16):

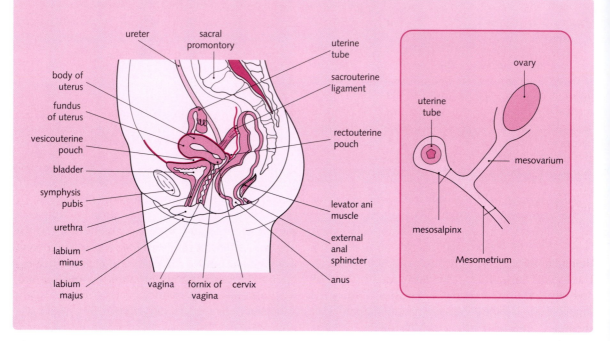

Fig. 5.15 Sagittal section through the female pelvis.

Fig. 5.16 Uterus and its blood supply.

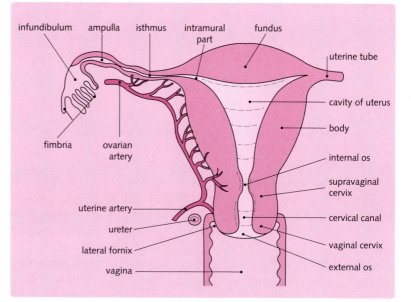

- The fundus lies above the entrance of the uterine tube.
- The body receives the uterine tubes. It is enclosed by peritoneum of the broad ligament. The cavity of the uterus occupies the body: slit-like in transverse section, triangular in longitudinal section.
- The cervix is the narrowest part of the uterus and is structurally and functionally distinct from it. It has a supravaginal part and a vaginal part. The vaginal fornix surrounds the cervix. The cervical canal is continuous with the uterine cavity at the internal os. It opens into the vagina at the external os.

The cervical canal is lined by columnar epithelium. Between the two regions is a transition zone where cervical carcinomas arise. A cervical smear attempts to identify premalignant lesions so they can be removed before cancers arise.

The upper anterior, superior and posterior surfaces of the uterus are covered by peritoneum. Posteriorly the peritoneum is reflected onto the rectum to form the rectouterine pouch (Fig. 5.15). The peritoneum continues from the lateral surface of the uterus to the pelvic side wall as the broad ligament.

Uterine (fallopian) tubes
The uterine tubes extend from the junction of the body and fundus of the uterus. They run in the upper edge of the broad ligament (see Fig. 5.16). The tubes are supported by a mesentery-like fold of peritoneum – the mesosalpinx.

The uterine tube is composed of the isthmus, the dilated ampulla, and the conical infundibulum which opens into the abdominal cavity. The outer end of the infundibulum is fimbriated. One of these fimbria, the ovarian fimbria, is attached to the ovary.

When the ovum is shed, it is taken up by the infundibulum and passed to the uterus.

Ligaments of the uterus
The broad ligament is a double fold of peritoneum that runs from the uterus to the pelvic wall on either

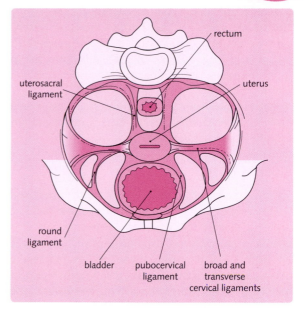

Fig. 5.17 Ligaments of the uterus, viewed from above.

side (Fig. 5.17). It forms the mesosalpinx for the uterine tubes, mesometrium for the uterus, and the mesovarium for the ovary. It helps to form the uterovesical pouch anteriorly and the rectouterine pouch posteriorly.

The suspensory ligament of the ovary contains the ovarian vessels and lymphatics. The round ligament of the uterus lies in the broad ligament's anterior margin. The mesovarium extends back from the posterior surface of the broad ligament to the ovary.

The round ligament extends from the body of the uterus to pass through the inguinal canal to the labium majus. It is the female remnant of the gubernaculum (see Testis, **p. 92**).

Transverse cervical (cardinal) ligaments are thickened connective tissue at the base of each broad ligament, extending from the cervix and vaginal fornix to the side wall of the pelvis. The uterosacral ligaments extend from the cervix to the fascia over piriformis, passing on either side of the rectum. The pubocervical ligaments extend from the cervix and upper vagina to the posterior aspect of the pubic bones. These stabilize the cervix.

The parametrium is the tissue lying between the two peritoneal layers of the broad ligament. It contains the uterine and ovarian vessels and lymphatics, the round ligament, and the suspensory ligament of the ovary.

Ectopic pregnancy

The fertilized ovum may implant ectopically, most commonly into the fallopian tube. If not diagnosed early, the tube may rupture and haemorrhage into the abdominal cavity. A ruptured tubal pregnancy on the right and the ensuing peritonitis may be mistaken for appendicitis.

Vessels of the uterus and uterine tubes

The uterine artery, a branch of the internal iliac artery, runs in the broad ligament. It anastomoses with branches of the ovarian artery. Each artery gives rise to tubal branches, which anastomose and supply the uterine tubes (Fig 5.16).

The venous drainage is into a uterine plexus. Two uterine veins arise from the plexus, and these drain into the internal iliac vein.

Ovary

The ovary is an ovoid organ lying in the ovarian fossa (in the angle between the internal and external iliac vessels), closely related to the obturator nerve. It produces the ova and steroid hormones.

The ovary is attached to the broad ligament by the mesovarium. It is attached to the uterus by the ligament of the ovary, which runs between the two layers of the broad ligament and is continuous with the round ligament, both being remnants of the gubernaculum.

Blood supply is from the ovarian artery, a branch of the abdominal aorta. It runs in the broad ligament and supplies the uterus and uterine tubes. It anastomoses with the uterine artery. An ovarian venous plexus communicates with the uterine venous plexus. Two ovarian veins follow the artery: the right ovarian vein drains into the inferior vena cava; the left vein drains into the left renal vein. Lymphatic drainage is to aortic nodes.

Positions of the uterus

The normal position of the uterus is anteflexed (the fundus and body bent forward from the cervix) and anteverted (the uterus leans forward from the vagina). In roughly 20% of women the uterus is retroverted (bent backwards) – this may cause discomfort during intercourse but has no affect on fertility. Usually the uterus falls into the anteverted position as it expands in pregnancy although in a small number of cases it becomes jammed in position against the sacrum.

The ovary is closely related to the obturator nerve in the ovarian fossa—disease of the ovary may cause referred pain to the medial aspect of the thigh and knee.

Vessels of the pelvis

These are principally the internal iliac arteries and the internal iliac veins. The external iliac artery is concerned mainly with the blood supply to the lower limb.

Internal iliac artery

The common iliac artery bifurcates at the pelvic brim opposite the sacroiliac joint into internal and external iliac arteries (Fig. 5.18). The internal iliac artery passes inferiorly and branches into anterior and posterior divisions. The branches may be divided into those supplying the body wall (iliolumbar, lateral sacral), those leaving the pelvis to supply the lower limb and gluteal region (obturator, internal pudendal and superior and inferior gluteal) and visceral branches (superior and inferior vesical, uterine, vaginal, middle rectal etc.).

Internal iliac vein

The internal iliac vein commences at the greater sciatic notch by the confluence of the gluteal veins and

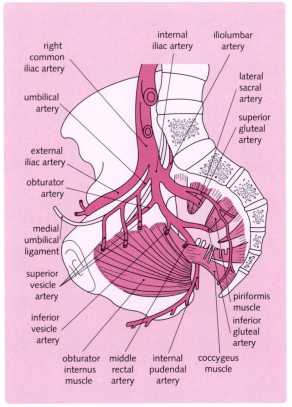

Fig. 5.18 Branches of the internal iliac artery.

others that accompany branches of the internal iliac arteries. It passes superiorly out of the pelvis, posterior to the artery on the medial surface of psoas major. Here, it joins the external iliac vein to form the common iliac vein.

Tributaries include:

- Veins corresponding to the arteries.
- The uterine and vesicoprostatic venous plexuses.
- The rectal venous plexuses.
- The lateral sacral veins (it communicates with the vertebral venous plexus via these veins).
- The obturator vein.

Nerves of the pelvis

Obturator nerve

The obturator nerve supplies the adductor compartment of the thigh by piercing the medial border of

psoas and passing on the lateral wall of the pelvis to the obturator foramen. It passes through the obturator foramen into the thigh with the obturator artery and vein below it.

Sacral plexus

The sacral plexus is formed by the anterior rami of L4 and L5 spinal nerves (the lumbrosacral trunk) and the anterior rami of S1–S4 spinal nerves (Fig. 5.19). The plexus lies on piriformis, covered by pelvic fascia. The lateral sacral arteries and veins lie anterior to the plexus. The sacral nerves and lumbosacral trunk give off branches and then divide into the anterior and posterior divisions.

Autonomic system

See **p. 107** for more detail.

If venous drainage of the lower limb becomes obstructed, the pelvic veins enlarge and provide an alternative route for venous return.

The obturator nerve may be damaged during ovary removal (oophrectomy). This results in the spasm of adductor muscles of the thigh and cutaneous sensory loss over the medial thigh and knee.

Fig. 5.19 Sacral plexus.

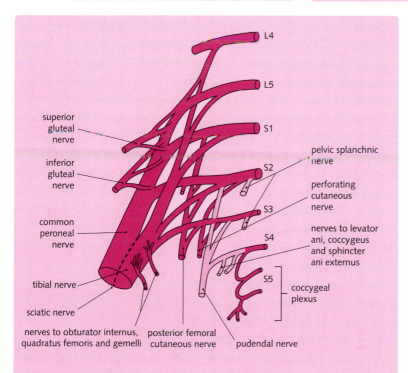

- L4
- L5
- S1
- S2
- S3
- S4
- S5

superior gluteal nerve
inferior gluteal nerve
common peroneal nerve
tibial nerve
sciatic nerve
nerves to obturator internus, quadratus femoris and gemelli
posterior femoral cutaneous nerve

pelvic splanchnic nerve
perforating cutaneous nerve
nerves to levator ani, coccygeus and sphincter ani externus
coccygeal plexus
pudendal nerve

Sacral sympathetic trunk

The sacral sympathetic trunk crosses the pelvic brim behind the common iliac vessels. There are four ganglia along each trunk and they unite in front of the coccyx at the ganglion impar. The sacral sympathetic trunk gives somatic branches to all the sacral nerves and visceral branches to the inferior hypogastric plexus.

Inferior hypogastric plexus

The right and left hypogastric plexuses comprise the pelvic plexuses (Fig. 5.20). They lie on the side wall of the pelvis, lateral to the rectum. They receive the right and left hypogastric nerves from the superior hypogastric plexus.

Branches

These are all visceral. Functions include the control of micturition, defaecation, erection, ejaculation and orgasm.

Lymphatic drainage of the pelvis

This is summarized in Figure 5.21.

THE PERINEUM

The perineum is the region of the trunk lying below the pelvic diaphragm, bounded by the pelvic outlet and divided into an anterior urogenital triangle and a posterior anal triangle. The term can be used to describe the superficial area between the thighs or the whole compartment. Figure 5.22 illustrates the perineum's boundaries.

All structures are supplied by the pudendal artery and nerve (S2, 3, 4).

Anal triangle

The anal triangle has an anterior boundary formed by an imaginary transverse line between the ischial tuberosities. The lateral boundaries are the sacrotuberous ligaments and the apex is the tip of the coccyx (Fig. 5.22). It contains the two ischioanal fossae; separated in the midline by the anal canal, the anococcygeal ligament, and the perineal body. The triangle slopes anteriorly and inferiorly from its apex. Muscles of the anal triangle are outlined in Fig. 5.23.

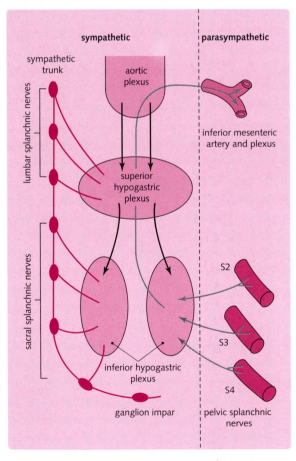

Fig. 5.20 Autonomic plexuses in the pelvis. (Adapted from *Anatomy as a Basis for Clinical Medicine*, by E C B Hall-Craggs. Courtesy of Williams & Wilkins.)

Fig. 5.21 Lymphatic drainage of the pelvis	
Structure	**Lymphatic drainage**
Anal canal	Superficial inguinal nodes
Bladder	Internal and external iliac nodes
Ovary	Aortic nodes
Rectum	Inferior mesenteric nodes Internal iliac nodes Pararectal nodes Preaortic nodes
Urethra	Internal iliac nodes Superficial inguinal nodes
Uterus and uterine tubes	External iliac nodes Internal iliac nodes Sacral nodes
Vagina	Internal and external iliac nodes Superficial inguinal nodes

Anal canal

The anal canal commences at the anorectal junction where the rectum passes through puborectalis (pelvic diaphragm). It extends for about 4 cm and ends at the anus.

Lining of the anal canal

The upper part of the anal canal is lined by epithelium thrown into folds—the anal columns. Inferiorly, these columns are linked by horizontal folds, forming the anal valves. The recesses between the columns and valves are the anal sinuses where the anal glands open. The lower margins of the anal valves form the pectinate line. The anocutaneous junction (white line), where the lining of the canal becomes true skin, is a short distance inferior to this.

Muscular wall of the anal canal

This surrounds the mucous membrane and it is composed of the internal and external anal sphincters (Fig. 5.24).

The internal anal sphincter is a continuation of the circular smooth muscle of the rectum. It surrounds the upper three-quarters of the anal canal and it ends at the white line.

At the anorectal junction the longitudinal muscle joins with puborectalis muscle fibres to form a descending fibroelastic sheet called the conjoint longitudinal coat. This runs between the internal and external anal sphincters piercing them to insert into the perianal skin and ischioanal fossa fat.

The external anal sphincter has subcutaneous, superficial and deep parts but these fuse together, forming a single muscular mass. The muscle is striated and under voluntary control via the perineal branch of S4 spinal nerve and the inferior rectal nerve (a branch of the pudendal nerve). The anorectal ring (the chief muscle of continence) is formed by the internal sphincter, the deep part of the external sphincter and the puborectalis part of levator ani.

Figure 5.25 shows the blood supply and lymphatic drainage of the anal canal. Veins anastomose freely, forming an internal rectal plexus inside the submucosa and an external rectal plexus outside the muscular wall.

Ischioanal fossa and pudendal canal

The ischioanal fossa lies lateral to the anal canal. It is filled with adipose tissue, and it contains the

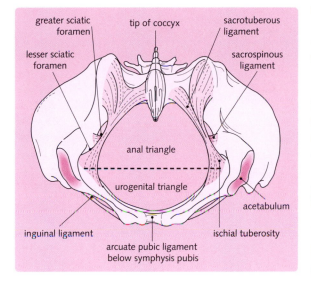

Fig. 5.22 Boundaries of the perineum.

Fig. 5.23 Muscles of the anal triangle. (Adapted from *Essential Clinical Anatomy*, 1996, by K L Moore. Williams & Wilkins.)			
Name of muscle (nerve supply)	**Origin**	**Insertion**	**Action**
External anal sphincter—subcutaneous part (inferior rectal nerve and perineal branch of fourth sacral nerve)	Encircles anal canal, no bony attachments		Voluntary sphincter of anal canal
External anal sphincter—superficial part (inferior rectal nerve and perineal branch of fourth sacral nerve)	Perineal body	Coccyx	
External anal sphincter—deep part (inferior rectal nerve and perineal branch of fourth sacral nerve)	Encircles anal canal	Coccyx	

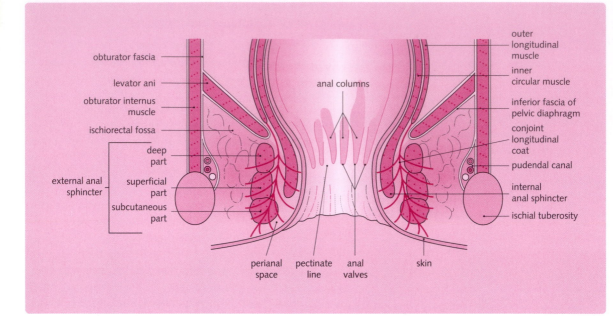

Fig. 5.24 Anal canal and ischioanal fossa.

Haemorrhoids

These are dilatations of the internal rectal venous plexus, usually due to straining at stool in chronic constipation but are also caused by pregnancy, familial predispositions and occasionally by portal hypertension.

- 1st degree haemorrhoids remain inside the anal canal and may cause bleeding.
- 2nd degree haemorrhoids prolapse temporarily during defecation.
- 3rd degree haemorrhoids prolapse permanently and may strangulate.

These typically appear at 3, 7 and 11 o'clock positions around the anus. They are typically painless until they extend below the pectinate line into the area of somatic innervation. Haemorrhoids are treated by injection with a sclerosing material or ligated with a rubber band.

The fat of the ischioanal fossa has a poor blood supply. Therefore, it is vulnerable to infection and abscess formation.

pudendal canal as well as the inferior rectal arteries and nerves (see Fig. 5.24). Its boundaries are detailed in Figure 5.26.

The pudendal canal lies on the lateral wall of the ischioanal fossa. The canal is roofed by fascia that is continuous with the obturator internus fascia above, and that fuses with the ischial tuberosity below. It contains the internal pudendal vessels and the pudendal nerve, which pass from the lesser sciatic foramen to the deep perineal pouch.

The male urogenital triangle

The male urogenital triangle is bounded posteriorly by an imaginary transverse line between the two ischial tuberosities. Its lateral boundaries are the ischiopubic rami, which meet at the apex—the pubic symphysis (Fig. 5.22).

Within the urogenital triangle is the deep perineal space, lying below the anterior part of the levator ani muscle. The deep perineal space contains striated muscle, 'sandwiched' between superior and inferior layers of fascia (Fig. 5.27).

Loose pelvic fascia forms the superior boundary to the deep space, which contains the deep transverse perineal muscles and the sphincter urethrae.

The inferior fascia forms the inferior boundary of the deep perineal space. This tough fascial layer is

Fig. 5.25 Blood supply, lymphatic drainage and nerve supply of the anal canal

	Above pectinate line	Below Pectinate line
Epithelium	Colummar (mucosa)	Stratified squamous
Arteries	Superior rectal (from inferior mesenteric)	Middle and inferior rectal (from internal iliac)
Lymph drainage	Internal iliac nodes	Superficial inguinal nodes
Nerve supply	Visceral—inferior hypogastric plexus. Sensitive to stretch	Somatic—inferior rectal from pudendal (S2, 3, 4). Sensitive to pain, touch, etc.

Fig. 5.26 Boundaries of the Ischioanal fossa

Boundary	Components
Base	Skin over anal region of perineum
Medial wall	Anal canal and levator ani
Lateral wall	Ischial tuberosity and obturator internus
Apex	Where levator ani is attached to its tendinous origins over obturator fascia
Anterior extension	Superior to deep perineal pouch

called the perineal membrane and it is attached to the ischiopubic rami, from just behind the pubic symphysis to the ischial tuberosities. In the anatomical position, it lies horizontally.

Between the superficial perineal fascia (of Colles) and perineal membrane is the superficial perineal space.

The urethra penetrates the deep perineal space and perineal membrane (Fig. 5.27).

Figure 5.28 outlines the muscles of the urogenital triangle. These muscles are involved in micturition, copulation, and support of the pelvic viscera.

Deep perineal space

The deep perineal space is the region above the perineal membrane. It contains the deep transverse perineal muscles, sphincter urethrae and the following structures:

- The membranous urethra.
- The bulbourethral glands.

- The pudendal vessels (continuing forward from the pudendal canal).
- The dorsal nerve of the penis.

The perineal membrane, sphincter urethrae and pelvic fascia together constitute the urogenital diaphragm. The bulbourethral glands are two small glands lying on either side of the membranous urethra (see Fig. 5.26) – their ducts pierce the perineal membrane to enter the spongy part of the urethra. Secretions contribute to the seminal fluid.

Superficial perineal space

The superficial perineal space is lined inferiorly by the superficial perineal fascia of Colles; it is continuous with the membranous superficial fascia (Scarpa's fascia) of the anterior abdominal wall, which descends to line the scrotum. It is attached to the ischiopubic rami, the posterior border of the perineal membrane, the perineal body, and the fascia lata of the thigh. The superficial perineal fascia extends into the penis as the superficial fascia of the penis (Buck's fascia), attaching to the glans penis.

Superiorly the space is limited by the perineal membrane. The contents of the space include the root of the penis, superficial transverse perineal, bulbospongiosus, and ischiocavernosus muscles. It also contains the perineal branches of the internal pudendal artery and pudendal nerve.

The male external genitalia

The male external genitalia consist of the penis and the scrotum. The scrotum is described in Chapter 4.

Fig. 5.27 Coronal section of the male perineum.

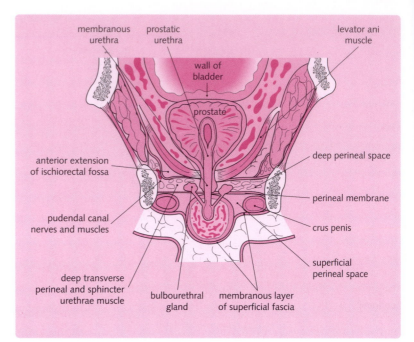

Penis

The penis is suspended from the symphysis pubis. It consists of the root, the shaft and the glans (Fig. 5.29).

The root is made up of three masses of erectile tissue: the bulb of the penis, and the right and left crura. The bulb and crura are partially surrounded by the bulbospongiosus and ischiocavernosus muscles. The superficial transverse perineal muscle is also closely related to these.

Distally, the crura become the corpora cavernosa and the bulb becomes the corpus spongiosum. These contain numerous spaces into which arteries empty. The urethra passes into the erectile tissue of the bulb and continues in the corpus spongiosum to the external urethral orifice.

The distal end of the corpus spongiosum expands to form the glans penis. The shaft is surrounded by thin loose skin. At the proximal part of the glans penis the skin is reflected upon itself to form the prepuce or foreskin, which covers the glans. The prepuce is attached to the ventral surface of the glans by a fold of skin, the frenulum of the prepuce, which contains a small artery.

A tough tunica albuginea surrounds the penis. The deep fascia of the penis encircles the tunica albuginea. Around this deep fascia runs the superficial fascia of the penis (Buck's fascia).

The crura and corpora cavernosa receive blood from the deep arteries of the penis. The bulb and corpus spongiosum are supplied by the artery to the bulb and the dorsal artery, which also supplies the skin and superficial layers.

These vessels allow rapid distension of the cavernous spaces to produce an erection.

Venous drainage is to the deep and superficial dorsal veins.

Parasympathetic (responsible for erection) and sensory fibres enter the penis via the pudendal nerves and their terminal branches, the dorsal nerves of the penis.

Vessels of the male urogenital triangle

The internal pudendal artery is a branch of the internal iliac artery. It exits the pelvis via the greater sciatic foramen to enter the pudendal canal, entering

Fig. 5.28 Muscles of the urogenital triangle. (Adapted from *Essential Clinical Anatomy*, 1996, by K L Moore. Williams & Wilkins.)

Name of muscle (nerve supply)	Origin	Insertion	Action
Superficial transverse perineal muscle (perineal branch of pudendal nerve)	Ischial tuberosity	Perineal body	Fixes perineal body
Bulbospongiosus (perineal branch of pudendal nerve)	Perineal body and median raphe in male, perineal body in female	Fascia of bulb of penis and corpora spongiosum and cavernosum in male, fascia of bulbs of vestibule in female	In male, empties urethra after micturition and ejaculation, and assists in erection of penis; in female, sphincter of vagina and assists in erection of clitoris
Ischiocavernosus (perineal branch of pudendal nerve)	Ischial tuberosity and ischial ramus in male and female	Fascia covering corpus cavernosum	Erection of penis or clitoris
Deep transverse perineal muscle (perineal branch of pudendal nerve)	Ramus of ischium	Perineal body	Fixes perineal body
Sphincter urethrae (perineal branch of pudendal nerve)	Pubic arch	Surrounds urethra	Voluntary sphincter of urethra, important muscle of urinary incontinence

the perineum via the lesser sciatic foramen at the ischial spine. At the anterior end of the canal it enters the deep perineal pouch and continues forward on the deep surface of the perineal membrane. It terminates by dividing into the dorsal and deep arteries of the penis or clitoris. Its branches are outlined in Figure 5.30.

The internal pudendal veins are the venae comitantes of the arteries. The deep dorsal vein of the penis drains into the prostatic plexus. The superficial dorsal vein of the penis drains to a superficial pudendal vein and then to the femoral vein.

The blood supply to the scrotum is described in Chapter 4 – it is a body wall structure, so has corresponding supply and drainage.

Lymphatics of the male urogenital triangle

The penis and scrotum drain into the superficial (skin) and deep (glans and corpora) inguinal nodes.

Nerves of the male urogenital triangle

The pudendal nerve (S2–S4) passes with the internal pudendal artery through the lesser sciatic foramen and the pudendal canal, where it gives rise to the inferior rectal nerve. The inferior rectal nerve supplies the external anal sphincter and the skin around the anus. At the posterior border of the perineal membrane the nerve divides into the perineal nerve and the dorsal nerve of the penis. The perineal nerve passes superficial to the perineal membrane. It supplies the scrotum posteriorly and all the remaining striated muscles of the perineum.

Note that spinal segments S2–S4 are therefore essential for continence.

The dorsal nerve of the penis runs with the dorsal artery of the penis. It passes over the dorsum of the penis lateral to the artery and terminates in the glans.

The nerve supply to the scrotum is described in Chapter 4.

To recall the pudendal nerve supplies levator ani remember S2, 3, 4 keep your guts off the floor.

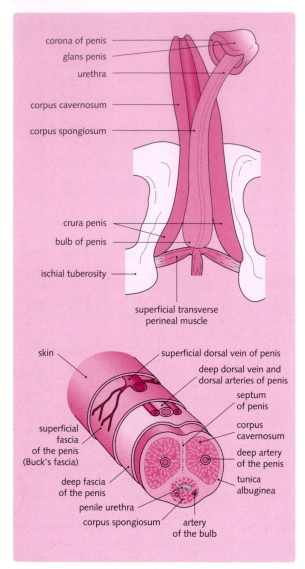

Fig. 5.30 Branches of internal pudendal artery	
Vessel (in female)	**Course and distribution**
Inferior rectal artery	Crosses the ischiorectal fossa to supply the muscles and skin of the anal canal
Perineal branch	Passes to the superficial perineal space to supply its muscles and the scrotum (or labia in female)
Artery to bulb of penis (or clitoris)	Supplies the erectile tissue of the bulb and corpus spongiosum
Deep artery of penis (or clitoris)	Supplies the corpus cavernosum
Dorsal artery of penis (or clitoris)	Passes to the dorsum of the penis (or clitoris). It supplies the erectile tissue of the corpus cavernosum and superficial structures
Urethral artery	Supplies the urethra

Fig. 5.29 Composition and structure of the penis.

The female urogenital triangle

The muscles, fasciae and spaces of the female urogenital triangle are similar to those of the male urogenital triangle. However, certain features differ because of the presence of the vagina and external female genitalia: the vagina pierces both superficial and deep perineal spaces.

The deep perineal space also lacks the female equivalent of the bulbourethral gland.

The superficial perineal space again is similar to that of the male, and it is lined by a less-defined superficial perineal fascia. However, it is full of fat; it is smaller; and it is found within the labia majora.

Perineal membrane

The perineal membrane is wider in the female since the pelvis is wider, and it is also weaker than in the male because of the presence of the vagina. As the urethra and vagina pierce the membrane their outer fascial covering fuses with it.

Perineal body

In the female, the perineal body lies between the vagina and the anal canal. The perineal body lacks support from the perineal membrane because of the presence of the vagina, so the perineal body in the female has greater mobility. The superficial and deep transverse perineal muscles, the pubovaginalis, bulbospongiosus, and the superficial part of the external anal sphincter are attached to the perineal body.

The external female genitalia

The external female genitalia consist of the mons pubis, external urethral orifice, clitoris, vagina, vestibule, bulb of the vestibule, greater vestibular glands, labia majora, and labia minora. Together these parts form the vulva (Fig. 5.31).

Mons pubis

In the adult (i.e. after puberty), this is the mound of coarse-haired skin and fat anterior to the pubic symphysis. The mons pubis extends posteriorly as the labia majora.

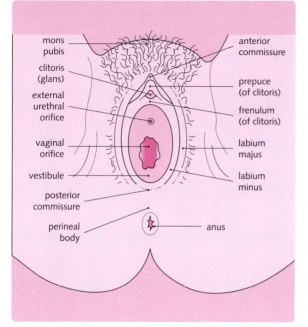

labels on figure:
mons pubis
clitoris (glans)
external urethral orifice
vaginal orifice
vestibule
posterior commissure
perineal body
anterior commissure
prepuce (of clitoris)
frenulum (of clitoris)
labium majus
labium minus
anus

Fig. 5.31 Female external genitalia.

Labia majora

These two fatty folds of skin are joined together anteriorly to form the anterior commissure, and they are continuous with the mons pubis. As the folds pass posteriorly they fade into the skin near the anus, forming the posterior commissure, which overlies the perineal body. The round ligament of the uterus ends in the labium majus.

Labia minora

These are fat free skin folds that lie within the labia majora and surround the vestibule of the vagina. They enclose the clitoris by forming the prepuce in front and the frenulum behind.

Clitoris

This homologue of the penis consists of two erectile crura attached to the perineal membrane and ischiopubic rami. Anteriorly, the crura become the corpora cavernosa. These are bound together by fascia to form the body of the clitoris. The glans surmounts the body. It is connected to the bulbs of the vestibule by erectile tissue. These lie on either side of the vaginal orifice.

Vestibule

This contains the openings of the greater vestibular glands, the vagina, and the external urethral orifice.

Bulb of the vestibule

This is the homologue of the penile bulb and corpus spongiosum. Posteriorly these two erectile masses, either side of the vagina, are attached to the perineal membrane. Anteriorly they join the glans of the clitoris. Each is covered by the bulbospongiosus muscle.

Greater vestibular glands

The homologues of the bulbourethral glands, these are found in the superficial perineal pouch in contact with the posterior end of the bulb of the vestibule. Their ducts open into the vestibule and lubricate the vagina in sexual arousal.

Vagina

Superiorly, the vagina passes through the pelvic floor surrounded by part of the puborectalis; anteriorly, it is closely related to the urethra; posteriorly, the perineal body separates it from the anal canal; inferiorly, it opens into the vestibule at the introitus. This opening is partially occluded by a thin membrane—the hymen—which is usually destroyed during sexual intercourse.

External urethral orifice

This lies in the vestibule posterior to the glans of the clitoris but anterior to the vagina.

Lymphatics of the female urogenital triangle

The lymph drains to the superficial inguinal lymph nodes.

Vessels and nerves of the female urogenital triangle

The internal pudendal artery has a similar course and distribution in the female as in the male, except:

- Posterior labial branches replace scrotal branches.

Pudendal nerve block

A pudendal nerve block relieves pain caused by perineal stretching in childbirth. The nerve is blocked where it crosses the sacrospinous ligament near the ischial spine: the ischial spine is palpated by a finger within the vagina and the needle is introduced transcutaneously.

- The artery to the bulb and vestibule and the dorsal arteries of the clitoris replace the arteries to the penis.

The blood supply to the external genitalia (e.g. the labia) is the same as for the scrotum. It receives the superficial and deep external pudendal arteries (from the femoral artery). It drains via corresponding veins into the great saphenous vein. The pudendal nerve has a similar distribution in both sexes. The only difference is in the naming of the nerves, in which labial replaces scrotal.

The nerve supply to the labia is the same as for the scrotum:

- The anterior third is supplied by the ilioinguinal nerve.
- The posterior two thirds are supplied by the posterior labial branch of the pudendal nerve (medially) and by the perineal branch of the posterior femoral cutaneous nerve (laterally).

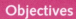

The lower limb

6

Objectives

In this chapter you will learn to:

- Describe the venous drainage of the lower limb and how varicose veins develop.
- Outline the cutaneous innervation of the lower limb.
- Understand the route of lymphatic drainage of the lower limb.
- Explain the skeleton of the hip joint and a femoral neck fracture.
- Describe the gluteal region muscles, contents and a site for intramuscular injections.
- State the boundaries and contents of the femoral triangle.
- Explain the arterial supply of the thigh and a site for pulse palpation.
- State the muscles of the thigh and their nerve supply.
- State the boundaries and contents of the popliteal fossa.
- Understand the anatomy of the knee joint, especially the ligaments.
- Outline the muscles of the leg and their nerve supply.
- Explain the antigravity action of the calf and its venous pump.
- Describe the arterial supply of the leg and a site for pulse palpation.
- Describe the skeleton of the foot and ankle joint, especially the ligaments.
- Describe the anatomy of the dorsum of the foot.
- State the intrinsic muscles of the foot.
- Describe the blood and nerve supply of the sole of the foot.
- List the structures that support the arches of the foot.
- Recognize the bony features of a normal radiograph of the lower limb.
- Have a method for reviewing an X-ray of the lower limb.

REGIONS AND COMPONENTS OF THE LOWER LIMB

The lower limb is built for support, locomotion and the maintenance of equilibrium. Weight is transferred from the rigid bony pelvis, through the acetabulum, to the lower limb. Propulsive movements are transmitted in a similar way but in the opposite direction.

The hip joint is formed by the acetabulum and the head of the femur. It is a very stable joint, with a good range of movement.

The femur articulates with the tibia at the knee joint. Only flexion and extension are possible at this joint. The superior part of the fibula serves for muscle attachment only, and it does not take part in the formation of the knee joint or in weight bearing.

Both the tibia and the fibula articulate with the talus to form the ankle joint, where only flexion and extension movements may occur.

The blood supply to the lower limb is from the external iliac artery. This becomes the femoral artery beneath the inguinal ligament, and it supplies the thigh. Behind the knee, the femoral artery becomes the popliteal artery, which supplies the leg and the foot.

The gluteal region is supplied by the superior and inferior gluteal arteries, branches of the internal iliac artery.

The lower limb is innervated by the lumbar and sacral plexuses via the femoral, obturator and sciatic nerves. The gluteal region is also supplied by the superior and inferior gluteal nerves.

SURFACE ANATOMY AND SUPERFICIAL STRUCTURES

Hip and thigh region

The iliac crest, tubercle, anterior superior and posterior superior iliac spines are palpable (Chapter 5). The pubic tubercle may be seen in thin subjects.

The femur is surrounded by muscle; thus, only the greater trochanter of the femur (the most lateral palpable structure in the hip region) and femoral epicondyles can be felt. The lateral condyle of the femur is more easily palpated than the medial due to the position of the vastus medialis muscle; however, the adductor tubercle can be identified on the medial condyle. In the flexed knee, the patellar surface of the femur is palpable.

Knee region

The patella is a sesamoid bone into which the quadriceps tendon inserts. Its borders can be palpated, with the apex inferiorly and base superiorly.

On the lateral side of the knee the head of the fibula is readily seen and palpable. The lateral condyle of the tibia articulates with the fibular head. Both femoral condyles are easily felt.

Posteriorly, the diamond-shaped popliteal fossa is seen when the knee is flexed against resistance. Its upper borders are formed by the hamstring muscles and the lower borders by the calf muscles; it contains the popliteal vessels, tibial and common peroneal nerves.

Leg region

The subcutaneous anteromedial surface of the tibia (shin bone) is easily felt. Anteriorly at the upper end of the tibia an oval tuberosity is felt. The tibial tuberosity is the site of attachment of the quadriceps tendon.

On the neck of the fibula, the common peroneal nerve can be palpated as it becomes superficial and runs from the popliteal fossa into the lateral compartment of the leg. It is vulnerable to injury at this point. The peroneal muscles lie laterally on the leg completely covering the fibula except distally where it forms the lateral malleolus.

Ankle

The malleoli are prominences medially and laterally. The distal part of the tibia forms the medial malleolus and the distal part of the fibula forms the lateral malleolus. These form a synovial (hinge) joint with the talus bone.

Foot

On the dorsal surface, the head of the talus is the only distinguishable feature on palpation. The other tarsal bones cannot be identified individually. The metatarsal bones and phalanges are easily identified and palpated along their length. The tendons of the extensor muscles are visible together with subcutaneous veins.

On the plantar surface, the calcaneum can be felt as the heel bone as well as the navicular tuberosity anterior to the medial malleolus. The base of the fifth metatarsal is felt laterally, but the other bones are covered by the plantar aponeurosis, intrinsic muscles and long flexor tendons.

Musculature

The rounded outline of the buttock is due to the gluteus maximus muscle mass and subcutaneous fat.

There are three muscular compartments in the thigh which are anterior (extensor), medial (adductor) and posterior (flexor). Each has a common nerve supply:

- The femoral nerve supplies the extensor compartment.
- The obturator nerve supplies the adductor compartment.
- The sciatic nerve supplies the flexor compartment.

Extensor compartment of the thigh

The large quadriceps muscle mass covers the anterior surface of the thigh. It inserts into the patella and, via the patellar ligament, into the tibial tuberosity. The rectus femoris component can be identified on muscle contraction. The vastus lateralis and vastus medialis muscle form the lateral and medial borders of the thigh. The vastus intermedius muscle lies deeply between them. Vastus medialis extends further distally forming a muscular prominence on the medial aspect of the knee.

When contracted the sartorius muscle forms an oblique ridge passing inferiorly on the medial side of the knee.

The greater part of gluteus maximus and tensor fasciae latae insert into the iliotibial tract on the lateral surface of the thigh. It is a thickening in the fascia lata which supports the knee.

Flexor compartment of the thigh

The three hamstrings lie in the posterior compartment of the thigh. They emerge from below gluteus maximus and can be demonstrated by flexing the knee against resistance. The biceps femoris tendon can be palpated and seen attaching to the fibular head. Semimembranosus and semitendinosus muscles are felt medially, the semimembranosus muscle being thick and rounded. The tendon of semitendinosus inserts with sartorius into the tibia.

Adductor compartment of the thigh

The adductor muscles are large and form the medial aspect of the thigh.

There are three muscular compartments in the leg which are anterior (extensor), lateral (peroneal) and posterior (flexor). Each has a common nerve supply:

- The deep peroneal nerve supplies the extensor compartment.
- The superficial peroneal nerve supplies the peroneal compartment.
- The tibial nerve supplies the flexor compartment.

Flexor compartment of the leg

The large gastrocnemius heads, with the medial and lateral borders of soleus muscles either side, are seen at the back of the leg during muscle action. These join to form the tendocalcaneus, which inserts into the calcaneum and are powerful plantarflexors of the ankle joint.

Peroneal compartment of the leg

Laterally the peroneal muscles are seen. The peroneus longus arises from the fibula above peroneus brevis. The peroneus longus tendon passes superficially over the peroneus brevis.

Extensor compartment of the leg

The anterior extensor muscles lie lateral to the tibia. The tibialis anterior muscle is most easily identified and its tendon can be traced inferiorly across the ankle into the foot. Tendons of the extensor muscles are easily identifiable from medial to lateral as tibialis anterior, extensor hallucis longus and extensor digitorum longus.

On the dorsal surface of the foot, extensor digitorum brevis causes an identifiable round muscle mass anterior to the lateral malleolus. The dorsal interossei can be seen between metatarsal bones.

Superficial fascia of the lower limb

The membranous superficial fascia (Scarpa's fascia) becomes fused with the fascia lata of the thigh as it extends inferiorly from the anterior abdominal wall. The position at which the fusion occurs is at a skin crease just below the inguinal ligament.

Fascia lata

The fascia lata is the deep fascia of the thigh. It lies deep to the skin and superficial fascia, and it encloses the compartments of the thigh like a stocking. Its attachments can be traced along the pelvis:

- Ilium, sacrum, and sacrotuberous ligament (posteriorly).
- Ischial tuberosity, ischiopubic ramus and body of the pubic bone (inferiorly).
- Pubic tubercle and pectinate line (anteriorly).
- Iliac crest (superiorly).

Inferiorly the fascia lata is attached to the tibia and fibula and continues below becoming the deep fascia of the calf.

The iliotibial tract is a thickening of the fascia lata. It begins at the level of the greater trochanter and it extends to the lateral condyle of the tibia. The tract helps to support the hyperextended knee when standing.

The thigh is divided into anterior, posterior and medial compartments by lateral, medial and intermediate intermuscular septa (Fig. 6.1), which are derived from the fascia lata.

Superficial veins

The foot drains into the dorsal venous arch, which drains laterally into the small saphenous vein and medially into the great saphenous vein.

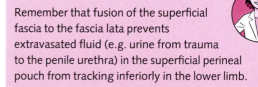

Remember that fusion of the superficial fascia to the fascia lata prevents extravasated fluid (e.g. urine from trauma to the penile urethra) in the superficial perineal pouch from tracking inferiorly in the lower limb.

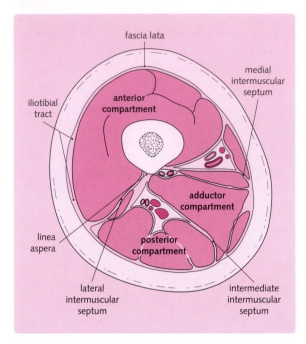

Fig. 6.1 Compartments of the left thigh.

Great saphenous vein

The great saphenous vein passes anterior to the medial malleolus, and it ascends in the subcutaneous tissue on the medial side of the leg and thigh until it reaches the saphenous opening in the fascia lata (Fig. 6.2A and inset). Here, it perforates the cribriform fascia covering the opening and joins the femoral vein. It communicates with the deep veins of the limb via perforating veins. Normally blood flows from the superficial veins to the deep veins.

The valves of the great saphenous vein allow the flow of blood in one direction only from distal to proximal.

Tributaries of the great saphenous vein arise from the anterior and medial aspects of the thigh and from the anterior abdominal wall. These include:

• The superficial circumflex iliac vein.
• The superficial epigastric vein.
• The external pudendal vein.

Small saphenous vein

The small saphenous vein passes posterior to the lateral malleolus and runs superiorly and posteriorly to pierce the deep fascia of the popliteal fossa, where it joins the popliteal vein (Fig. 6.2B). It drains the lateral part of the leg and communicates with the deep veins of the leg via perforating veins.

Lymphatic drainage of the lower limb

Lymphatics from the superficial tissues of the lower limb drain into the superficial inguinal lymph nodes (Fig. 6.3). These lie superficial to the fascia lata along the inguinal ligament and around the termination of the saphenous vein. They also receive lymph from the perineum, the abdominal wall, and the buttock.

The superficial nodes drain to deep nodes lying alongside the femoral vessels in the femoral canal. The deep nodes drain the deep tissues of the lower limb and their efferent vessels drain centrally into nodes lying alongside the external iliac vessels.

Cutaneous innervation of the lower limb

Figures 6.4 and 6.5 illustrate the dermatomes of the lower limb and its cutaneous innervation, respectively.

The superficial inguinal lymph nodes drain a variety of structures. On palpating enlarged nodes in the groin it is important to remember that they drain: lower limb (cellulitus), perineum (syphilis), buttock (abscess) and the abdominal wall inferior to the umbilicus.

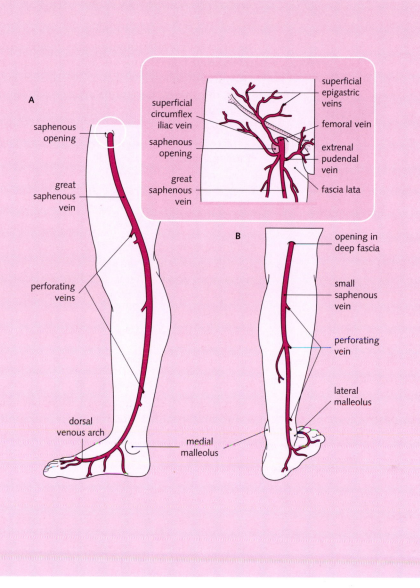

Fig. 6.2 Great (A) and small (B) saphenous veins and their tributaries. Inset shows tributaries of great saphenous vein.

THE GLUTEAL REGION, HIP AND THIGH

Skeleton of the hip and thigh

Pelvic girdle

The pelvic girdle protects the pelvic cavity and supports the body weight. It transmits load to the lower limbs via the sacrum, hip bone, and hip joint (see Chapter 5).

Femur

The femur is the long bone of the thigh. The bone and its muscle attachments are illustrated in Figure 6.6.

Gluteal region

The gluteal region, or buttock, lies behind the pelvis and extends from the iliac crest to the fold of the buttock. The greater and lesser sciatic foramina in this region are formed anteriorly by the greater and lesser

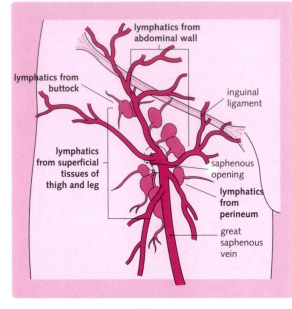

Fig. 6.3 Superficial inguinal lymph nodes.

sciatic notches, and posteriorly are completed by the sacrotuberous and sacrospinous ligaments. The muscles, vessels, and nerves that exit or enter the sciatic foramina and supply the gluteal region, are shown in Figures 6.7–6.10. The piriformis muscle is the key to understanding this region because vessels and nerves either pass superior or inferior to it.

Neurology

Damage to the superior gluteal nerve, as occurred in polio cases or in multiple sclerosis, causes gluteus medius and minimus paralysis. Gluteus medius and minimus abduct the hip while walking to allow the opposite limb to swing forward without hitting the ground. When a patient stands on one leg, if the hip drops or dips down on the contralateral side, then it is the abductor muscles on the Stance side are paralysed (Trendelenburg's sign).

The gluteal region is an intramuscular injection site. Each buttock is divided into quadrants. A vertical line midway between the natal cleft and lateral aspect of thigh and a horizontal line midway between the gluteal fold and iliac crest. The supero-lateral quadrant is a safe site for injections.

Anterior compartment of the thigh

The anterior compartment of the thigh is enclosed by the fascia lata. The medial intermuscular septum separates it from the medial compartment, and the lateral intermuscular septum separates the anterior compartment from the posterior compartment (Fig. 6.1.)

The muscles of the anterior compartment are described in Figure 6.11.

Factors stabilizing the patella

Due to the width of the pelvis, the quadriceps lies obliquely in the thigh. This causes the pull of the quadriceps tendon to be oblique; however, the pull of the patella ligament is vertical. As the quadriceps muscle contracts the patella has the tendency to move laterally as a result of these two vectors. This is prevented by three factors:

- The lateral condyle of the femur projects further anteriorly (see Fig. 6.20).
- The lowest fibres of vastus medialis insert into the patella directly, and they are approximately horizontal. Contraction pulls the patella medially.
- Tension in the medial patella retinaculum.

Femoral triangle

The femoral triangle contains the femoral artery, vein, and nerve (Fig. 6.12). These all lie superficially just beneath the skin, superficial fascia and fascia lata.

The femoral artery, vein and femoral canal are enclosed by the femoral sheath, which is a continuation of the transversalis and iliac fasciae into the thigh. The femoral nerve is separated from the femoral sheath by the iliopsoas fascia.

Femoral canal

The femoral canal contains efferent lymphatics passing from the deep inguinal nodes to the abdomen

The arrangement of the femoral vessels and nerve as they pass inferiorly from behind the inguinal ligament into the femoral triangle can be remembered (from lateral to medial) as 'NAVY' (nerve, artery, vein, Y-fronts).

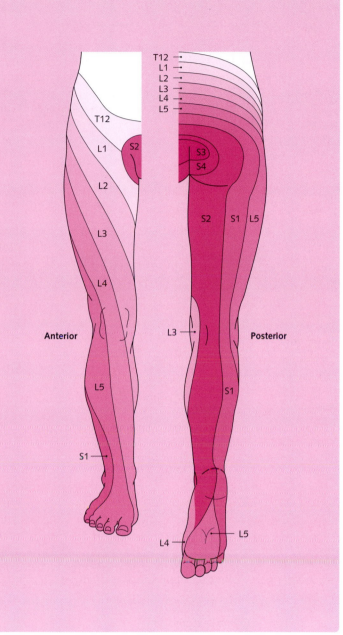

Fig. 6.4 Dermatomes of the lower limb.

(see Fig. 6.12). It provides space for expansion of the femoral vein during times of increased venous return from the lower limb. Its proximal boundaries, i.e. the femoral ring, are the lacunar ligament (medially), the medial part of the inguinal ligament (anteriorly), the femoral vein (laterally), and pectineus lying upon the superior pubic ramus (posteriorly).

Adductor canal

At the apex of the femoral triangle, the femoral vessels disappear beneath sartorius and follow the muscle to the medial aspect of the thigh in a channel—the adductor canal. It is bounded laterally by the vastus medialis and posteromedially by the adductor longus

147

Fig. 6.5 Cutaneous innervation of the lower limb.

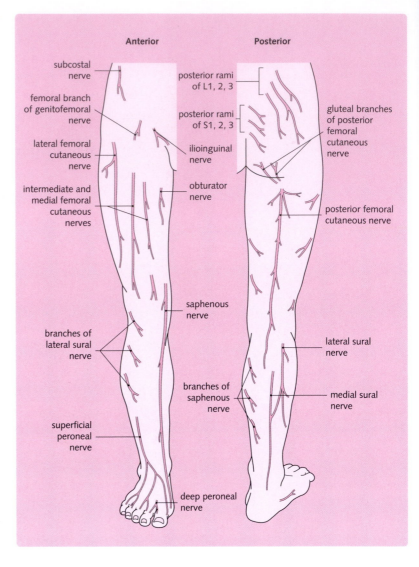

and adductor magnus. Its anterior boundary is sartorius and a fascial thickening. The contents are the nerve to vastus medialis, the saphenous nerve, femoral artery and vein.

Vessels of the thigh

Figure 6.13 outlines the arterial supply of the thigh.

Cruciate anastomosis

The cruciate anastomosis provides an alternative circulation should the femoral artery be obstructed. It is made up of:

- The inferior gluteal branch of the internal iliac artery.

- The medial and lateral circumflex femoral arteries (branches of profunda femoris).

> **Clinical examination**
>
> The femoral pulse is one of four main pulses that can be palpated. The femoral artery lies at the mid-inguinal point, half way between the anterior superior iliac crest and pubic symphysis. The artery is a cannulation site for arteriograms. Other pulses include the popliteal pulse, palpated with the knee flexed to reduce tension in the fascial stocking that covers the popliteal fossa and allows the artery to be compressed against tibia. The posterior tibial artery passes posteriorly to the medial malleolus.

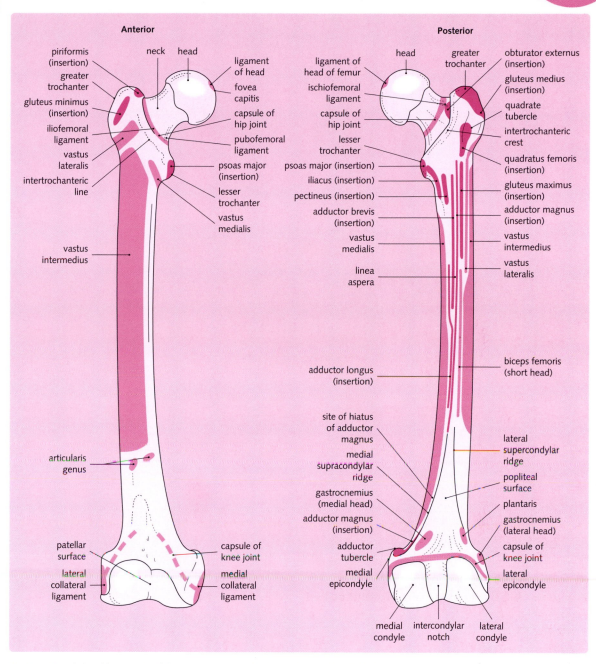

Fig. 6.6 Muscles and ligaments of the anterior and posterior surfaces of the right femur.

- The first perforating artery (branch of profunda femoris).

All the perforating arteries of profunda femoris anastomose with each other and with the muscular branches of the popliteal artery. In this way the internal iliac artery and the popliteal artery are linked. Note that the profunda femoris and its branches supply the thigh.

Femoral vein

The femoral vein lies posterior to the artery in the adductor canal. Below the inguinal ligament the vein lies medial to the artery in the femoral sheath. It passes posterior to the inguinal ligament to become the external iliac vein. It receives the corresponding branches of the profunda femoris artery and the great

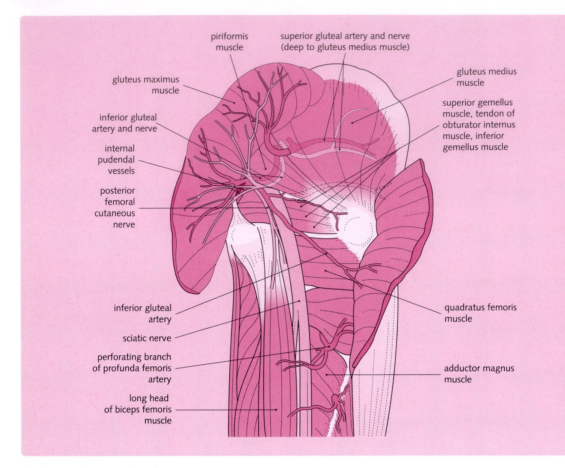

Fig. 6.7 Right gluteal region showing the main nerves and vessels.

saphenous vein (whose tributaries correspond to branches of the femoral artery).

Nerves of the thigh

The nerves of the thigh region are outlined in Figure 6.14.

Adductor compartment of the thigh

The muscles of the adductor compartment are outlined in Figure 6.15. All are supplied by the obturator nerve except for the part of the adductor magnus muscle that belongs to the posterior compartment, which is supplied by the sciatic nerve.

The perforating branches of the profunda femoris artery and the muscular branches of the femoral artery provide the majority of the blood supply to the adductor compartment. Proximally, the obturator artery also contributes to the blood supply of this region.

Posterior compartment of the thigh

The muscles of the posterior compartment are outlined in Figure 6.16 and illustrated in Figure 6.17. They are all supplied by the sciatic nerve (see Fig. 6.14).

Blood supply to the posterior compartment is mainly from the perforating branches of the profunda femoris, with a small contribution from the inferior gluteal artery.

Hip joint

The hip joint is a ball-and-socket synovial joint comprising articulation between the acetabulum and the head of the femur. It is a very stable joint (unlike the shoulder joint) and it exhibits a high degree of mobility.

Fig. 6.8 Muscles of the gluteal region

Name of muscle (nerve supply)	Origin	Insertion	Action
Tensor fasciae latae (superior gluteal nerve)	Iliac crest	Iliotibial tract	Extends knee joint Tenses iliotibial tract
Gluteus maximus (inferior gluteal nerve)	Ilium, sacrum, coccyx, and sacrotuberous ligament	Iliotibial tract and gluteal tuberosity of femur	Extends and laterally rotates thigh at hip joint; extends knee joint
Gluteus medius (superior gluteal nerve)	Ilium	Greater trochanter of femur	Abducts thigh at hip joint and tilts pelvis when walking
Gluteus minimus (superior gluteal nerve)	Ilium	Greater trochanter of femur	As gluteus medius and medially rotates thigh
Piriformis (S1, S2 nerves)	Anterior surface of sacrum	Greater trochanter of femur	All these muscles rotate thigh laterally at hip joint and stabilize the hip joint
Obturator internus (sacral plexus)	Inner surface of obturator membrane	Greater trochanter of femur	
Gemellus inferior (sacral plexus)	Ischial tuberosity	Greater trochanter of femur	
Gemellus superior (sacral plexus)	Ischial spine	Greater trochanter of femur	
Quadratus femoris (sacral plexus)	Ischial tuberosity	Quadrate tubercle on femur	

Fig. 6.9 Arteries of the gluteal region

Artery	Course and distribution
Internal pudendal	Passes through the greater sciatic foramen to enter the gluteal region, then passes into the perineum via the lesser sciatic foramen; supplies the muscles of the pelvic region and the external genitalia
Superior gluteal	Enters the gluteal region through the greater sciatic foramen; supplies gluteus maximus, medius and minimus, and tensor fasciae latae
Inferior gluteal	Passes through the greater sciatic foramen to enter the gluteal region; supplies gluteus maximus, obturator internus, and quadratus femoris

Stability is mainly achieved from the close fit between the femoral head and the acetabulum. Great mobility is achieved because the femoral neck is much narrower than the diameter of the head so that considerable movement may occur in all directions before the neck impinges on the acetabular labrum.

The C-shaped articular surface of the acetabulum is covered by hyaline cartilage. The peripheral edge of this surface is deepened by a rim of fibrocartilage—the acetabular labrum. The labrum thus contributes further to joint stability. The labrum bridges across the acetabular notch as the transverse ligament.

The articular surface of the head of the femur is also covered by hyaline cartilage. The non-articular convexity of the head is excavated into a pit (fovea) for attachment of the ligament of the head of the femur.

The capsule is attached around the labrum and transverse ligament and the neck of the femur. Synovial membrane lines its internal surface. The capsule is reflected proximally onto the femoral neck, binding blood vessels that supply the head tightly to the neck. A femoral neck fracture can damage these vessels. The capsule is loose and strong. The capsule is reinforced by three strong ligaments that extend from the pelvic bone to the femur:

Fig. 6.10 Nerves of the gluteal region

Nerve (origin)	Course and distributions
Inferior gluteal (anterior rami of L5–S2)	Leaves pelvis through greater sciatic foramen below piriformis, and supplies gluteus maximus
Superior gluteal (anterior rami of L4–S1)	Leaves pelvis through greater sciatic foramen above piriformis and passes between gluteus medius and minimus to supply these muscles and tensor fasciae latae
Nerve to quadratus femoris (anterior rami of L4, L5, and S1)	Leaves pelvis through greater sciatic foramen below piriformis to supply the hip joint, inferior gemellus, and quadratus femoris
Nerve to obturator internus (anterior rami of L5, S1, and S2)	Enters gluteal region through greater sciatic foramen below piriformis descends posterior to ischial spine, enters lesser sciatic foramen. It supplies obturator internus and superior gemellus muscles
Posterior femoral cutaneous (sacral plexus—S1–S3)	Leaves pelvis through greater sciatic foramen, below piriformis, runs deep to gluteus maximus. It emerges from its inferior border to supply skin of buttock (gluteal branches) and then surface skin over posterior of thigh and calf
Pudendal (anterior rami of S2–S4)	Enters gluteal region through greater sciatic foramen below piriformis, descends posteriorly over the sacrospinous ligament, entering perineum through lesser sciatic foramen to supply it
Sciatic (lumbo sacral plexus—L4–S3)	Leaves pelvis through greater sciatic foramen below piriformis, to enter gluteal region—it has no motor branches in the gluteal region

Fig. 6.11 Muscles of the anterior compartment of the thigh

Name of muscle (nerve supply)	Origin	Insertion	Action
Quadriceps femoris—rectus femoris; vastus lateralis, medialis, and intermedius (femoral nerve)	Ilium and upper part of femur	Quadriceps tendon into patella then patellar ligament onto tibia	Extends leg at knee joint; flexes hip joint
Sartorius (femoral nerve)	Anterior superior iliac spine	Shaft of tibia	Flexes, abducts, and laterally rotates thigh at hip joint; flexes and medially rotates leg at knee joint
Psoas major (lumbar plexus, L1–L3 nerves)	T12 body, transverse processes, bodies, and intervertebral discs L1–L5	Lesser trochanter of femur (together with iliacus muscle)	Flexes thigh on trunk
Iliacus (femoral nerve)	Iliac fossa of hip bone	Lesser trochanter of femur	Flexes thigh on trunk
Pectineus (femoral nerve and obturator nerve)	Superior ramus of pubis	Upper shaft of femur	Flexes and abducts thigh at hip joint

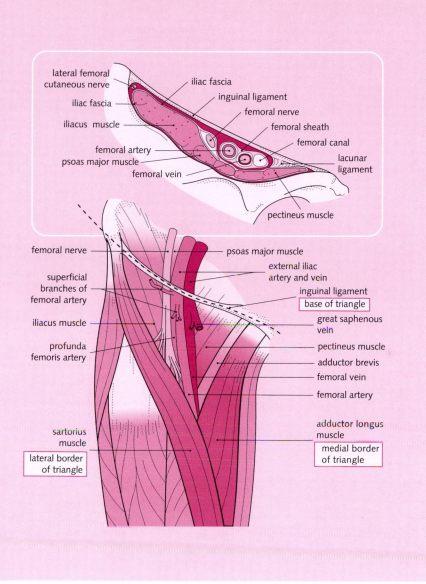

Fig. 6.12 Right femoral triangle and its contents. Inset shows inferior view of femoral canal.

- The pubofemoral ligament—lies inferiorly and prevents excessive abduction and hyperextension.
- The ischiofemoral ligament—lies posteriorly and prevents excessive medial rotation and hyperextension.
- The iliofemoral ligament—lies anteriorly and prevents hyperextension and lateral rotation.

Blood supply is from arteries that anastomose freely around the joint and are:

- The medial and lateral circumflex femoral arteries.
- The superior gluteal artery.
- The inferior gluteal artery.
- The obturator artery.

The trochanteric anastomosis lies near the trochanteric fossa and supplies blood vessels along the femoral neck which supply the head of the femur. It is formed by the superior and inferior gluteal arteries, and lateral and medial circumflex femoral arteries.

Nerve supply comprises the following:

- The femoral nerve.
- The sciatic nerve.
- The obturator nerve.

Fig. 6.13 Arterial supply to the thigh

Artery	Origin	Course and distribution
Femoral	Continuation of external iliac artery distal to inguinal ligament	Descends through femoral triangle, enters the adductor canal and ends by passing through the adductor hiatus; supplies anterior and anteromedial surfaces of the thigh
Profunda femoris	Femoral artery	Passes inferiorly, deep to adductor longus, to supply posterior compartment of thigh
Lateral circumflex femoral	Profunda femoris; may arise from femoral artery	Passes laterally deep to sartorius and rectus femoris to supply anterior part of gluteal region, and femur and knee joint
Medial circumflex femoral	Profunda femoris	Passes medially and posteriorly between pectineus and iliopsoas, and enters gluteal region; supplies head and neck of femur
Obturator	Internal iliac artery	Passes through obturator foramen and enters medial compartment of thigh; supplies obturator externus, pectineus, adductors of thigh, and gracilis—muscles attached to ischial tuberosity and head of femur

Movements of the hip joint

The muscles involved and factors that restrict movements are described in Fig. 6.18.

THE KNEE AND POPLITEAL FOSSA

Popliteal fossa

The diamond-shaped popliteal fossa is bordered by the biceps femoris, semitendinosus and semimembranosus muscles superiorly and by the gastrocnemius muscle inferiorly (Fig. 6.19). It is roofed by the deep

Orthopaedics

A dislocated hip causes the leg to shorten and become medially rotated as the femoral head lies upon the ilium. Conversely, a fracture of the femoral neck causes the leg to shorten and become laterally rotated. This is due to the axis of rotation moving from the femoral head to the femoral shaft. The medial hip rotators (e.g. iliopsoas) now cause lateral rotation. It is important to determine whether the fracture is within the joint capsule (intracapsular) or outside (extracapsular). Intracapsular fractures may interrupt the blood supply to the femoral head causing avascular necrosis.

fascia, which is pierced by the small saphenous vein and lymphatics. The floor is formed by the femur, the oblique popliteal ligament, capsule of the knee joint and the popliteus muscle.

Contents of the popliteal fossa

From deep to superficial include:

Popliteus muscle

- Proximal attachment—lies within the capsule of the knee joint from a pit just below the lateral epicondyle of the femur and the lateral meniscus of the knee joint.
- Distal attachment—popliteal surface of the tibia.
- Nerve supply—tibial nerve.
- Action—'unlocks' the knee and draws the lateral meniscus posteriorly.

Popliteal artery

This is the continuation of the femoral artery as it passes through the adductor hiatus. It is the deepest structure and lies in direct contact with the capsule of the knee joint and popliteal surface of the femur. It terminates at the lower border of popliteus, where it divides into the anterior and posterior tibial arteries.

It gives off superior, middle and inferior genicular arteries and muscular branches. Anastomoses of the genicular vessels with descending branches of the femoral and profunda femoris arteries and with

Fig. 6.14 Nerves of the thigh

Nerve (origin)	Course and distribution
ilioinguinal (lumbar plexus—L1)	Supplies skin over femoral triangle
Genitofemoral (lumbar plexus—L1–L2)	Descends on anterior surface of psoas major and divides into genital and femoral branches: femoral branch supplies skin over femoral triangle; genital branch supplies scrotum or labia majora
Lateral femoral cutaneous (lumbar plexus—L2–L3)	Passes deep to inguinal ligament, 2–3 cm medial to anterior superior iliac spine; supplies skin on anterior and lateral aspects of thigh
Medial and intermediate femoral cutaneous (femoral nerve)	Arise in femoral triangle and pierce fascia lata of thigh; supply skin on medial and anterior aspect of thigh
Posterior femoral cutaneous (sacral plexus—S2–S3)	Passes through greater sciatic foramen below piriformis; supplies skin over posterior aspect of thigh, buttock, and proximal leg
Femoral (lumbar plexus—L2–L4)	Passes deep to inguinal ligament; supplies anterior thigh muscles, hip and knee joints, and skin on anteromedial side of thigh
Obturator (lumbar plexus—L2–L4)	Enters thigh through obturator foramen and divides: anterior branch supplies adductor longus, adductor brevis, gracilis, and pectineus; posterior branch supplies obturator externus and adductor magnus
Sciatic (sacral plexus—L4–S3)	Enters gluteal region through greater sciatic foramen below or through piriformis, descends along posterior aspect of thigh, and divides proximal to the knee into tibial and common peroneal nerves; innervates hamstrings by its tibial division (except for short head of biceps femoris—innervated by common peroneal division) and has articular branches to hip and knee joints

Fig. 6.15 Muscles of the adductor compartment of the thigh

Name of muscle (nerve supply)	Origin	Insertion	Action
Adductor brevis (obturator nerve)	Inferior ramus of pubis	Posterior surface of femur	Adducts thigh at hip joint
Adductor longus (obturator nerve)	Body of pubis	Posterior surface of femur	Adducts thigh at hip joint
Adductor magnus (adductor part—obturator nerve; hamstring part—sciatic nerve)	Ischiopubic ramus	Posterior surface of femur, adductor tubercle of femur	Adducts thigh at hip joint; hamstring part extends thigh at hip joint
Gracilis (obturator nerve)	Ischiopubic ramus	Upper part of tibia	Adducts thigh at hip joint and flexes leg at knee joint
Obturator externus (obturator nerve)	Outer surface of obturator membrane	Greater trochanter of femur	Lateral rotation of thigh at hip joint

Fig. 6.16 Muscles of the posterior compartment of the thigh

Name of muscle (nerve supply)	Origin	Insertion	Action
Biceps femoris: Long head (tibial division of sciatic) Short head (common peroneal division of sciatic)	Ischial tuberosity Linea aspera	Head of fibula (both heads)	Flex leg at knee joint and extend thigh at hip joint
Semitendinosus (tibial division of the sciatic)	Ischial tuberosity	Upper part of tibial shaft	Flex leg at knee joint and extend thigh at hip joint
Semimembranosus (tibial division of sciatic)	Ischial tuberosity	Medial condyle of the tibia, forms the oblique popliteal ligament	Flex leg at knee joint and extend thigh at hip joint

Fig. 6.17 Structure of the posterior aspect of the right thigh.

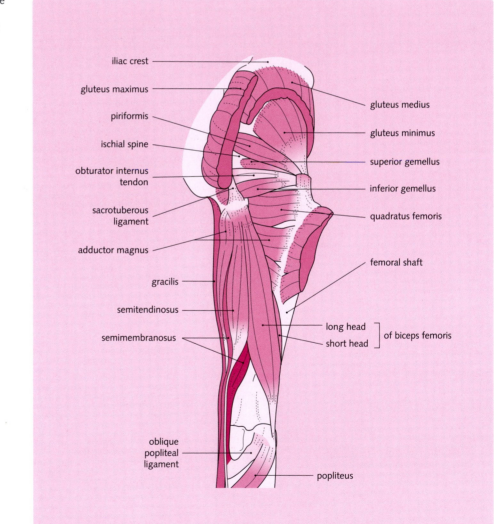

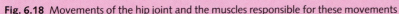

Fig. 6.18 Movements of the hip joint and the muscles responsible for these movements

Movement of the thigh on the trunk	Movement at the hip joint	Muscles involved	Factors limiting movement
Flexion	Head of the femur moves about a transverse axis passing through both acetabula and causes the shaft to swing anteriorly	Psoas major, iliacus, tensor fasciae latae, pectineus, sartorius	Thigh touching abdomen, hamstring muscle tension if leg is extended
Extension	As flexion but opposite direction	Gluteus maximus, hamstrings	Iliofemoral ligament, pubofemoral ligament
Abduction	Head of the femur moves in the acetabulum about an anteroposterior axis and causes the femoral neck and shaft to swing laterally	Gluteus medius, gluteus minimus	Abductor muscle tension, pubofemoral ligament
Adduction	As abduction but opposite direction	Adductors, gracillis	Gluteus medius, gluteus minimus, other leg
Medial rotation	Rotation of the femoral head in the acetabulum about a vertical axis that passes through the femoral head and medial condyle. The neck of the femur swings anteriorly	Tensor fasciae latae, gluteus medius, gluteus minimus, iliopsoas, pectineus, adductor longus	Ischiofemoral ligament
Lateral rotation	As medial rotation but opposite direction	Obturator internus, obturator externus, piriformis, gemelli, quadratus femoris, gluteus maximus	Iliofemoral ligament

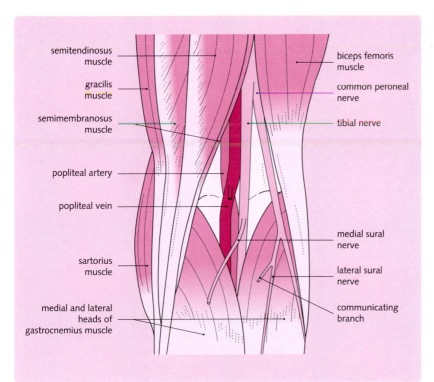

Fig. 6.19 Right popliteal fossa and its contents.

ascending branches of the tibial arteries form an important collateral supply if the main vessels become occluded.

Popliteal vein

This passes superiorly in the popliteal fossa, first medial to, and then superficial to, the artery before entering the adductor hiatus. It receives the small saphenous vein together with veins corresponding to the arterial branches.

Common peroneal nerve

This lies posterior to the tendon of biceps femoris in the popliteal fossa until it reaches the head of the fibula. Branches in the popliteal fossa include:

- The lateral sural nerve, which supplies the skin of the calf.
- A communicating branch with the medial sural nerve.
- Branches to the knee joint.

Tibial nerve

This is superficial and bisects the popliteal fossa vertically. Branches in the fossa include:

- Articular branches to the knee.
- Muscular branches to soleus, gastrocnemius, plantaris, and popliteus.
- The medial sural cutaneous nerve, which joins the communicating branch of the lateral sural cutaneous nerve to form the sural nerve. The sural nerve supplies the lateral side of the calf and heel.

Knee joint

The main features of the bones that articulate at the knee are illustrated in Figure 6.20.

The knee joint is an articulation between the femur and the tibia, with the patella articulating with the femur anteriorly. It is a synovial hinge joint that allows some rotation.

The articular surfaces are covered by hyaline cartilage and consist of the femoral condyles, the patella, and the superior surface of the tibial condyles.

Capsule

The capsule encloses the articular surfaces posteriorly, but it is incomplete:

- anterosuperiorly, to allow communication between the joint cavity and the suprapatellar bursa;

- posteroinferiorly, to allow entry of the popliteus tendon.

Anteriorly it is replaced by the articular surface of the patella.

The capsule is strengthened anteriorly by the patellar retinacula—expansions of the tendons of the vastus medialis and lateralis. It is also reinforced by the quadriceps tendon, the patella, and the patellar ligament.

Synovial membrane

The synovial membrane lines the capsule (Fig. 6.21). Superiorly it becomes continuous with the suprapatellar bursa. The cruciate ligaments and popliteus tendon lie outside the synovial cavity.

Bursae around the knee joint

The bursae around the knee joint include:

- The suprapatellar bursa.
- The prepatellar bursa.
- The superficial and deep infrapatellar bursae.

Ligaments

Ligaments play a major role in stabilizing the knee joint (Fig. 6.22). The cruciate ligaments keep the articular surfaces applied to each other throughout the range of movement and prevent the femur sliding on the tibial plateau.

The two cruciate ligaments cross each other, forming the letter X. The anterior cruciate ligament runs between the lateral femoral condyle and the anterior intercondylar area of the tibia. The posterior

Orthopaedics

Around the knee there are several bursae (fluid filled pouches continuous with joint space). Kneeling for repeated prolonged periods may cause inflammation (bursitis) and localized swelling (increased synovial fluid), e.g. clergyman's knee (prepatella bursitis) or housemaid's knee (infrapatella bursitis). Inflammation of the joint can spread to suprapatellar bursa through its communication. The knee joint can be aspirated to obtain a fluid sample for analysis by advancing a needle placed in the centre of a triangle formed by the patellar apex, lateral tibia condyle and femoral epicondyle in a slightly flexed knee.

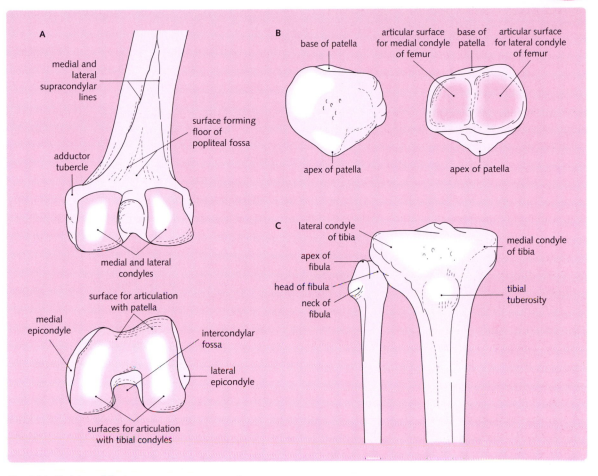

Fig. 6.20 Skeleton of the knee.

(A) Posterior and inferior aspects of the lower end of the right femur.
(B) Anterior and posterior aspects of the patella.
(C) Anterior aspect of the upper end of the right tibia and fibula.

cruciate ligament runs between the medial femoral condyle and the posterior intercondylar area of the tibia. The anterior cruciate ligament prevents posterior displacement of the femur on the tibia, as well as limiting extension of the lateral femoral condyle. In knee joint extension it forms the axis of medial rotation for the femur which locks the joint on standing. The posterior cruciate ligament prevents the femur from anterior displacement on the tibia.

Menisci

The menisci are two crescentic plates of fibrocartilage (Fig. 6.23). The horns of the menisci are attached to the intercondylar area of the tibia. At the periphery they are loosely attached via the coronary ligament to the capsule. The medial meniscus is firmly attached to the deep part of the tibial collateral ligament. They increase the congruity of the articular surfaces.

Movements at the knee joint

The movements at the knee joint are outlined in Figure 6.24. The 'locking of the knee joint' puts the knee into a slightly hyperextended position, and it is an extremely stable platform upon which the femur stands.

As the knee extends, the anterior cruciate ligament becomes taut and it stops the lateral condyle of the femur from extending further. However, due to a larger surface area of the medial condyle (see Fig. 6.20) extension continues medially around the anterior cruciate ligament. This produces medial rotation of the femur upon the tibia, and causes the

Fig. 6.21 Synovial membrane and its ligaments.

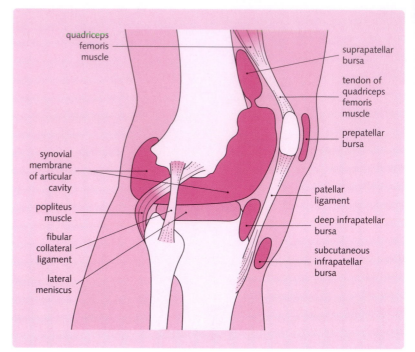

Fig. 6.22 Ligaments of the knee joint

Ligament	Attachment
Patellar (often called patella tendon)	The termination of the quadriceps tendon running from the patella to the tibial tuberosity; its tension is controlled by the quadriceps muscle, which stabilizes the joint through its full range of movement
Tibial or medial collateral	From the medial femoral epicondyle to the tibia
Fibular or lateral collateral	From the lateral femoral epicondyle to the fibular head
Oblique popliteal	Expansion of the semi-membranosus tendon, which reinforces the knee joint capsule posteriorly
Anterior cruciate	From the anterior part of the intercondylar area of the tibia to the medial surface of the lateral femoral condyle
Posterior cruciate	From the posterior part of the intercondylar area of the tibia to the lateral surface of the medial femoral condyle

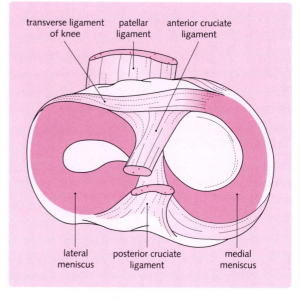

Fig. 6.23 Menisci and their ligaments.

The knee joint must be unlocked before flexion can occur. This is performed by the popliteus muscle, which laterally rotates the femur and loosens the ligaments.

Blood and nerve supply of the knee joint

Blood supply comes from the genicular branches of the popliteal artery. The nerve supply comprises

oblique, popliteal, medial collateral and lateral collateral ligaments to tighten together. At the end of this movement the knee becomes locked.

Fig. 6.24 Movements at the knee joint

Movement	Muscle
Flexion	Hamstrings, gastrocnemius, gracilis
Extension	Quadriceps femoris
Medial and lateral rotation of flexed knee	Hamstrings
Unlocking of knee	Popliteus
Locking of knee—a passive rotation of the femur upon the tibia	Is caused at the end of extension by the anterior cruciate ligament becoming taut and the femoral medial condyle moving round this ligament

the articular branches of the sciatic, femoral and obturator nerves.

THE LEG AND FOOT

Skeleton of the leg

Important features of the bones of the leg are illustrated in Figure 6.25.

The interosseous membrane is a tough band of tissue linking the interosseous borders of the tibia and fibula. It is pierced superiorly by the anterior tibial artery and inferiorly by branches of the peroneal artery.

Superior tibiofibular joint

This is an articulation between the head of the fibula and the lateral condyle of the tibia. It is a synovial joint stabilized by the anterior superior and posterior superior tibiofibular ligaments. It allows a slight gliding movement.

Inferior tibiofibular joint

This is an articulation between the lower end of the tibia and fibula. It is a fibrous joint stabilized by the anterior inferior and posterior inferior tibiofibular ligaments. It allows little movement, and it stabilizes the ankle joint by keeping the lateral malleolus clasped against the lateral surface of the talus.

Compartments of the leg

The leg is divided into anterior, posterior and lateral (peroneal) compartments (Fig. 6.26). The muscles of the posterior compartment are divided into superficial and deep groups by the deep transverse crural fascia.

Anterior (extensor) compartment of the leg

Muscles of the anterior compartment are shown in Figures 6.27 and 6.28.

Vessels of the anterior compartment

The anterior tibial artery is the vessel of the anterior compartment (Figs 6.29 and 6.30). It is a terminal branch of the popliteal artery.

Nerves of the anterior compartment

The common peroneal nerve (L4–L5, S1–S2) leaves the popliteal fossa to enter the lateral compartment of the leg by winding around the neck of the fibula

Clinical examination

The intramuscular septa of the leg are unyieldingly strong. Inflammation or haemorrhage in the anterior compartment can compress the anterior tibial artery and deep peroneal nerve. This is compartment syndrome and is characterized by 6 Ps: (i) Pain (especially on activity due to ischaemia and lactic acid build up), (ii) Pulselessness (arterial compression causes unpalpable dorsalis pedis artery), (iii) Paralysis (of extensor muscles if untreated), (iv) Paraesthesia (in first interdigital cleft due to nerve compression), (v) Perishingly cold (poor perfusion of foot), (vi) Pallor (pale skin due to reduced perfusion).

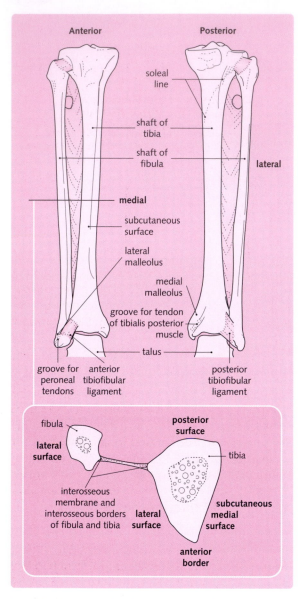

Fig. 6.25 Anterior and posterior features of the right tibia and fibula, and the relationship of the two bones and the interosseous membrane in cross-section.

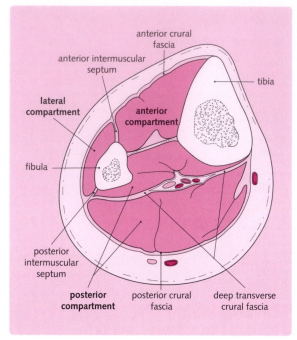

Fig. 6.26 Compartments of the left leg.

Dorsum of the foot

The structures from the anterior compartment pass onto the dorsum of the foot. The extensor digitorum longus tendons pass to the lateral four digits of the foot and join an extensor expansion. These expansions have the same arrangement as those found in the medial four digits of the hand. Over the proximal phalanx each expansion splits into three slips. An axial (central) slip inserts into the middle phalanx. Two collateral slips insert into the distal phalanx. Each expansion receives interossei and lumbrical muscle attachments.

The extensor digitorum brevis and extensor hallucis brevis muscles are the only muscles intrinsic to the dorsum of the foot. Arising from the calcaneum, the three tendons of extensor digitorum brevis join the lateral sides of the extensor digitorum longus tendons for the middle three toes over the metatarsophalangeal joint. From a similar origin, the extensor hallucis brevis tendon inserts into the proximal phalanx of the hallux (great toe). The muscle belly of this tendon is usually separate from the rest of the muscle. The nerve supply is by the deep peroneal nerve and the muscle extends the digits (toes).

(Fig. 6.31). Here, it divides into the superficial and deep peroneal nerves. It is superficial and vulnerable to damage in sporting injuries.

The deep peroneal nerve supplies the extensor muscles in the leg and it terminates as the cutaneous supply to the cleft of skin between the first and second toes. The superficial peroneal nerve supplies the lateral compartment of the leg and skin on the dorsum of the foot.

Fig. 6.27 Muscles of the anterior compartment of the leg

Name of muscle (nerve supply)	Origin	Insertion	Action
Extensor digitorum longus (deep peroneal nerve)	Fibula and interosseous membrane	Extensor expansion of lateral four toes	Extends toes and dorsiflexes foot at ankle joint
Extensor hallucis longus (deep peroneal nerve)	Fibula and interosseous membrane	Base of distal phalanx of great toe	Extends big toe, and dorsiflexes foot at ankle joint
Peroneus tertius (deep peroneal nerve)	Fibula and interosseous membrane	Base of 5th metatarsal bone	Dorsiflexes and everts foot
Tibialis anterior (deep peroneal nerve)	Tibia and interosseous membrane	Medial cuneiform and base of 1st metatarsal bone	Dorsiflexes and inverts foot

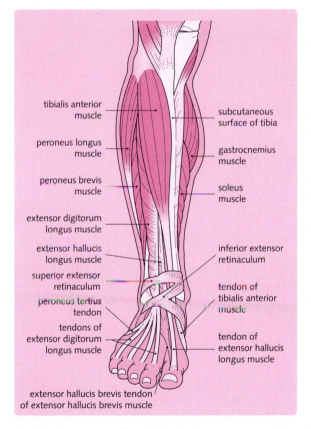

tibialis anterior muscle

peroneus longus muscle

peroneus brevis muscle

extensor digitorum longus muscle

extensor hallucis longus muscle

superior extensor retinaculum

peroneus tertius tendon

tendons of extensor digitorum longus muscle

extensor hallucis brevis tendon of extensor hallucis brevis muscle

subcutaneous surface of tibia

gastrocnemius muscle

soleus muscle

inferior extensor retinaculum

tendon of tibialis anterior muscle

tendon of extensor hallucis longus muscle

Fig. 6.28 Extensor muscles of the anterior compartment of the right leg.

Extensor retinacula

The superior and inferior extensor retinacula keep the extensor tendons firmly bound down to the dorsum of the foot (Fig. 6.32). The retinacula are derived from the anterior crural fascia.

The superior band passes from the anterior border of the tibia to the anterior border of the fibula. The inferior band is Y-shaped, and it runs from the calcaneus to the medial malleolus and plantar fascia.

Nerves and vessels of the dorsum of the foot

The deep peroneal nerve and anterior tibial artery enter the foot beneath the extensor retinacula. The anterior tibial artery continues as the dorsalis pedis artery (see Fig. 6.30). It can be palpated between the tendons of extensor hallucis longus and extensor digitorum longus.

Cutaneous innervation of the dorsum of the foot is from the superficial peroneal nerve, the deep peroneal nerve, the sural nerve, and the saphenous nerve.

Lateral compartment of the leg

The composition of the lateral compartment is shown in Figure 6.33. Its muscles are outlined in Figure 6.34 and are innervated by the superficial peroneal nerve.

Posterior compartment of the leg

Figure 6.35 outlines the muscles of the posterior compartment. Soleus is an antigravity muscle that contracts alternately with the extensor muscles of the leg on standing and maintains balance. It is a slow plantar flexor of the ankle joint unlike gastrocnemius which causes rapid flexion. Soleus contraction helps to initiate walking by overcoming the inertia of the body's weight. Gastrocnemius contraction increases the speed of movement.

Soleus and gastrocnemius contraction aid venous return from the lower limb to the heart.

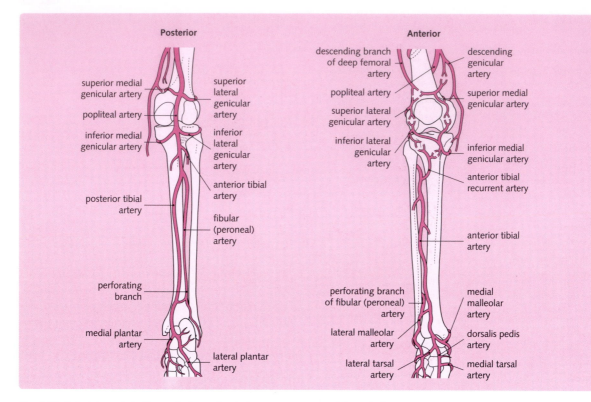

Fig. 6.29 Arterial supply to the posterior and anterior compartments of the right leg.

Fig. 6.30 Arterial supply to the leg		
Artery (origin)	**Course**	**Distribution**
Popliteal (continuation of femoral artery at adductor hiatus)	Passes through popliteal fossa to leg; ends at lower border of popliteus muscle by dividing into anterior and posterior tibial arteries	Superior, middle, and inferior genicular arteries to both lateral and medial aspects of knee
Anterior tibial (popliteal artery)	Passes into anterior compartment through gap in superior part of interosseous membrane and descends on this membrane	Anterior compartment of leg
Dorsalis pedis (continuation of anterior tibial artery distal to extensor retinaculum)	Runs on the dorsum of the foot and gives tarsal, arcuate and first dorsal metatarsal arteries before descending into the first interosseous space to join plantar arch	Muscles on dorsum of foot; pierces first dorsal interosseous muscle to contribute to formation of plantar arch
Posterior tibial (popliteal artery)	Passes through posterior compartment of leg and terminates distal to flexor retinaculum by dividing into medial and lateral plantar arteries	Posterior and lateral compartments of leg; nutrient artery passes to tibia, contributes to knee anastomoses
Peroneal (posterior tibial artery)	Descends in posterior compartment adjacent to posterior intermuscular septum	Posterior compartment of leg; perforating branches supply lateral compartment of leg

Fig. 6.31 Nerves of the leg

Nerve (origin)	Course and distribution
Common peroneal (sciatic nerve)	Arises at apex of popliteal fossa and follows medial border of biceps femoris and its tendon; passes over posterior aspect of head of fibula and then winds around neck of fibula, deep to peroneus longus, where it divides into deep and superficial peroneal nerves; supplies skin on posterolateral part of leg via its branch—lateral sural cutaneous nerve
Deep peroneal (common peroneal nerve)	Arises between peroneus longus and neck of fibula; descends on interosseous membrane and enters dorsum of foot; supplies anterior muscles of leg, and skin of first interdigital cleft
Saphenous (femoral nerve)	Descends with femoral vessels and the great saphenous vein to supply skin on medial side of leg and foot
Superficial peroneal (common peroneal nerve)	Arises between peroneus longus and neck of fibula and descends in lateral compartment of leg; supplies peroneus longus and brevis and skin on anterior surface of leg and dorsum of foot
Sural (usually arises from both tibial and common peroneal nerves)	Descends between heads of gastrocnemius and becomes superficial at middle of leg; supplies skin on posterolateral aspects of leg and lateral side of foot
Tibial (sciatic nerve)	Descends through popliteal fossa and lies on popliteus; then runs inferiorly with posterior tibial vessels and terminates beneath flexor retinaculum by dividing into medial and lateral plantar nerves; supplies posterior muscles of leg, knee joint, skin, and muscles of the sole of the foot

Flexor retinaculum

The flexor retinaculum runs from the medial malleolus to the calcaneus and plantar fascia (Fig. 6.36). The deep flexor muscles pass beneath the retinaculum, surrounded by synovial sheaths, together with the tibial nerve and the posterior tibial artery.

Skeleton of the foot

The skeleton of the foot consists of the tarsals, the metatarsals and the phalanges (Fig. 6.37).

The body weight is transferred from the tibia and fibula to the talus and calcaneus, and then across the remaining tarsal and metatarsal bones. The weight is transferred to the ground via the calcaneus and the heads of the metatarsals. The metatarsal bones are composed of a base proximally, a body, and a distal head. The great toe (the hallux) has two phalanges; the other digits have three (proximal, middle and distal).

Ankle joint

The ankle joint is the articulation between the superior surface of the talus and the inferior end of the tibia and fibula, including the medial and lateral malleoli. It is a synovial hinge joint that allows only flexion and extension. Dorsiflexion (extension) involves tibialis anterior, extensor digitorum longus, and extensor hallucis longus. Plantarflexion (flexion) involves gastrocnemius, soleus, flexor digitorum longus, flexor hallucis longus and tibialis posterior.

The joint is surrounded by a capsule that is lax anteroposteriorly and reinforced by strong medial and lateral ligaments. The medial (deltoid) ligament runs from the medial malleolus to the tuberosity of

For the structures passing behind the medial malleolus remember the mnemonic: Tom, Dick And Very Naughty Harry (tibialis posterior, flexor digitorum longus, artery, vein, nerve, flexor hallucis longus).

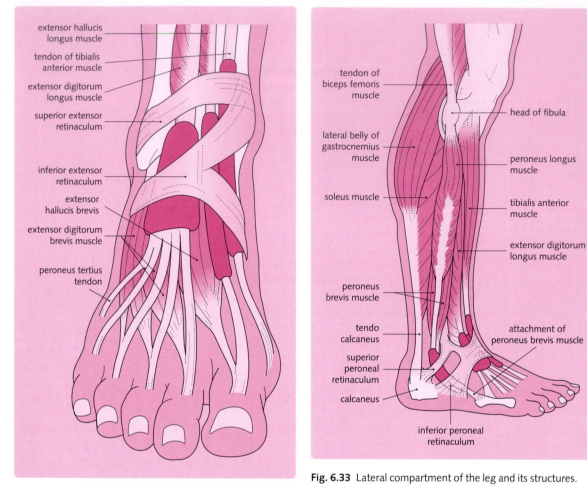

Fig. 6.32 Structures of the extensor retinacula.

Fig. 6.33 Lateral compartment of the leg and its structures.

Fig. 6.34 Muscles of the lateral compartment of the leg			
Name of muscle (nerve supply)	**Origin**	**Insertion**	**Action**
Peroneus longus (superficial peroneal nerve)	Fibula	1st metatarsal and medial cuneiform	Plantarflexes and everts the foot
Peroneus brevis (superficial peroneal nerve)	Fibula	5th metatarsal bone	Plantarflexes and everts the foot

the navicular bone, the sustentaculum tali, and the medial tubercle of the talus. The lateral ligament arises from the lateral malleolus, and it is inserted into the neck of the talus, the calcaneus, and the lateral tubercle of the talus (it is the most commonly injured ligament and results in a sprained ankle).

The articular surface of the talus is wedge shaped, having a wider anterior surface and a narrower posterior surface. As a result the ankle joint is most stable in dorsiflexion because the wider anterior border is 'driven' between the two malleoli, which clasp it.

Fig. 6.35 Muscles of the posterior compartment of the leg

Superficial group			
Name of muscle (nerve supply)	**Origin**	**Insertion**	**Action**
Plantaris (tibial nerve)	Lateral supracondylar ridge of femur	Calcaneus	These muscles plantarflex the foot at the ankle joint
Soleus (tibial nerve)	Tibia and fibula	Via tendo calcaneus (Achilles tendon) into calcaneus	
Gastrocnemius (tibial nerve)	Medial and lateral condyles of femur	Via tendo calcaneus (Achilles tendon) into calcaneus	
Deep group			
Name of muscle (nerve supply)	**Origin**	**Insertion**	**Action**
Flexor digitorum longus (tibial nerve)	Tibia	Distal phalanges of lateral four toes	Flexes lateral four toes; plantarflexes foot
Flexor hallucis longus (tibial nerve)	Fibula	Distal phalanx of big toe	Flexes big toe; plantarflexes foot
Tibialis posterior (tibial nerve)	Tibia and fibula and interosseous membrane	Navicular bone and surrounding bones	Plantarflexes and inverts foot

Fig. 6.36 Flexor retinaculum.

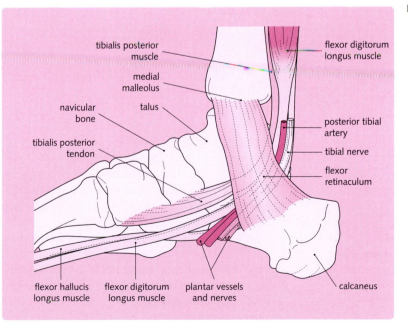

167

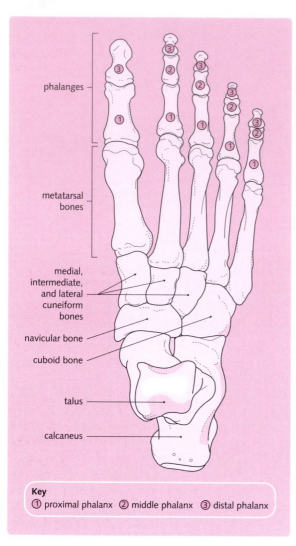

phalanges

metatarsal bones

medial, intermediate, and lateral cuneiform bones

navicular bone

cuboid bone

talus

calcaneus

Key
① proximal phalanx   ② middle phalanx   ③ distal phalanx

Fig. 6.37 Skeleton of the foot.

Blood supply is from the anterior and posterior tibial arteries.

Nerve supply is from the tibial and deep peroneal nerves.

Orthopaedics

The ankle is a frequently injured joint due to forced inversion. The lateral ligament consists of three bands and is weaker than the medial (deltoid) ligament. As a result the lateral ligament is more prone to tearing in ankle sprains. There are three grades of sprain: (i) stretching of ligament, (ii) partial tear (not all the way through ligament), and (iii) complete tear. Damage to the ligament causes an unstable ankle that is prone to invert involuntarily.

Intertarsal joints of the foot

The intertarsal joints of the foot are formed by the articulating tarsal bones. All are synovial joints except the cuboidonavicular joint, which is a fibrous joint.

Subtalar (talocalcaneal) joint

The subtalar joint is formed by the talus articulating with the calcaneum. It is strengthened by the talocalcaneal ligaments. Inversion and eversion movements occur at this joint (see Chapter 1 for a description of these movements).

Midtarsal joints

The midtarsal joints include the talocalcaneonavicular and the calcaneocuboidal joints. The talocalcaneonavicular joint is formed by the talus, calcaneus and navicular bones. It is strengthened by the spring (calcaneonavicular) ligament. The calcaneocuboidal joint is formed by the calcaneus and cuboid bones. It is strengthened by the bifurcate ligament, and long and short plantar ligaments. Movements at these joints are inversion and eversion.

Other tarsal joints

The cuneonavicular, cuboideonavicular, intercuneiform and cuneocuboidal joints are strengthened by dorsal, plantar and interosseous ligaments. There is very little movement in these joints, and it is only a slight gliding movement.

Arches of the foot

Each foot has a lateral and medial longitudinal arch. If the feet are placed together they form a transverse arch. These arches support the weight of the body, and they are maintained by bone shape, muscles and ligaments.

The medial is higher than the lateral arch, and it consists of the calcaneus, talus, navicular and cuneiform bones and the medial three metatarsals. The talus acts as a keystone in the centre of the arch. The plantar calcaneonavicular (spring), long and short plantar ligaments, and strong dorsal ligaments tie the bones together. The plantar aponeurosis, abductor and flexor muscles in the first and third layers, and the flexor digitorum longus tendon, support the arch. Finally, the tibialis muscles and deltoid ligament suspend the arch from a bone through their attachments, superiorly.

The lateral arch consists of the calcaneus, the cuboid and the lateral two metatarsals. This is maintained by the long and short (calcaneocuboidal) plantar ligaments, the plantar aponeurosis, muscles of the first layer of the foot and the peroneus longus tendon.

Each foot contains half of the transverse arch. Each half consists of the metatarsal bases, cuboid, and the three cuneiforms. It is maintained by the wedge-shaped cuneiform bones and metatarsal bases, the strong long and short plantar ligaments, as well as the deep transverse ligaments. The peroneus longus and brevis tendons suspend and tie the arch ends together.

Sole of the foot

The sole bears the weight of the body. The skin is thick and hairless. Fibrous septa divide the subcutaneous fat into small loculi, and they anchor the skin to the deep fascia or plantar aponeurosis (Fig. 6.38). This makes subcutaneous injections difficult.

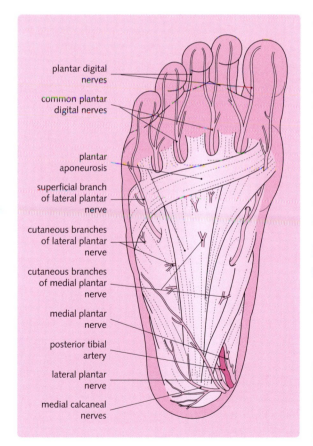

plantar digital nerves

common plantar digital nerves

plantar aponeurosis

superficial branch of lateral plantar nerve

cutaneous branches of lateral plantar nerve

cutaneous branches of medial plantar nerve

medial plantar nerve

posterior tibial artery

lateral plantar nerve

medial calcaneal nerves

Fig. 6.38 Plantar fascia and cutaneous innervation of the sole of the foot.

The plantar aponeurosis extends from the calcaneal tuberosity and divides into five bifurcating slips that insert into the flexor fibrous sheaths at the base of the toes. The bifurcation allows passage of the flexor tendons. It is very strong; it supports the longitudinal arch and protects the underlying muscles, vessels and nerves. It is perforated by the cutaneous nerves supplying the sole of the foot.

The muscles of the sole of the foot are in four layers (see Fig. 6.39). The axis of abduction and adduction passes through the second digit. Therefore, digits either move towards (adduction) or away (abduction) from the second digit.

Nerves of the foot

The nerves of the foot are described in Figures 6.40 and 6.41.

Blood supply to the foot

The posterior tibial artery terminates by dividing into the medial and lateral plantar arteries under the flexor retinaculum (Fig. 6.42).

The medial plantar artery passes forward with the medial plantar nerve. It gives off muscular branches and terminates as a plantar digital branch to the medial side of the big toe and has branches that join the plantar metatarsal branches of the plantar arch.

The lateral plantar artery crosses the sole of the foot, and it gives off muscular and cutaneous branches. At the level of the base of the fifth metatarsal, the artery passes medially and anastomoses with the dorsalis pedis artery to form the plantar arch. From this arch plantar metatarsal arteries arise and these form the plantar digital arteries for the toes.

Fibrous flexor and flexor synovial sheaths

Fibrous flexor sheaths in the foot are similar to those of the hand. They run from the head of the metatarsal

Note that the lateral plantar nerve in the foot has a similar distribution to the ulnar nerve in the hand (both have a superficial and a deep branch) and that the medial plantar nerve in the foot has a similar distribution to the median nerve in the hand.

Fig. 6.39 Intrinsic plantar muscles of the foot. (IP, interphalangeal joint; PIP, proximal interphalangeal joint; DIP, distal interphalangeal joint; MTP, metatarsophalangeal joint.)

Muscle (nerve supply)	Origin	Insertion	Action
First layer			
Abductor hallucis (medial plantar nerve)	Calcaneus, flexor retinaculum, plantar aponeurosis	Proximal phalanx of hallux	Abduct hallux (great toe)
Flexor digitorum brevis (medial plantar nerve)	Calcaneus, plantar aponeurosis	Each tendon bifurcates and inserts into the middle phalanx of the lateral four digits	Flexes lateral four digits
Abductor digiti minimi (lateral plantar nerve)	Calcaneus, plantar aponeurosis	Proximal phalanx of digitus minimus	Abducts digitus minimus (little toe)
Second layer			
Flexor accessorius or Quadratus plantae (lateral plantar nerve)	Calcaneus	Tendon of flexor digitorum longus	Pulls on the tendon of flexor digitorum longus and takes up the slack of this tendon when the ankle is plantarflexed. This allows the digits to be flexed in this position
Lumbricals (first medial lumbrical—medial plantar nerve; lateral three lumbricals—lateral plantar nerve)	Tendons of flexor digitorum longus	Extensor expansions of lateral four digits	Maintains extension of the digits at DIP and PIP joints while flexor digitorum longus tendons are flexing the lateral four digits at the MTP
Third layer			
Flexor hallucis brevis (medial plantar nerve)	Cuboid and three cuneiforms	Proximal phalanx of hallux	Flexes hallux (great toe)
Adductor hallucis: (lateral plantar nerve) Oblique head	Second to fourth metatarsal bases and plantar ligament	Both heads insert into the proximal phalanx of the hallux	Adducts hallux towards second toe
Transverse head	Deep transverse ligament		
Flexor digiti minimi brevis (lateral plantar nerve)	Fifth metatarsal	Proximal phalanx of digitus minimus	Flexes digitus minimus (little toe)
Fourth layer			
Palmar interossei (lateral plantar nerve)	Third, fourth, fifth metatarsals	Proximal phalanx of digits and their extensor expansions	Adduct digits towards second digit.
Dorsal interossei (lateral plantar nerve)	First and second; second and third; third and fourth; fourth and fifth metatarsals	Proximal phalanx of digits and their extensor expansions	Abduct digits away from second digit. With palmar interossei and lumbricals they extend the DIP, PIP joints and flex the MTP joint.

bone to the base of the distal phalanx and surround the synovial sheaths. The sheath has anular (ring) fibres over the bones and cruciate (criss-cross) fibres over the joints (to allow movement).

The synovial sheaths for the flexor digitorum longus tendons surround them from just above the fibrous flexor retinaculum to the navicular bone. The tendon of flexor hallucis longus is covered by a synovial sheath from above the retinaculum to the base of the first metatarsal. As the above mentioned tendons enter their fibrous flexor sheath, they are again covered by a synovial sheath. The synovial sheath for tibialis posterior extends from the flexor retinaculum to the tendons insertion into the navicular bone.

Functions of the feet

The feet serve to:

- Support the body weight.
- Maintain balance and allow movement on uneven surfaces.
- Act as propulsive levers, e.g. in walking and running.

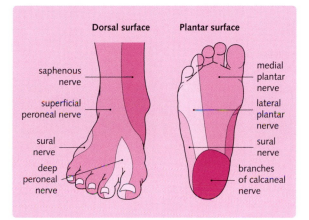

Fig. 6.40 Distribution of nerves of the foot.

RADIOLOGICAL ANATOMY

Imaging of the bones and joints

When there are symptoms and/or signs of joint problems or a fracture, an X-ray is the first imaging investigation to be performed. Two images are taken that are 90° to each other and, in some cases, include the joint above and below the injury, especially if the forearm or lower leg is involved. Information not only about the bones or joints can be gained but also on the tissues surrounding them, e.g. calcification may suggest a tumour or endocrine problem.

Normal radiographic anatomy

See Chapter 2 for description of normal limb radiographic anatomy.

Figures 6.43, 6.44 and 6.45 show the normal articulation of the hip, knee and foot. The osteology of the lower limb is demonstrated.

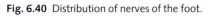

Fig. 6.41 Outline of the nerves of the foot	
Nerve (origin)	**Distribution**
Saphenous (femoral nerve)	Supplies skin on medial side of foot as far anteriorly as head of 1st metatarsal
Superficial peroneal (common peroneal nerve)	Supplies skin on dorsum of foot and all digits, except adjoining sides of first and second digits
Deep peroneal (common peroneal nerve)	Supplies extensor digitorum brevis, extensor hallucis brevis and skin on contiguous sides of first and second digits
Medial plantar (larger terminal branch of the tibial nerve)	Supplies skin of medial side of sole of foot and plantar surfaces of first three and one half digits; also supplies abductor hallucis, flexor digitorum brevis, flexor hallucis brevis, and first lumbrical
Lateral plantar (smaller terminal branch of tibial nerve)	Supplies quadratus plantae, abductor digiti minimi and flexor digiti minimi brevis; deep branch supplies plantar and dorsal interossei, lateral three lumbricals, and adductor hallucis; supplies skin on sole lateral to a line splitting fourth digit
Sural (tibial and common peroneal nerves)	Lateral aspect of foot
Calcaneal nerves (tibial and sural nerves)	Skin of heel

Fig. 6.42 Blood and nerve supply to the sole of the foot.

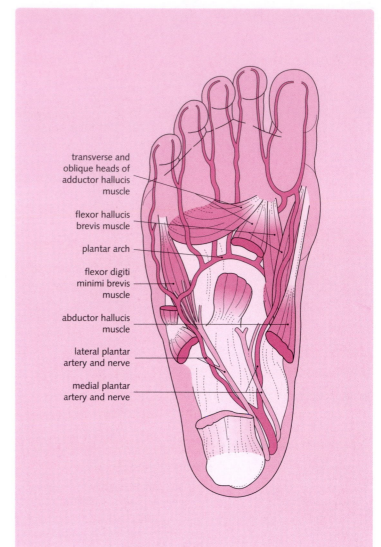

transverse and oblique heads of adductor hallucis muscle

flexor hallucis brevis muscle

plantar arch

flexor digiti minimi brevis muscle

abductor hallucis muscle

lateral plantar artery and nerve

medial plantar artery and nerve

Orthopaedics

In osteoarthritis classical joint changes can be seen. These include narrowing of the joint space, subchondral sclerosis (bone appears whiter under joint hyaline cartilage), bone cysts (seen as darkened areas within bone adjacent to joint) and osteophytes (smooth spur-like bony growths).

On a normal hip X-ray a smooth curved line can be traced with your finger. Starting at the shaft of the femur, medially, trace proximally across the femoral neck (medially) to the superior pubic ramus (anterior border). This is known as Shenton's line and any disruption to its smooth convex course suggests a femoral neck fracture.

How to examine an X-ray methodically

See Chapter 2 for the description of a method for examining a radiograph of the lower limb, it applies to the lower limb as well as the upper limb.

Angiography of the limbs

In Figures 6.46, 6.47 and 6.48, arteriography highlights the arterial supply to the hip, thigh, knee, leg and foot.

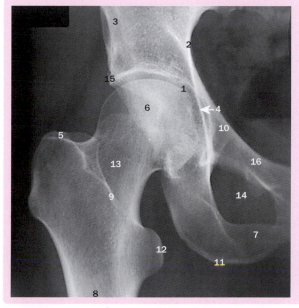

1	Acetabulum
2	Arcuate line
3	Ilium
4	Fovea
5	Greater trochanter of femur
6	Head of femur
7	Inferior ramus of pubis
8	Shaft of the femur
9	Intertrochanteric line
10	Ischial spine
11	Ischial tuberosity
12	Lesser trochanter
13	Neck of femur
14	Obturator foramen
15	Rim of the acetabulum
16	Superior ramus of pubis

Fig. 6.43 An anterioposterior radiograph of the right hip.

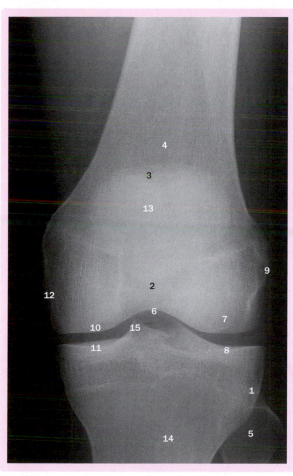

1	Apex (styloid process of fibula)
2	Apex of the patella
3	Base of the patella
4	Femur
5	Head of fibula
6	Intercondylar fossa
7	Lateral condyle of femur
8	Lateral condyle of tibia
9	Lateral epicondyle of femur
10	Medial condyle of femur
11	Medial condyle tibia
12	Medial epicondyle of femur
13	Patella
14	Tibia
15	Tubercles of intercondylar eminence

Fig. 6.44 An anterioposterior radiograph of the knee.

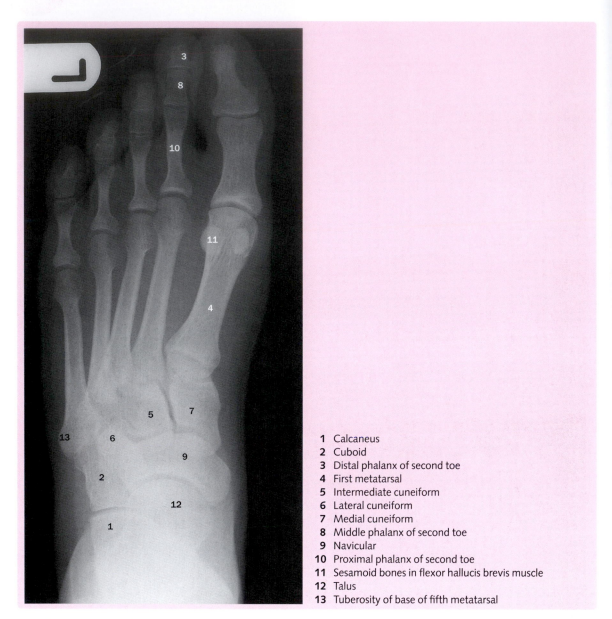

Fig. 6.45 A radiograph of the foot.

1 Calcaneus
2 Cuboid
3 Distal phalanx of second toe
4 First metatarsal
5 Intermediate cuneiform
6 Lateral cuneiform
7 Medial cuneiform
8 Middle phalanx of second toe
9 Navicular
10 Proximal phalanx of second toe
11 Sesamoid bones in flexor hallucis brevis muscle
12 Talus
13 Tuberosity of base of fifth metatarsal

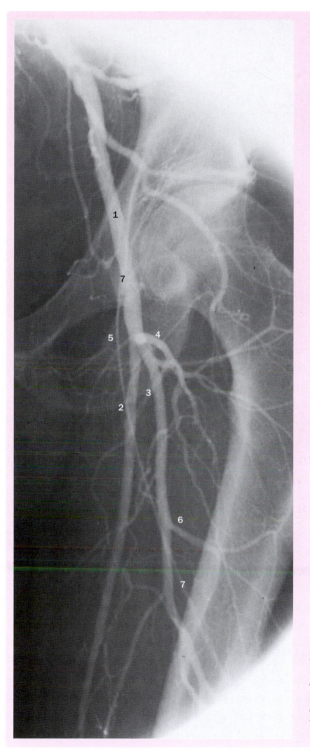

Fig. 6.46 A femoral arteriogram.

1 Profunda femoris artery
2 Common femoral artery
3 Superficial femoral artery
4 Lateral circumflex artery
5 Medial circumflex artery
6 Perforating artery
7 Catheter introduced into distal abdominal aorta via femoral artery

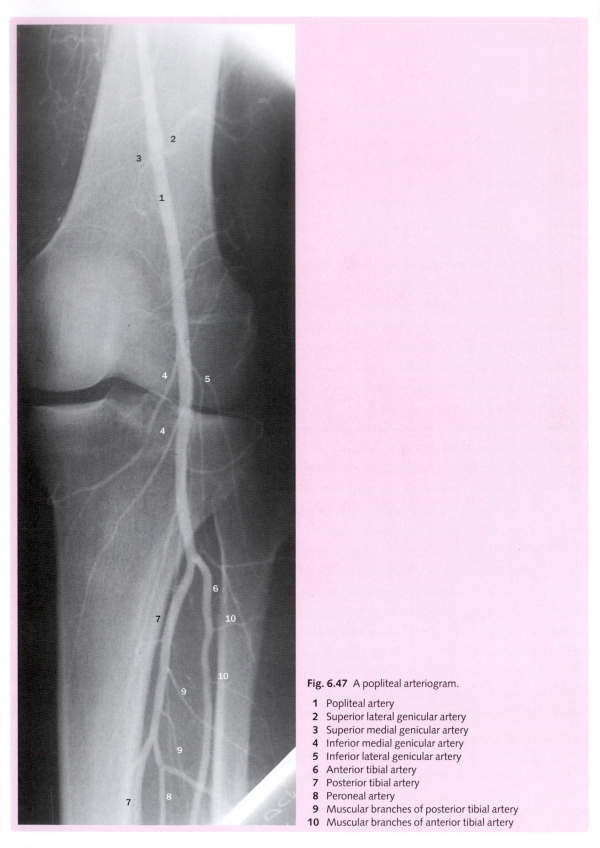

Fig. 6.47 A popliteal arteriogram.

1 Popliteal artery
2 Superior lateral genicular artery
3 Superior medial genicular artery
4 Inferior medial genicular artery
5 Inferior lateral genicular artery
6 Anterior tibial artery
7 Posterior tibial artery
8 Peroneal artery
9 Muscular branches of posterior tibial artery
10 Muscular branches of anterior tibial artery

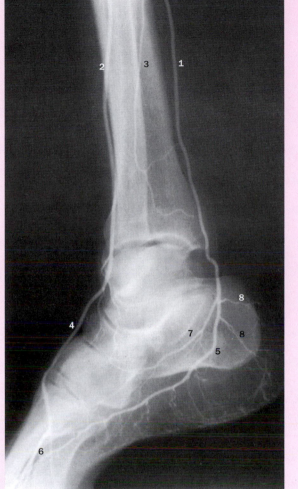

1 Posterior tibial artery
2 Anterior tibial artery
3 Peroneal artery
4 Dorsalis pedis artery
5 Lateral plantar artery
6 Plantar arch
7 Medial plantar artery
8 Medial calcaneal artery

Fig. 6.48 A foot arteriogram.

REGIONS AND COMPONENTS OF THE HEAD AND NECK

Skull

The skull is composed of a number of different bones joined at sutures. The bones of the skull may be divided into:

- The cranium (made of outer and inner tables of bone, separated by diploë – see Fig. 7.10)
- The facial skeleton.

The cranium is subdivided into:

- An upper part—the vault.
- A lower part—the base of the skull.

Norma verticalis

Superior view – illustrated in Figure 7.1.

Norma occipitalis

Posterior view – Figure 7.2. The mastoid process of the temporal bone and the external occipital protuberance, a midline elevation from the occipital bone from which the superior nuchal line extends laterally, are important muscle attachments.

Norma frontalis

Anterior view – Figure 7.3. The frontal bones form the forehead and the superior margin of the orbits (the other boundaries are described on **page 195**). They articulate with the nasal bones and the frontal process of the maxilla (upper jaw). The mandible (lower jaw) lies below the maxilla. Both mandible and maxilla bear teeth.

Norma lateralis

Lateral view – Figure 7.4. The parietal bone articulates with the greater wing of the sphenoid bone and

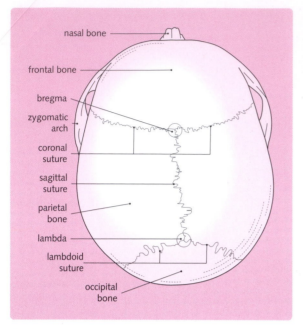

Fig. 7.1 Skull viewed from above.

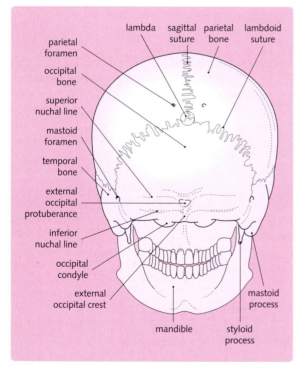

Fig. 7.2 Skull viewed from behind.

the temporal bone. At a point called the pterion, the middle meningeal artery lies just deep to this point.

A fracture at the pterion can rupture the middle meningeal artery causing an extradural haematoma (see **page 190**).

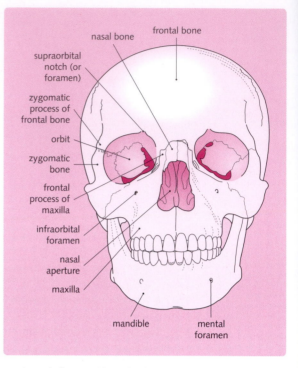

Fig. 7.3 Skull viewed from the front.

The zygomatic arch is formed by the zygomatic process of the temporal bone and the temporal process of the zygomatic bone.

Norma basalis

Inferior view – Figure 7.5. The palate is formed by the palatine process of the maxilla and the horizontal processes of the palatine bones. The alveolar process of the maxilla surrounds the palate.

Openings in the skull

Figures 7.6 and 7.16 show important openings in the base of the skull and their contents.

Fetal skull

The fetal skull differs from the adult skull in the following ways:

- The facial skeleton is proportionately smaller.
- Several protuberances (e.g. the mastoid process) are unformed.
- There is a midline suture between frontal bones: the metopic suture, which usually disappears at 6 years.

Fig. 7.4 Lateral view of the skull.

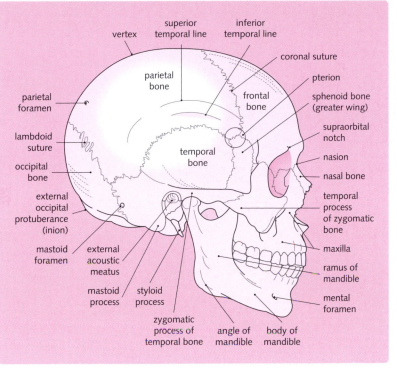

- There are two fibrous defects between bones – fontanelles. The anterior fontanelle is at the bregma (closes in the first 6 months of life); the posterior at the lambda (closes 18–24 months).

Cervical vertebrae

There are seven cervical vertebrae forming the skeleton of the neck, covered in greater detail in Chapter 8. All except C1 (atlas), C2 (axis), and C7 are typical vertebrae (Figs 7.7 and 7.8). C7 possesses a longer spinous process, which is usually the most superior spinous process palpable.

Atlanto-occipital joint

The atlanto-occipital joint is between the articular surfaces of the lateral masses of C1 vertebra and the occipital condyles. It is a synovial joint surrounded by a loose capsule. Flexion and extension (nodding movements) are allowed at this joint, but no rotation.

Atlanto-axial joints

There are two lateral synovial joints between the articular surfaces of the lateral masses of the axis and atlas (Fig. 7.9) and a median joint between the dens (odontoid process) of the axis and the anterior arch of the atlas. These joints allow rotational (shaking) movements of the head where the skull and the atlas rotate as a unit on the axis. Alar ligaments prevent excess rotation.

The transverse ligament of the atlas holds the dens against the anterior arch of the atlas.

Hangman's fracture

Rupture of this ligament, e.g. during head trauma, allows the dens to impinge on the cervical spinal cord, causing paralysis of the body below the neck. If the dens compresses the medulla, the patient may die.

THE FACE AND SCALP

Scalp

The scalp consists of five layers (Fig. 7.10), and it has a very rich blood supply (Fig. 7.11). The scalp veins closely mirror the arterial supply and connect with the diploic veins in the skull bones and the intracranial venous sinuses by valveless emissary veins.

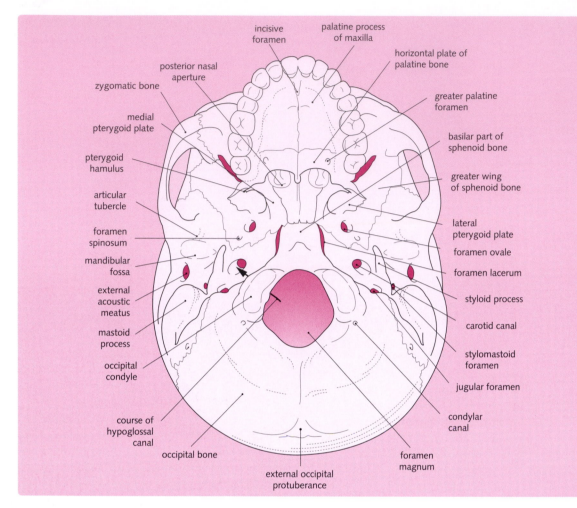

Fig. 7.5 Skull seen from below.

The order of the layers of the scalp are:
S   Skin
C   Connective tissue
A   Aponeurosis
L   Loose connective tissue
P   Pericranium (periostium)

Infections of the scalp are, therefore, potentially very serious as they may spread intracranially.

Sensory nerve supply to the scalp is shown in Figure 7.11. The muscles of the scalp and external ear are supplied by the facial nerve.

Face

The skin of the face is connected to the facial bones by loose connective tissue, in which the muscles of

Scalp laceration

The scalp has a very rich blood supply and bleeds profusely – blood vessels run in the connective tissue layer, which holds them open. A wound that passes transversely through the aponeurotic layer will gape, but one that runs longitudinally or is superficial will not. Another important fact to remember is that the arterial supply of the scalp travels up from below – this will dictate whether or not a flap of scalp retains its blood supply.

facial expression lie. There is no deep fascia. Like the scalp, the skin of the face is very sensitive and very vascular.

Sensory innervation of the face is from the trigeminal nerve (V). It has three divisions: the ophthalmic

Fig. 7.6 The important openings in the base of the skull and the structures that pass through them

Opening in skull	Structures transmitted
Anterior cranial fossa	
Cribriform plate	Olfactory nerve
Middle cranial fossa	
Foramen ovale	V_3 (mandibular division of trigeminal nerve), lesser petrosal nerve
Foramen rotundum	V_2 (maxillary division of trigeminal nerve)
Foramen spinosum	Middle meningeal artery and vein
Foramen lacerum (upper part only)	Internal carotid artery, greater petrosal nerve
Optic canal	Optic nerve, ophthalmic artery
Superior orbital fissure	Lacrimal, frontal and nasociliary branches of V_1 (ophthalmic branch of trigeminal nerve); oculomotor, abducent, and trochlear nerves; superior ophthalmic vein
Posterior cranial fossa	
Foramen magnum	Medulla oblongata, spinal part of accessory nerve, upper cervical nerves; right and left vertebral arteries
Hypoglossal canal	Hypoglossal nerve
Internal acoustic meatus	Facial, vestibulocochlear nerves; labyrinthine artery
Jugular foramen	Glossopharyngeal, vagus, accessory nerves; sigmoid sinus becomes internal jugular vein

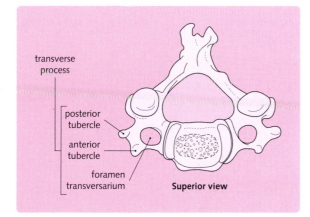

transverse process

posterior tubercle

anterior tubercle

foramen transversarium

Superior view

Fig. 7.7 Typical cervical vertebra.

Subaponeurotic haematoma

Bleeding below the aponeurosis, e.g. from a blow to the back of the head or a scalp laceration, can track forward underneath the aponeurosis to the orbital region, resulting in black eyes.

Fig. 7.8 Distinctive characteristics of a typical cervical vertebra

Part	Characteristics
Body	Small; longer from side to side than anteroposteriorly; superior surface is concave, inferior surface is convex
Vertebral foramen	Large and triangular
Transverse processes	Foramina transversaria (small or absent in C7)
Articular processes	Superior facets directed superoposteriorly, inferior facets directed inferoanteriorly
Spinous processes	Short and bifid in C3 to C5, long in C6, and longer in C7

(V_1), the maxillary (V_2), and the mandibular (V_3) nerves which supply the upper, middle and lower thirds of the face, respectively (Fig. 7.12).

183

Muscles of the face

Most of the muscles of facial expression are attached to the overlying skin (Fig. 7.13). They are all supplied by the facial nerve (VII).

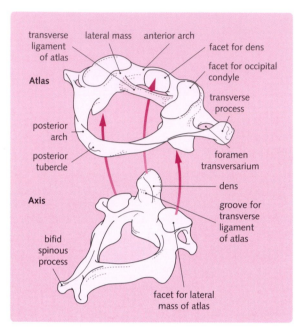

Fig. 7.9 Atlas and axis (showing their articulations).

Occipitofrontalis

This is formed by two frontal bellies on the forehead and two occipital bellies at the back, joined by a flat, aponeurotic tendon that is part of the scalp. It raises the eyebrows.

Orbicularis oculi

This consists of orbital (closes the eye) and palpebral (blinking of the eyelids) parts – connected to bone via the medial palpebral ligament at the medial angle of the eye.

Buccinator

This muscle lies in the cheek – it forces food out of the cheeks and into the vestibule of the mouth.

Obicularis oris

This lies around the mouth and closes/purses the lips.

Motor nerve supply to the face

This is from the facial nerve (VII). It exits the skull through the stylomastoid foramen to lie between the ramus of the mandible and the mastoid process. It enters the parotid gland and divides into its five groups of terminal branches that supply the muscles of facial expression (see Fig. 7.12).

Before entering the parotid gland the facial nerve gives off the posterior auricular nerve and a muscular branch, which supplies the occipital belly of

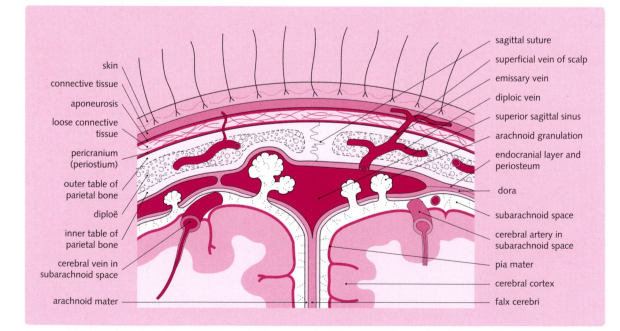

Fig. 7.10 Layers of the scalp.

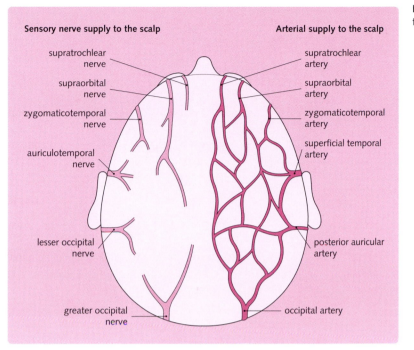

Fig. 7.11 Nerve and arterial supply to the scalp.

Sensory nerve supply to the scalp

supratrochlear nerve

supraorbital nerve

zygomaticotemporal nerve

auriculotemporal nerve

lesser occipital nerve

greater occipital nerve

Arterial supply to the scalp

supratrochlear artery

supraorbital artery

zygomaticotemporal artery

superficial temporal artery

posterior auricular artery

occipital artery

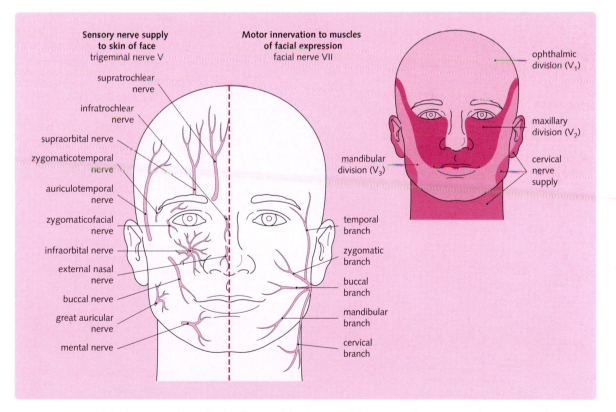

Sensory nerve supply to skin of face
trigeminal nerve V

supratrochlear nerve

infratrochlear nerve

supraorbital nerve

zygomaticotemporal nerve

auriculotemporal nerve

zygomaticofacial nerve

infraorbital nerve

external nasal nerve

buccal nerve

great auricular nerve

mental nerve

Motor innervation to muscles of facial expression
facial nerve VII

mandibular division (V₃)

temporal branch

zygomatic branch

buccal branch

mandibular branch

cervical branch

ophthalmic division (V₁)

maxillary division (V₂)

cervical nerve supply

Fig. 7.12 Nerves of the face. Inset shows the distribution of the divisions of the trigeminal nerve. Note the great auricular nerve is not part of the trigeminal nerve.

Fig. 7.13 Muscles of the face.

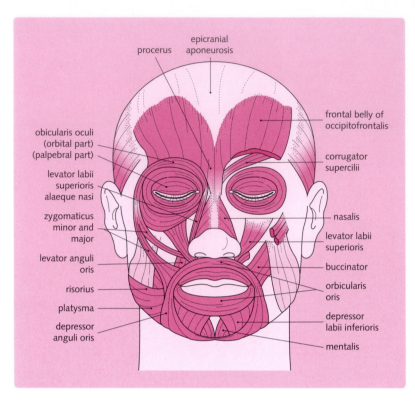

Labels on figure:
- procerus
- epicranial aponeurosis
- frontal belly of occipitofrontalis
- obicularis oculi (orbital part) (palpebral part)
- corrugator supercilii
- levator labii superioris alaeque nasi
- nasalis
- zygomaticus minor and major
- levator labii superioris
- levator anguli oris
- buccinator
- risorius
- orbicularis oris
- platysma
- depressor labii inferioris
- depressor anguli oris
- mentalis

occipitofrontalis, stylohyoid and the posterior belly of digastric.

Vessels of the face

The face has a very rich blood supply, mainly from the facial and superficial temporal arteries, both of which are branches of the external carotid artery (Fig. 7.14).

The facial artery ascends deep to the submandibular gland, winds around the inferior border of the mandible, and enters the face. It gives off the inferior labial, superior labial and lateral nasal arteries then terminates as the angular artery at the medial canthus of the eye.

The supraorbital and supratrochlear arteries are terminal branches of the ophthalmic artery—a branch of the internal carotid artery.

Of the veins (Fig. 7.14):

- The supraorbital and supratrochlear veins unite to form the facial vein, which descends in the face, receiving tributaries corresponding to the branches of the artery.
- The superficial temporal and maxillary veins form the retromandibular vein in the parotid salivary gland.
- The posterior auricular and posterior division of the retromandibular veins form the external jugular vein.
- Occipital veins drain into the suboccipital venous complex.
- The facial vein and the anterior division of the retromandibular vein drain into the internal jugular vein.

For branches of the facial nerve to the face use the following mnemonic: Ten Zulus Bought My Cat (temporal, zygomatic, buccal, mandibular, cervical).

While the facial artery is a branch of the external carotid artery, the facial vein drains into the internal jugular vein.

Fig. 7.14 Blood supply to the face.

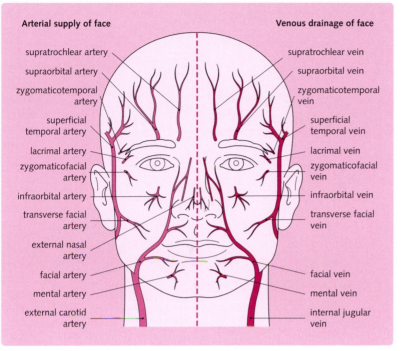

Arterial supply of face

- supratrochlear artery
- supraorbital artery
- zygomaticotemporal artery
- superficial temporal artery
- lacrimal artery
- zygomaticofacial artery
- infraorbital artery
- transverse facial artery
- external nasal artery
- facial artery
- mental artery
- external carotid artery

Venous drainage of face

- supratrochlear vein
- supraorbital vein
- zygomaticotemporal vein
- superficial temporal vein
- lacrimal vein
- zygomaticofacial vein
- infraorbital vein
- transverse facial vein
- facial vein
- mental vein
- internal jugular vein

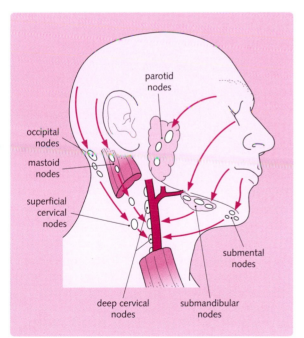

- parotid nodes
- occipital nodes
- mastoid nodes
- superficial cervical nodes
- submental nodes
- deep cervical nodes
- submandibular nodes

Fig. 7.15 Lymphatic drainage of the face. (Adapted from *Anatomy as a Basis for Clinical Medicine*, by E C B Hall-Craggs. Courtesy of Williams & Wilkins.)

Lymphatic drainage of the face

The lymph vessels of the face all eventually drain into the deep cervical chain of lymph nodes (Fig. 7.15).

THE CRANIAL CAVITY AND MENINGES

The cranium protects the brain and its surrounding meninges. The cranium is covered by periosteum: pericranium on the outer surface and endocranium on the inner surface. The two layers are connected at the sutures of the skull.

The cranial bones consist of outer and inner tables of compact bones separated by cancellous bone containing red marrow—the diploë (see Fig. 7.10).

The base of the skull's internal surface may be divided into the anterior, middle and posterior cranial fossae (Fig. 7.16). The foramina in the cranial fossae and their main contents are outlined in Fig. 7.6.

Fig. 7.16 Internal surface of the base of the skull, showing the cranial fossae.

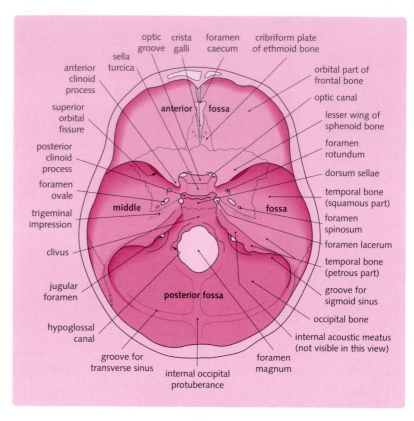

Cranial fossae

Anterior cranial fossa

The anterior cranial fossa contains the frontal lobes of the brain and the olfactory bulbs. It contains the cribriform plate (perforated by the olfactory nerves) and the vertical crista galli of the ethmoid bone.

Middle cranial fossa

A shallow depression (trigeminal impression) near the apex of the petrous temporal bone houses the sensory ganglion of the trigeminal nerve.

The middle cranial fossa contains the temporal lobes of the cerebral hemispheres, the floor of the forebrain, the optic chiasma, the termination of the internal carotid arteries, and the pituitary gland.

The optic chiasma lies above (not in!) the optic groove, with the optic canals at either end of the groove. The pituitary gland lies in the pituitary fossa or sella turcica, below the optic chiasma.

Posterior cranial fossa

The posterior cranial fossa is roofed by the tentorium cerebelli layer of the dura mater. It contains the pons, the medulla, the cerebellum and the midbrain.

Pituitary tumour

A tumour of the pituitary gland may compress the optic chiasma. As this carries fibres from the temporal fields, the patient will complain of 'tunnel vision' or a bitemporal hemianopia.

Meninges

There are three meningeal layers surrounding the brain and spinal cord (see Fig. 7.10): dura, arachnoid and pia.

Dura mater

The dura mater is made up of dense fibrous tissue firmly adherent to the endocranium. It is continuous with the dura mater of the spinal cord through the foramen magnum. The dura sends sleeves around the cranial nerves, which fuse with the epineurium of the nerves outside the skull.

The dura gives rise to four septa that support the brain and restrict its movement:

Falx cerebri

This is a sickle-shaped fold of dura lying in the midline between the two cerebral hemispheres

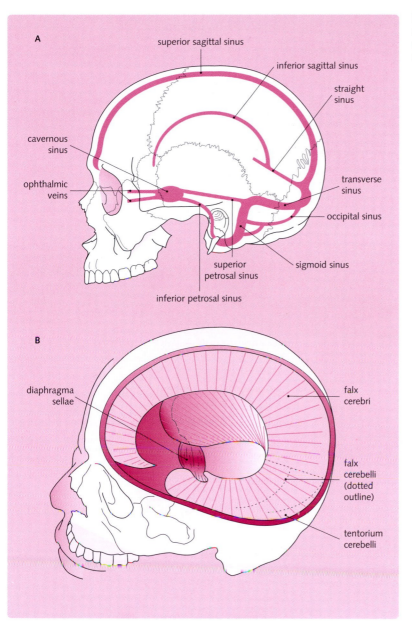

Fig. 7.17 (A) The positions of the cranial venous sinuses. (B) The falx cerebri, falx cerebelli, diaphragma sellae, and tentorium cerebelli.

A

superior sagittal sinus

inferior sagittal sinus

straight sinus

cavernous sinus

ophthalmic veins

transverse sinus

occipital sinus

superior petrosal sinus

sigmoid sinus

inferior petrosal sinus

B

diaphragma sellae

falx cerebri

falx cerebelli (dotted outline)

tentorium cerebelli

Some anatomists refer to the dura as the 'meningeal layer of dura' and the endocranial layer of periosteum as the 'periosteal layer of dura'.

(Fig. 7.17). It is attached anteriorly to the crista galli. Posteriorly, it blends with the tentorium cerebelli.

The superior sagittal sinus runs in its superior margin (its attachment to the vault of the skull). The inferior sagittal sinus runs in its free inferior margin.

The straight sinus runs along its attachment to the tentorium cerebelli.

Tentorium cerebelli

This is a crescent-shaped fold of dura mater that roofs the posterior cranial fossa (see Fig. 7.17). It covers the cerebellum, and it supports the occipital lobes of the cerebral hemispheres.

The tentorium has an attachment that begins on either side at the posterior clinoid process, passes back along the petrous temporal bone and curves around the inner aspect of the occipital bone. Posteriorly the falx cerebri and falx cerebelli are attached to its upper and lower surfaces. Its free margin is anchored to the anterior clinoids, forming the tentorial notch through which the midbrain passes.

The superior petrosal and transverse venous sinuses run along its attachment to the petrous and occipital bones, respectively.

Falx cerebelli

This projects forward in between the two cerebellar hemispheres, attached to the internal occipital crest. Its posterior margin contains the occipital sinus.

Diaphragma sellae

This is a small circular fold of dura forming the roof of the pituitary fossa.

Arachnoid mater

The arachnoid mater lies against but is not attached to the dura and it is separated from the pia mater by the subarachnoid space, containing cerebrospinal fluid.

Where the arachnoid bridges major irregularities of the brain surface, the subarachnoid space expands to form subarachnoid cisterns.

Pia mater

The pia mater closely invests the brain surface. It continues as a sheath around the small vessels entering the brain.

Nerve supply of the meninges

Dura mater in the anterior and middle cranial fossae is supplied by the trigeminal nerve. The posterior fossa is supplied by the upper three cervical nerves, vagal and hypoglossal meningeal nerve branches.

Cranial venous sinuses

The cranial venous sinuses lie between endocranium and dura, are lined by endothelium, and are valveless (see Figs 7.10 and 7.17). Veins from the various parts of the brain and from the diploë, the orbit, and the inner ear drain into these sinuses.

Neck pain can be referred to the head due to the upper three cervical nerves supplying the dura mater posteriorly.

Intracranial haemorrhages

- Extradural (epidural) – due to bleeding from the branches of the middle meningeal artery (e.g. due to a fracture of the pterion), causing blood to collect between the periosteum and dura. Brief unconsciousness is followed by a lucid interval of several hours then drowsiness and unconsciousness.
- Subdural – the veins leading from the brain to the dural venous sinuses may tear in sudden movement or trauma, causing bleeding into the potential space between dura and arachnoid.
- Subarachnoid – an artery in the subarachnoid space (e.g. part of the circle of Willis) ruptures, bleeding into the CSF. This results in severe headache, loss of consciousness and death.

Superior sagittal sinus

The superior sagittal sinus runs in the upper border of the falx cerebri. It commences at the foramen caecum and passes backwards, grooving the vault of the skull. At the internal occipital protuberance, it forms the confluence of the sinuses, and it continues as a transverse sinus (usually the right). It receives numerous cerebral veins and several accumulations of arachnoid granulations (see Fig. 7.10).

Inferior sagittal sinus

The inferior sagittal sinus lies in the free margin of the falx cerebri. It drains into the straight sinus.

Straight sinus

The straight sinus lies between the falx cerebri and tentorium cerebelli and is formed by the junction of the inferior sagittal sinus and the great cerebral vein. It ends by turning to form (usually the left) transverse sinus.

Transverse sinuses

The transverse sinuses commence at the internal occipital protuberance and run in the attachment of the tentorium cerebelli. They end by turning inferiorly as the sigmoid sinuses. They receive the superior petrosal sinuses and the cerebral cerebellar, and diploic veins.

Sigmoid sinuses

Each sigmoid sinus turns downward and medially to groove the mastoid process. It then turns downward through the posterior part of the jugular foramen to become continuous with the internal jugular vein.

Occipital sinus

The occipital sinus lies in the attached margin of the falx cerebelli. It drains into the bases of the sigmoid sinuses.

Cavernous sinuses

The cavernous sinuses lie on either side of the body of the sphenoid, and they extend from the superior orbital fissure anteriorly to the apex of the petrous temporal bone posteriorly.

They receive:

- The superior and inferior ophthalmic veins.
- The cerebral veins.
- The sphenoparietal sinus.
- The central vein of the retina.

They drain posteriorly into the superior and inferior petrosal sinuses and inferiorly into the pterygoid venous plexus. The two sinuses communicate via anterior and posterior intercavernous sinuses.

Relations of the cavernous sinuses

The internal carotid artery and its sympathetic nerve plexus and the abducens nerve run through the sinus (Fig. 7.18). The oculomotor and trochlear nerves and the ophthalmic and maxillary divisions of the trigeminal nerves lie in the lateral wall of the sinus, between the endothelium and the dura.

Spread of infection from the face

The facial vein connects with the cavernous sinus in the skull via the superior ophthalmic vein, and it provides a path for spread of infection and clotted blood from the face to the cavernous sinus. This gives rise to the 'danger area of the face' – a triangular region with its base at the top lip and its apex at the bridge of the nose from which infection may spread. Infection obstructs the venous drainage from the orbit, causing oedema and papilloedema and is very difficult to treat.

Superior and inferior petrosal sinuses

The superior and inferior petrosal sinuses emerge from the cavernous sinus and lie at the superior and inferior borders of the petrous temporal bone, respectively.

The superior sinus drains into the transverse sinus and the inferior into the internal jugular vein.

Arteries of the cranial cavity

The brain is supplied by the two internal carotid arteries and the two vertebral arteries.

Internal carotid artery

The internal carotid artery is a terminal branch of the common carotid artery (Fig. 7.19). It enters the skull through the carotid canal and enters the middle

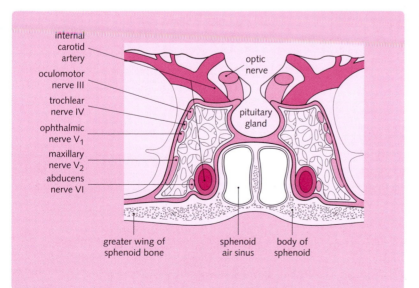

Fig. 7.18 A coronal section of the cavernous sinus showing its relations.

internal carotid artery
optic nerve
oculomotor nerve III
trochlear nerve IV
ophthalmic nerve V$_1$
maxillary nerve V$_2$
abducens nerve VI
pituitary gland
greater wing of sphenoid bone
sphenoid air sinus
body of sphenoid

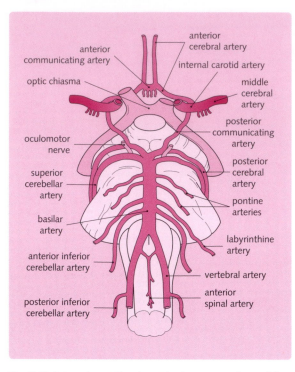

Fig. 7.19 Internal carotid and vertebral arteries on base of the brain.

cranial fossa through the foramen lacerum in the floor of the cavernous sinus. The artery runs forward in the cavernous sinus, turning superiorly to pierce the roof at the anterior end. It then enters the sub-arachnoid space and gives off the ophthalmic artery, turning backwards to the region of the anterior perforated substance of the brain at the medial end of the lateral cerebral sulcus. Here, it gives off the anterior cerebral and posterior communicating arteries then continues as the middle cerebral artery.

Vertebral artery

On either side, a vertebral artery arises from the first part of the subclavian artery. It ascends in the foramina of the upper six cervical vertebra transverse processes (Fig 7.7) and enters the skull through the foramen magnum. It passes upwards on the medulla oblongata (see Fig. 7.19), and it joins the vessel from the opposite side to form the basilar artery.

Cranial branches of the vertebral artery include:

- The meningeal arteries.
- The anterior and posterior spinal arteries.
- The posterior inferior cerebellar artery.
- The medullary arteries.

Basilar artery

The basilar artery ascends on the anterior surface of the pons (see Fig. 7.19). At the upper border of the pons, it divides into the posterior cerebral arteries. It also gives off branches to the pons, cerebellum and internal ear.

Circle of Willis

The circulus arteriosus is an anastomosis between branches of the internal carotid arteries and the vertebral arteries (see Fig. 7.19), allowing blood entering either artery to flow to any part of both cerebral hemispheres. An anterior communicating artery connects the two anterior cerebral arteries and posterior communicating arteries connect the internal carotid to the posterior cerebral artery. It lies in the interpeduncular fossa beneath the forebrain.

Cranial nerves

The cranial nerves are summarized in Figure 7.20.

THE ORBIT

The eyeball and its associated structures are protected by the bony orbital cavity. The eyelids protect the eyes anteriorly.

Stroke (cerebrovascular accident)

Strokes are common in Western countries, commonly arising because of blockage of one of the major arteries, usually the middle cerebral (but also may be due to cerebral haemorrhage). The anastomosis between the cerebral vessels is not sufficient to supply the affected tissue, resulting in death of that part of the brain.

Subclavian steal syndrome

Where the two vertebral arteries join to form the basilar artery there is potential for anastomosis – should the first part of the subclavian artery become blocked, blood will backflow down the vertebral artery on that side to supply the upper limb. This causes light headedness when using the affected arm due to a diminished blood flow to the brain.

Fig. 7.20 Summary of cranial nerves

Nerve	Distribution and functions
Olfactory (I)	Smell from nasal mucosa of roof of each nasal cavity
Optic (II)	Vision from retina
Oculomotor (III)	Motor to superior, medial and inferior oblique; parasympathetic innervation to sphincter pupillae and ciliary muscle (constricts pupil and accommodates lens of eye) carries sympathetic nerve fibres (from carotid plexus) to smooth muscle part of levator palpebrae superioris
Trochlear (IV)	Motor to superior oblique
Trigeminal (V)—ophthalmic division (V_1)	Sensation from upper third of face, including cornea, scalp, eyelids, and paranasal sinuses
Trigeminal (V)—maxillary division (V_2)	Sensation from the middle third of face, including upper lip, maxillary teeth, mucosa of nose, maxillary sinuses, and palate; supplies dura mater anteriorly
Trigeminal (V)—mandibular division (V_3)	Motor to muscles of mastication, mylohyoid, anterior belly of digastric, tensor veli palatini and tensor tympani; sensation from lower third of face, including temporomandibular joint, and mucosa of mouth and anterior two thirds of tongue, supplies dura mater anteriorly
Abducent (VI)	Motor to lateral rectus
Facial (VII)	Motor to muscles of facial expression and scalp, stapedius, stylohyoid, and posterior belly of digastric; taste from anterior two thirds of tongue, floor of mouth, and palate; sensation from skin of external acoustic meatus; parasympathetic innervation to submandibular and sublingual salivary glands, lacrimal gland, and glands of nose and palate
Vestibulocochlear (VIII)	Vestibular sensation from semicircular ducts, utricle, and saccule; hearing from spiral organ
Glossopharyngeal (IX)	Motor to stylopharyngeus, parasympathetic innervation to parotid gland; visceral sensation from parotid gland, carotid body and sinus, pharynx, and middle ear; taste and general sensation from posterior third of tongue
Vagus (X)	Motor to constrictor muscles of pharynx, intrinsic muscles of larynx, and muscles of palate (except tensor veli palatini) and superior two thirds of oesophagus; parasympathetic innervation to smooth muscle of trachea, bronchi, digestive tract, and cardiac muscle of heart; visceral sensation from pharynx, larynx, trachea, bronchi, heart, to the splenic flexure oesophagus, stomach, and intestine; taste from epiglottis and palate; sensation from auricle, external acoustic meatus, and dura mater of posterior cranial fossa
Accessory (XI) cranial root spinal root	Motor to striated muscles of soft palate, pharynx, and larynx via fibres that join X in jugular foramen Motor to sternocleidomastoid and trapezius
Hypoglossal (XII)	Sensory to dura mater, posteriorly; motor to intrinsic and extrinsic muscles of tongue (except palatoglossus)

Eyelids

The superficial surface of the lids is covered by the skin; the deep surface is covered by mucosa—the conjunctiva, which reflects at the superior and inferior fornices onto the anterior surface of the eyeball; the space between eyeball and eyelid is called the conjunctival sac (Fig. 7.21). The opening between the eyelids is the palpebral fissure.

The fibrous framework of the eyelids is formed by the orbital septum (Figs 7.21 and 7.23). This is thickened at the lid margins to form the tarsal plates, which medially and laterally form the medial and lateral palpebral ligaments. The tarsal plates contain tarsal glands that empty at the margins of the eyelids and levator palpebrae superioris muscle is attached to the superior tarsal plate.

Sebaceous and ciliary glands also empty onto the eyelid.

The lacrimal gland lies at the upper lateral part of the orbit, wrapped around the tendon of levator

Fig. 7.21 Conjunctival sac, upper and lower lids, and cornea.

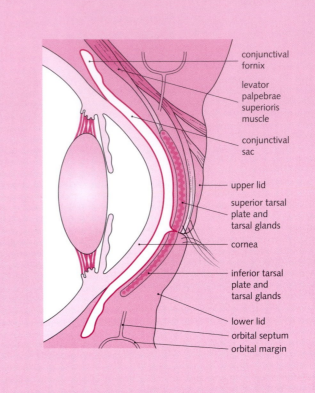

- conjunctival fornix
- levator palpebrae superioris muscle
- conjunctival sac
- upper lid
- superior tarsal plate and tarsal glands
- cornea
- inferior tarsal plate and tarsal glands
- lower lid
- orbital septum
- orbital margin

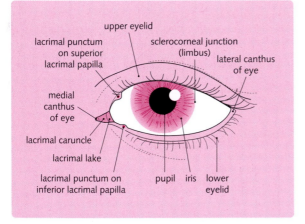

Fig. 7.22 Eyelids, palpebral fissure and eyeball.

upper eyelid
lacrimal punctum on superior lacrimal papilla
sclerocorneal junction (limbus)
lateral canthus of eye
medial canthus of eye
lacrimal caruncle
lacrimal lake
lacrimal punctum on inferior lacrimal papilla
pupil   iris   lower eyelid

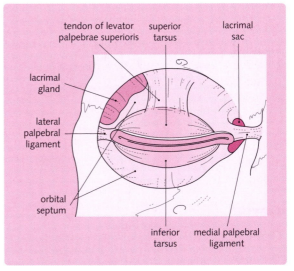

Fig. 7.23 Orbital septum, tarsi and palpebral ligaments.

tendon of levator palpebrae superioris   superior tarsus   lacrimal sac
lacrimal gland
lateral palpebral ligament
orbital septum
inferior tarsus   medial palpebral ligament

palpebrae superioris. It has numerous ducts opening into the conjunctival sac. The nerve supply to the lacrimal gland is parasympathetic secretomotor, originating in the lacrimal nucleus. Parasympathetic fibres travel in the facial nerve, greater petrosal nerve, and synapse in the pterygopalatine ganglion. The postganglionic fibres now join the zygomaticotemporal nerve (a V_2 branch), then the lacrimal nerve (a V_1 branch) before supplying the lacrimal gland.

The space between the medial part of the eyelids and the eyeball is called the lacrimal lake. It contains an elevation—the lacrimal caruncle. Tears produced by the lacrimal gland are continually spread over the conjunctiva and cornea by blinking, preventing dehydration of the conjunctiva. They then pass towards the lacrimal lake and into the lacrimal punctum to enter the lacrimal canaliculi, which drain into the lacrimal sac. This sac is the upper end of the nasolacrimal duct, which drains the tears into the inferior meatus of the nose.

Orbital cavity

Figure 7.24 illustrates the bony components of the orbital cavity. The bony walls of the orbital cavity are:

- Superiorly (roof)—frontal (orbital part), lesser wing of sphenoid.
- Medial wall—maxilla, lacrimal, ethmoid, body of sphenoid.
- Inferiorly (floor)—maxillary, zygomatic, palatine.
- Lateral wall—zygomatic (frontal process), greater wing of sphenoid.

Figure 7.25 lists the orbital openings and their contents.

Muscles of the orbit

The muscles of the orbit are outlined in Figure 7.26 and illustrated in Figure 7.27.

Vessels of the orbit

Figure 7.28 shows the arterial supply to the orbit. Note that the ophthalmic artery initially lies within the subarachnoid space of the optic nerve and pierces its dural sheath.

The superior ophthalmic vein communicates anteriorly with the facial vein and, posteriorly, it drains to the cavernous sinus. The inferior ophthalmic vein communicates via the inferior orbital fissure with the pterygoid venous plexus (a route for transmission of infection).

Nerves of the orbit

Optic nerve (II)

The optic nerve is surrounded by the three meningeal layers as it enters the orbit. It runs forward and laterally within the cone of rectus muscles and pierces the sclera. The meningeal layer fuses with the sclera here. The nerve carries afferent fibres from the retina.

Oculomotor nerve (III)

The oculomotor nerve is divided into superior and inferior divisions:

- The superior division supplies superior rectus and levator palpebrae superioris.
- The inferior division supplies inferior rectus, medial rectus, and inferior oblique.
- The nerve to inferior oblique sends a branch to the ciliary ganglion. This carries parasympathetic fibres to the sphincter pupillae and ciliary muscle.

Trochlear nerve (IV)

The trochlear nerve leaves the lateral wall of the cavernous sinus to enter the orbit. It runs forward and medially across the origin of levator palpebrae superioris to supply the superior oblique muscle.

Ophthalmic division of trigeminal nerve (V1)

This runs in the lateral wall of the cavernous sinus and gives three branches that pass through the superior orbital fissure to the orbit (see Fig. 7.24):

Lacrimal nerve

This passes along the upper part of the lateral rectus muscle to supply the skin and conjunctiva of the upper lid laterally. It is joined by a branch of the zygomaticotemporal nerve carrying parasympathetic fibres to the lacrimal gland.

> **Oculomotor nerve palsy**
>
> This results in ptosis (loss of innervation of levator palpebrae superioris), a dilated pupil (loss of parasympathetic innervation) and a lateral squint (unopposed lateral rectus and superior oblique). Compare this to ptosis and a constricted pupil in Horner's syndrome (**p. 217**).

> The superior oblique is the 'poor man's muscle' – always looking down and out.

> Motor innervation of the extraocular muscles is from the oculomotor nerve except for SO 4 and LR 6 (superior oblique—IV nerve; lateral rectus—VI nerve).

Fig. 7.24 Bones of the orbit and structures in the back of the orbit.

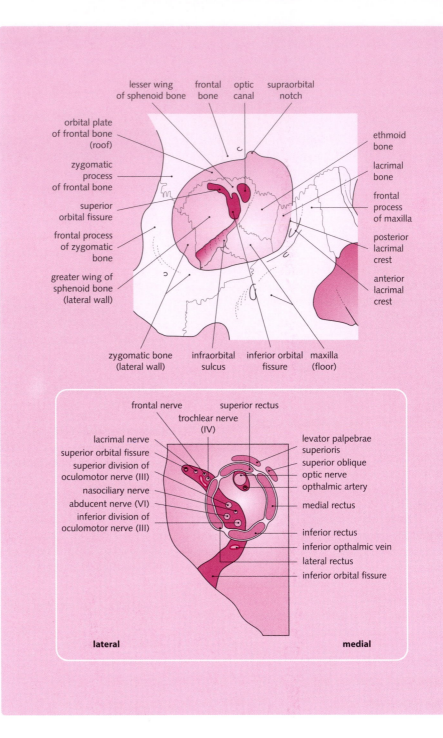

The following labels appear in the figure:

- lesser wing of sphenoid bone
- frontal bone
- optic canal
- supraorbital notch
- orbital plate of frontal bone (roof)
- zygomatic process of frontal bone
- superior orbital fissure
- frontal process of zygomatic bone
- greater wing of sphenoid bone (lateral wall)
- ethmoid bone
- lacrimal bone
- frontal process of maxilla
- posterior lacrimal crest
- anterior lacrimal crest
- zygomatic bone (lateral wall)
- infraorbital sulcus
- inferior orbital fissure
- maxilla (floor)

- frontal nerve
- superior rectus
- trochlear nerve (IV)
- lacrimal nerve
- superior orbital fissure
- superior division of oculomotor nerve (III)
- nasociliary nerve
- abducent nerve (VI)
- inferior division of oculomotor nerve (III)
- levator palpebrae superioris
- superior oblique
- optic nerve
- opthalmic artery
- medial rectus
- inferior rectus
- inferior opthalmic vein
- lateral rectus
- inferior orbital fissure

lateral   medial

Note that the pterygopalatine ganglion, NOT the ciliary ganglion, supplies the lacrimal gland.

Frontal nerve

This passes forward on the superior surface of levator palpebrae superioris. Before it reaches the orbital margin it divides into supraorbital and supratrochlear

Fig. 7.25 Orbital openings and their contents

Openings	Bones	Contents
Supraorbital notch (foramen)	Orbital plate of the frontal bone	Supraorbital nerve and vessels
Infraorbital groove and canal	Orbital plate of the maxilla	Infraorbital nerve and vessels
Inferior orbital fissure	Maxilla and greater wing of the sphenoid bone	Communicates with the pterygopalatine fossa and transmits the maxillary nerve and its zygomatic branch, the inferior ophthalmic vein, and sympathetic nerves
Superior orbital fissure	Greater and lesser wing of the sphenoid bone	Lacrimal, frontal, trochlear, oculomotor, abducens, and nasociliary nerves, and superior ophthalmic vein
Optic canal	Lesser wing of the sphenoid bone	Optic nerve and ophthalmic artery
Zygomaticotemporal and zygomaticofacial foramina	Zygomatic bone	Zygomaticotemporal and zygomaticofacial nerves
Anterior and posterior ethmoidal foramina	Ethmoid bone	Anterior and posterior ethmoidal nerves and vessels

nerves, which supply the skin of the forehead and scalp, and the frontal sinus.

Nasociliary nerve

This enters the orbit and crosses above the optic nerve to reach the medial wall of the orbit. It runs forward on the upper margin of medial rectus, gives the posterior ethmoidal branch and it ends by dividing into the anterior ethmoidal and infratrochlear nerves (Fig. 7.29).

Abducent nerve (VI)

The abducent nerve enters the orbit and supplies the lateral rectus muscle.

Ciliary ganglion

The ciliary ganglion is a parasympathetic ganglion situated posteriorly in the orbit, lateral to the optic nerve.

Preganglionic parasympathetic fibres from the Edinger–Westphal nucleus pass to synapse in the ganglion via the oculomotor nerve.

> ### Abducent nerve palsy
>
> The long intracranial course of the abducent nerve makes it vulnerable to damage. This causes a medial squint (loss of innervation of lateral rectus).

Postganglionic parasympathetic fibres pass to the back of the eyeball via the short ciliary nerves to supply the constrictor pupillae and ciliary muscle.

Sympathetic fibres (from the internal carotid plexus) pass through the ganglion to enter the short ciliary nerves to supply the dilator pupillae. General sensory fibres enter the ganglion via the nasociliary nerve. The long ciliary nerve also carries sympathetic (vasoconstrictor) and sensory fibres to the eyeball.

THE PAROTID REGION

Parotid gland

The parotid gland is the largest salivary gland. It lies between the ramus of the mandible and the sternocleidomastoid muscle (Fig. 7.30).

The gland is surrounded by a capsule derived from the investing layer of deep cervical fascia. The free edge of the deep layer forms the stylo-mandibular ligament, running from the mandibular angle to the styloid process and separating parotid and submandibular glands.

The parotid duct emerges from the anterior border of the gland. It passes over masseter and, at the anterior border of this muscle, it turns medially to pierce the buccal fat pad and buccinator to open into the oral cavity opposite the upper second molar tooth.

Fig. 7.26 Muscles of the eyeballs and eyelids

Extrinsic muscles of eyeball (striated skeletal muscle)			
Name of muscle (nerve supply)	Origin	Insertion	Action
Superior rectus (III nerve)	Common tendinous ring on posterior wall of orbital cavity	Superior surface of eyeball just posterior to corneoscleral junction	Raises cornea upward and medially
Inferior rectus (III nerve)	Common tendinous ring on posterior wall of orbital cavity	Inferior surface of eyeball just posterior to corneoscleral junction	Depresses cornea downward and medially
Medial rectus (III nerve)	Common tendinous ring on posterior wall of orbital cavity	Medial surface of eyeball just posterior to corneoscleral junction	Rotates eyeball so that cornea looks medially
Lateral rectus (VI nerve)	Common tendinous ring on posterior wall of orbital cavity	Lateral surface of eyeball just posterior to corneoscleral junction	Rotates eyeball so that cornea looks laterally
Superior oblique (IV nerve)	Body of sphenoid bone	Passes through trochlea and is attached to superior surface of eyeball beneath superior rectus, behind the equator	Rotates eyeball so that cornea looks downward and laterally
Inferior oblique (III nerve)	Floor of orbital cavity, anteriorly and medially	Lateral surface of eyeball deep to lateral rectus	Rotates eyeball so that cornea looks upward and laterally
Intrinsic muscles of eyeball (smooth muscle)			
Name of muscle (nerve supply)	Origin	Insertion	Action
Sphincter pupillae of iris (parasympathetic via III nerve)	Ring of smooth muscle passing circumferentially around pupil	–	Constricts pupil
Dilator pupillae of iris (sympathetic)	Ciliary body	Sphincter pupillae	Dilates pupil
Ciliary muscle (parasympathetic via III nerve)	Corneoscleral junction	Ciliary body	Controls shape of lens; in accommodation, makes lens more globular
Muscles of eyelids			
Name of muscle (nerve supply)	Origin	Insertion	Action
Orbicularis oculi (VII nerve)	Medial palpebral ligament, lacrimal bone	Skin around orbit, tarsal plates	Closes eyelids (helps spread tears across conjunctiva)
Levator palpebrae superioris (striated muscle: III nerve; smooth muscle: sympathetic)	Lesser wing of sphenoid bone	Superior tarsal plate	Raises upper lid

Structures within the parotid gland

The structures of the parotid gland are shown in Figure 7.31. From superficial to deep:

Facial nerve (VII)

Divides into its five terminal branches in the parotid gland.

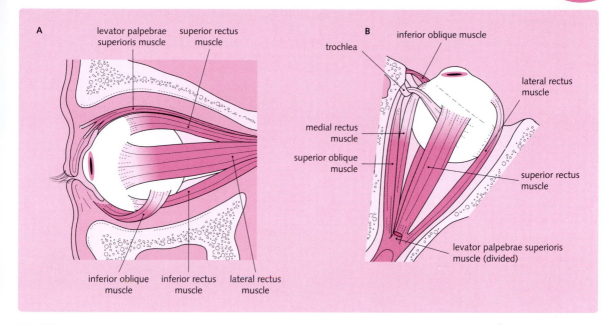

Fig. 7.27 Muscles of the orbit seen laterally (A) and from above (B).

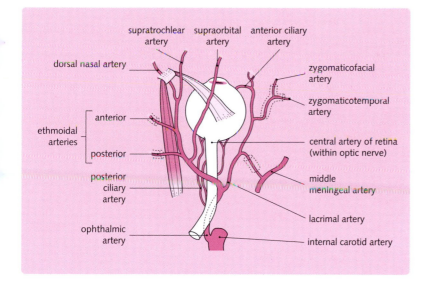

Fig. 7.28 Arterial supply to the orbit. Branches of the ophthalmic artery.

Retromandibular vein

The retromandibular vein is formed in the gland by the union of the superficial temporal and maxillary veins. It divides into anterior and posterior divisions, which leave the lower border of the gland. The anterior division joins the facial vein to drain into the internal jugular vein; the posterior division joins with the posterior auricular vein to form the external jugular vein.

External carotid artery

Divides into its two terminal branches at the neck of the mandible—the maxillary and superficial temporal arteries.

Parotid tumour

Parotid tumours are usually benign but may compress the facial nerve, weakening the facial muscles ipsilaterally (Bell's palsy). The corner of the mouth and eye droop – a patient cannot blow out their cheeks or keep their eye closed against resistance. When resecting the gland to remove a tumour, an electrical stimulator is used to find branches of the facial nerve.

Parotid duct stone

A stone in the parotid duct causes intense pain on salivation (i.e. during eating). Treatment is surgical.

Blood supply, lymphatic drainage and innervation of the parotid gland

Blood supply is from the external carotid artery and its terminal branches.

Parasympathetic secretomotor fibres from the glossopharyngeal nerve (IX) pass to the otic ganglion via the tympanic branch of the glossopharyngeal nerve and the lesser petrosal nerve. Postganglionic fibres pass to the parotid via the auriculotemporal nerve (a branch of V_3). The great auricular nerve supplies sensory fibres to the gland capsule. The auriculotemporal nerve supplies sensory fibres to the gland itself.

Parotid lymph nodes drain the gland to the deep cervical nodes.

Fig. 7.29 Branches of the nasociliary nerve	
Branch	**Action**
Communicating branch	Communicates with the ciliary ganglion—general sensory fibres from the eyeball pass to the ciliary ganglion via the short ciliary nerves and then to the nasociliary nerve via the communicating branch
Long ciliary nerve	2–3 branches containing sympathetic fibres for the dilator pupillae—runs with the short ciliary nerves and pierces the sclera to reach the iris
Posterior ethmoidal nerve	Exits through the posterior ethmoidal foramen to supply the ethmoidal and sphenoidal air sinuses
Infratrochlear nerve	Passes below the trochlea to supply the skin over the upper eyelid
Anterior ethmoidal nerve	Exits via the anterior ethmoidal foramen and enters the anterior cranial fossa on the cribriform plate of the ethmoid; then enters the nasal cavity via an opening opposite the crista galli to supply the mucosa of the nose; then supplies the skin of the nose as the external nasal nerve

Fig. 7.30 Parotid gland and its relations. (Adapted from *Clinical Anatomy For Medical Students*, 4th edn, by R S Snell. Little Brown & Co.)

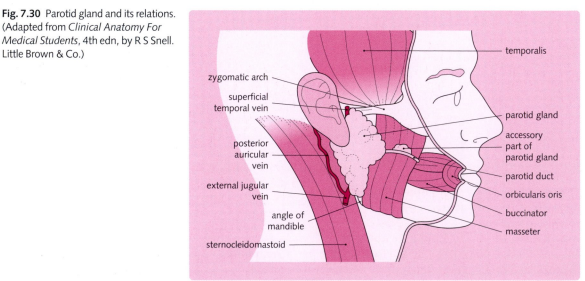

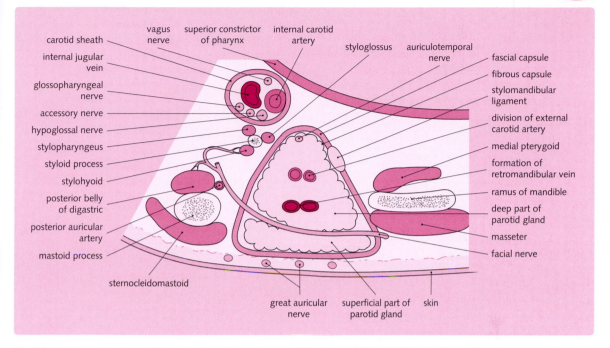

Fig. 7.31 Horizontal section of the neck, showing structures within the parotid gland. (Adapted from *Clinical Anatomy for Medical Students*, 4th edn, by R S Snell. Little Brown & Co.)

THE TEMPORAL AND INFRATEMPORAL FOSSAE

Temporal fossa

The temporal fossa lies on the lateral aspect of the skull. It is bounded by the superior temporal line of the temporal bone superiorly, by the frontal process of the zygomatic bone anteriorly, and by the zygomatic arch inferiorly.

Contents of the temporal fossa are:

- The temporalis muscle.
- Temporal fascia – the temporal fascia attaches inferiorly to the zygomatic arch and superiorly to the superior temporal line, covering temporalis in this region.
- The deep temporal nerves and vessels – from the mandibular nerve (V_3) and the maxillary artery respectively, they emerge from the border of lateral pterygoid to supply temporalis.
- The auriculotemporal nerve – from the mandibular nerve (V_3), supplies the skin of the auricle, the external auditory meatus, and the scalp over the temporal region.

- The superficial temporal artery – emerges from behind the temporomandibular joint, crosses the zygomatic arch, and ascends to the scalp.

Infratemporal fossa

The infratemporal fossa lies beneath the base of the skull between the pharynx and the ramus of the mandible (Fig. 7.32). It communicates with the temporal region deep to the zygomatic arch.

The infratemporal fossa contains (Fig. 7.33) the medial and lateral pterygoid muscles, branches of the mandibular nerve, the otic ganglion, the chorda tympani, the maxillary artery and the pterygoid venous plexus – detailed below.

Muscles of mastication

There are four muscles of mastication (see Fig. 7.34), all supplied by V_3. They can be clinically tested by asking the patient to:

- Clench the teeth (masseter and temporalis muscles).
- Move the chin from side to side in a chewing motion (lateral and medial pterygoid muscles).

Mandible

Important features of the mandible are shown in Figure 7.35. The two halves of the mandible unite at the midline symphysis menti.

Temporomandibular joint

The temporomandibular joint is the articulation between the condylar head of the mandible and the mandibular fossa of the temporal bone (Figs 7.36 and 7.37). It is a synovial joint, the joint space divided into upper and lower compartments by a fibrocartilaginous articular disc attached to the lateral pterygoid muscle anteriorly, and to the capsule of the joint.

The capsule surrounds the joint, and is attached to the margins of the mandibular fossa and the neck of the mandible. It is strengthened by the lateral (temporomandibular) ligament (lying laterally). The sphenomandibular and stylomandibular ligaments are also functionally associated with the joint.

Hinge-like movements (elevation and depression) take place in the lower joint space (between the condyle and the articular disc). When the mouth is opened widely, a gliding movement occurs in the upper joint space as the head and disc are pulled forward (protracted) by the medial pterygoid.

Mandibular nerve

V_3 exits the skull through the foramen ovale to enter the infratemporal fossa, where it immediately

Fig. 7.32 Boundaries of the infratemporal fossa	
Boundary	**Components**
Anterior	Posterior surface of the maxilla
Posterior	Styloid process
Superior	Infratemporal surface of the greater wing of the sphenoid bone
Medial	Lateral pterygoid plate
Lateral	Ramus of the mandible

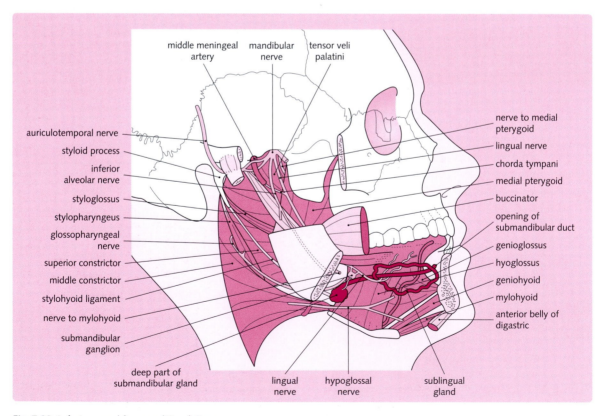

Fig. 7.33 Infratemporal fossa and its relations.

Fig. 7.34 Muscles of mastication

Muscle (nerve supply)	Origin	Insertion	Action
Temporalis (V_3 nerve)	Temporal fossa floor up to inferior temporal line	Coronoid process	Elevates mandible; posterior fibres retract a protruded mandible
Masseter (V_3 nerve)	Lower border and deep surface of zygomatic arch	Lateral surface of ramus of mandible	Elevates and protrudes mandible
Lateral pterygoid (V_3 nerve)			
Superior head	Infratemporal surface of sphenoid bone	Neck of the mandible	Acting together they protrude the mandible and pull the articular disc anteriorly; acting alone on one side produces deviation of mandible to contralateral side
Inferior head	Lateral surface of lateral pterygoid plate	Articular disc	
Medial pterygoid (V_3 nerve)			
Superficial head	Tuberosity of maxilla	Medial surface of ramus and angle of the mandible	Acting together they elevate the mandible; acting alone on one side produces deviation of mandible to contralateral side
Deep head	Medial surface of lateral pterygoid plate		

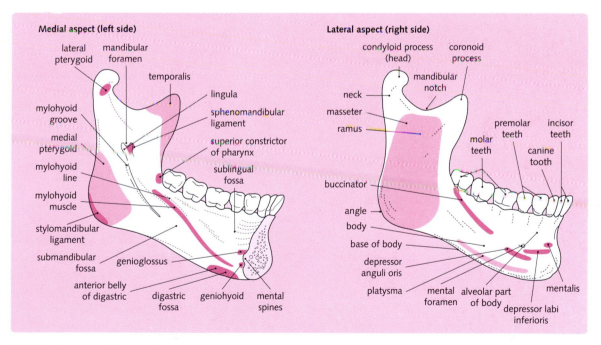

Fig. 7.35 Features of the mandible.

joins the motor root of the trigeminal nerve. Below the foramen ovale, the nerve is separated from the pharynx by the tensor veli palatini muscle and is deep to the superior head of the lateral pterygoid muscle. It divides into anterior and posterior divisions (Fig. 7.38).

Remember, the anterior division of the mandibular nerve is concerned with supplying the muscles of mastication except for its buccal branch which is sensory to the cheek skin, mucosa and gingivae.

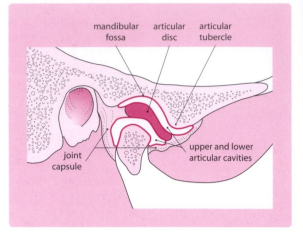

Fig. 7.37 Temporomandibular joint (lateral view).

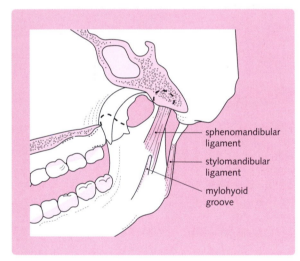

Fig. 7.36 Ligaments of the temporomandibular joint (medial view).

Otic ganglion

This is a parasympathetic ganglion lying below the foramen ovale.

Preganglionic secretomotor fibres from the inferior salivary nucleus of the glossopharyngeal nerve (IX) are carried in the tympanic branch to the tympanic plexus and tympanic membrane and then from here in the lesser petrosal nerve to enter the otic ganglion. The fibres synapse and postganglionic fibres hitchhike on the auriculotemporal nerve to enter the parotid gland.

Postganglionic sympathetic and sensory fibres also pass through the ganglion, without synapse.

Chorda tympani

The chorda tympani is a branch of the facial nerve in the temporal bone. It enters the infratemporal fossa via the petrotympanic fissure and joins the lingual nerve. It transmits preganglionic parasympathetic secretomotor fibres to the submandibular ganglion and taste fibres from the anterior two thirds of the tongue via the lingual nerve.

Maxillary artery

The maxillary artery is the large terminal branch of the external carotid artery in the parotid gland. It runs forward medial to the neck of the mandible to the lower border of lateral pterygoid, entering the infratemporal fossa. It then passes between the heads of lateral pterygoid and enters the pterygopalatine fossa through the pterygomaxillary fissure. Figure 7.39 lists the branches of the maxillary artery.

Pterygoid venous plexus

The pterygoid venous plexus lies around the muscles of mastication in the infratemporal fossa. It drains veins from the orbit, oral cavity and nasal cavity. It communicates with the cavernous sinus and with the facial vein.

THE EAR AND VESTIBULAR APPARATUS

The ear is the organ of hearing and balance. It may be divided into the external ear, the middle ear, and the internal ear.

Fig. 7.38 Branches of the mandibular nerve and the areas they supply.

Branch	Area supplied
Main trunk	
Meningeal branch	Re-enters cranial cavity via foramen spinosum
Nerve to medial pterygoid	Medial pterygoid and a branch that passes through otic ganglion to supply tensor tympani and tensor veli palatini
Anterior division (motor except the buccal nerve)	
Deep temporal nerves	Two or three nerves emerge from the upper border of lateral pterygoid—enter and supply temporalis
Masseteric nerve	Passes through mandibular notch to supply masseter muscle
Nerve to lateral pterygoid	Enters deep surface of lateral pterygoid and supplies it
Buccal nerve	Passes anteriorly between heads of lateral pterygoid to appear at anterior border of masseter; is sensory to skin of cheek and underlying buccal mucosa and gingiva
Posterior division (mainly sensory)	
Lingual nerve	Appears at lower border of lateral pterygoid and runs over superior surface of medial pterygoid to lie just beneath mucosa lining inner aspect of mandible adjacent to 3rd molar tooth (its subsequent course is described with the mouth); deep to lateral pterygoid, the nerve receives the chorda tympani
Inferior alveolar nerve	Runs parallel with lingual nerve over medial pterygoid; enters mandibular foramen and supplies teeth of lower jaw; at mental foramen, a branch of the nerve, the mental nerve, exits mandible to supply lower lip and chin region; mylohyoid nerve arises from inferior alveolar nerve just above mandibular foramen to supply mylohyoid and anterior belly of digastric
Auriculotemporal nerve	Emerges from behind the temporomandibular joint, crosses the root of the zygomatic arch behind the superficial temporal artery; supplied the skin of the auricle, the external auditory meatus, and scalp over the temporal region

The pterygoid venous plexus is devoid of valves, as are all veins of the head and neck.

External ear

Auricle

The auricle is a double layer of skin reinforced by cartilage. It collects sound and conducts it to the tympanic membrane.

External auditory (acoustic) meatus

The external auditory meatus extends from the auricle to the tympanic membrane (Fig. 7.40). The lateral third is cartilaginous and the medial two thirds are bony. It is lined by a layer of thin skin. Ceruminous and sebaceous glands produce cerumen (wax).

Tympanic membrane

The tympanic membrane is a thin membrane lying between the external and middle ears (see Fig. 7.40).

Fig. 7.39 Branches of the maxillary artery

Branch	Site of origin	Area supplied
Deep auricular artery	Behind neck of mandible	External auditory meatus and outer surface of eardrum
Anterior tympanic artery	Behind neck of mandible	Inner surface of eardrum via petrotympanic fissure
Middle meningeal artery	Infratemporal fossa	Enters cranial cavity via foramen spinosum to supply meninges
Inferior alveolar artery	Infratemporal fossa	Follows inferior alveolar nerve into mandibular canal and supplies lower jaw and teeth, and surrounding mucosa
Deep temporal arteries Masseteric artery Pterygoid branches	Infratemporal fossa	Muscles of mastication
Posterior superior alveolar artery	Pterygopalatine fossa	Enters posterior aspect of maxilla to supply molar and premolar teeth of maxilla
Infraorbital artery	Pterygopalatine fossa	Accompanies infraorbital nerve through infraorbital foramen onto face; reaches foramen by passing forward in infraorbital canal in orbital floor
Anterior superior alveolar artery	Infraorbital canal	Incisor and canine teeth
Palatine Sphenopalatine Pharyngeal branches	Pterygopalatine fossa	Described with the nasal cavity

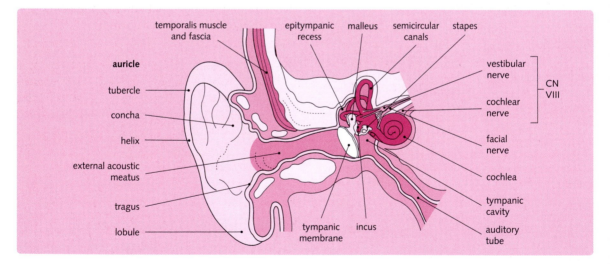

Fig. 7.40 External auditory meatus.

It is covered by skin externally and by mucous membrane internally. The membrane is outwardly concave, with a central depression—the umbo.

The membrane moves in response to air vibration. Movements are transmitted by three small bones, the ossicles across the middle ear to the internal ear.

The auriculotemporal nerve supplies the external surface of the tympanic membrane. The glossopharyngeal nerve supplies the internal surface.

Middle ear

The middle ear lies in the petrous temporal bone. It consists of the tympanic cavity and the epitympanic recess, which lies superior to the tympanic cavity. It is connected to the nasopharynx via the auditory tube and to the mastoid air cells via the mastoid antrum. The mucosa lining the tympanic cavity is continuous with that of the auditory tube, mastoid cells, and the mastoid antrum.

The middle ear contains:

- The ossicles (malleus, incus and stapes).
- Stapedius and tensor tympani muscles.
- The chorda tympani.
- The tympanic plexus of nerves.

Figure 7.41 describes the walls of the middle ear.

Mastoid antrum

The aditus to the antrum connects the mastoid antrum to the epitympanic recess of the tympanic cavity. The tegmen tympani separates the antrum from the middle cranial fossa. The floor of the antrum communicates with the mastoid air cells via several openings. The antrum and air cells are lined by

Fig. 7.41 Walls of the middle ear

Wall	Components
Roof (tegmental wall)	Tegmen tympani (thin plate of bone): separates cavity from dura in floor of middle cranial fossa
Floor (jugular wall)	A layer of bone separates tympanic cavity from superior bulb of internal jugular vein
Lateral wall (membranous)	Tympanic membrane with epitympanic recess superiorly
Medial wall (labyrinthine)	Separates tympanic cavity from inner ear
Anterior wall (carotid)	Separates tympanic cavity from carotid canal; superiorly lies opening of auditory tube and canal for tensor tympani
Posterior wall	Connected by aditus to mastoid antrum and air cells

mucosa. Anteroinferiorly the antrum is related to the canal for the facial nerve.

Auditory tube

The auditory tube connects the tympanic cavity to the nasopharynx. The posterior third is bony and the remainder is cartilaginous. The mucosa is continuous with that of the tympanic cavity and nasopharynx.

It allows pressure in the middle ear to equalize with atmospheric pressure, allowing free movement of the tympanic membrane. Pressure changes, e.g. during flying, can be equalized by swallowing or chewing—these movements open the auditory tubes.

Nerve supply is from the tympanic plexus (mainly tympanic branch IX).

Ossicles

The ossicles are the incus, malleus and stapes. The malleus is attached to the tympanic membrane. The incus connects the malleus to the stapes, which is attached to the oval window (Fig. 7.42). The ossicles transmit vibration from the tympanic membrane to the oval window.

There are two muscles associated with the ossicles: tensor tympani (medial pterygoid nerve – V_3) dampens vibration of the tympanic membrane, and stapedius (VII) dampens vibration of the stapes.

Internal ear

This lies in the petrous temporal bone (Fig. 7.43). It consists of a bony labyrinth and a membranous labyrinth. The two are separated by a space containing fluid called perilymph, which resembles cerebrospinal fluid (CSF).

Bony labyrinth

Vestibule

The central vestibule contains the utricle and saccule, components of the balance system. It is continuous with the cochlea anteriorly, with the semicircular canals posteriorly, and with the posterior cranial fossa by the aqueduct of the vestibule. The aqueduct

---

Auditory tube and infection

The auditory tube provides a passage for infection to spread from the nasopharynx to the tympanic cavity (middle ear).

extends to the posterior surface of the petrous temporal bone to open into the internal auditory meatus. It contains the endolymphatic ducts and blood vessels.

Cochlea

This contains the cochlear duct, and it is concerned with hearing. It makes 2.5 turns about a bony core—the modiolus. The large basal turn of the cochlea produces the promontory on the medial wall of the tympanic cavity.

Semicircular canals

These three lie perpendicular to one other. At one end of each canal is a swelling—the ampulla. The semicircular ducts lie in the canals.

Membranous labyrinth

This is a series of ducts and sacs in the bony labyrinth, which contain endolymph.

Saccule and utricle

These contain receptors that respond to linear acceleration and the static pull of gravity.

Cochlear duct

This accommodates the cochlear duct (of Corti), which contains the receptors of the auditory apparatus. The spiral organ lies between the scala vestibuli and the scala tympani, both of which are filled with perilymph and which communicate with each other at the tip of the cochlea.

Semicircular ducts

These contain receptors that respond to rotational acceleration in three different planes.

Endolymphatic duct

This duct opens into the endolymphatic sac. Endolymph has a composition similar to that of intracellular fluid.

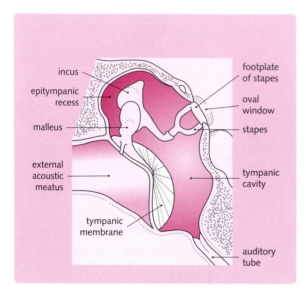

Fig. 7.42 Coronal section of the tympanic cavity showing the ossicles in situ.

Fig. 7.43 Internal ear.

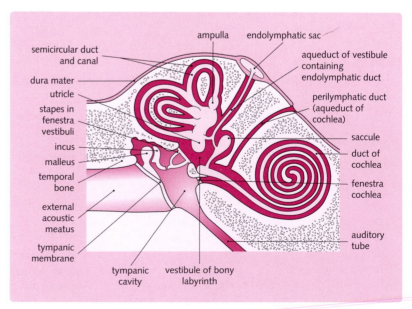

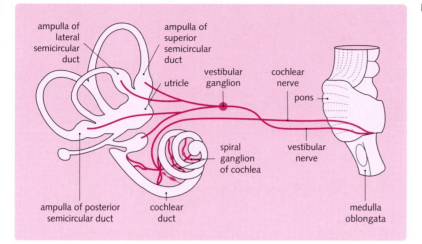

Fig. 7.44 Vestibulocochlear nerve.

Labels on figure:
ampulla of lateral semicircular duct
ampulla of superior semicircular duct
utricle
vestibular ganglion
cochlear nerve
pons
spiral ganglion of cochlea
vestibular nerve
ampulla of posterior semicircular duct
cochlear duct
medulla oblongata

Vestibulocochlear nerve (VIII)

Near the lateral end of the internal auditory meatus this nerve divides into an anterior cochlear nerve (hearing) and a posterior vestibular nerve (balance) (Fig. 7.44). The vestibular nerve enlarges to form the vestibular ganglion, and its fibres supply receptors in the semicircular ducts, the saccule and the utricle. The cochlear nerve forms the spiral ganglion and supplies the spiral organ.

Facial nerve in the temporal bone

The facial nerve (VII) and its sensory root—the nervus intermedius—enter the internal auditory meatus together with the vestibulocochlear nerve. The two roots fuse and enter the facial canal to pass above the internal ear to reach the medial wall of the middle ear. The nerve then turns sharply posteriorly above the promontory (the sensory geniculate ganglion lies at this sharp bend) and passes posteriorly to the posterior wall, where it turns downwards to leave the temporal bone through the stylomastoid foramen.

Branches in the temporal bone

Branches in the temporal bone comprise:

- The greater petrosal nerve – branches off at the geniculate ganglion and enters the middle cranial fossa. It is joined by the deep petrosal nerve (sympathetic) to form the nerve of the pterygoid canal.
- The nerve to stapedius.
- The chorda tympani. This is given off just above the stylomastoid foramen. It passes to the lateral wall of the middle ear, crosses the deep surface of the tympanic membrane, and enters a canal leading to the petrotympanic fissure. It joins the lingual nerve in the infratemporal fossa.

THE SOFT TISSUES OF THE NECK

The neck is the region between the head and the thorax.

Fascial layers of the neck

The fascial layers of the neck are illustrated in Figure 7.45.

Superficial fascia

The superficial fascia is a thin layer that encloses the platysma muscle. The cutaneous nerves, superficial vessels and superficial lymph nodes lie in the fascia.

Deep fascia

The deep fascia lies beneath the superficial fascia. It condenses to form the following:

Investing layer of deep cervical fascia

This completely encircles the neck, splitting to enclose the sternocleidomastoid and trapezius muscles. Posteriorly it is attached to the ligamentum nuchae. Superiorly, it is attached to the lower border of the mandible, the zygomatic arch and the base of the skull. It splits to enclose the parotid and submandibular glands and attaches to the hyoid.

Inferiorly the fascia is attached to the acromion, clavicle and sternum. It attaches to the anterior and

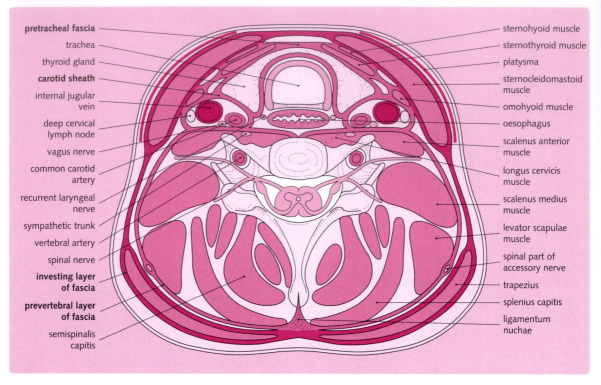

Fig. 7.45 Fascial layers of the neck.

posterior borders of the manubrium to form the suprasternal space, containing the jugular arch.

Pretracheal fascia

The pretracheal fascia is attached superiorly to the thyroid and cricoid cartilages. Inferiorly, it enters the thorax to blend with the fibrous pericardium. Laterally, it blends with the carotid sheath. It encloses the thyroid and parathyroid glands, and lies deep to the infrahyoid muscles.

Prevertebral fascia

This fascia covers the vertebral column and its associated muscles (Fig 7.45), attaching posteriorly to the ligamentum nuchae. It forms the axillary sheath around the axillary artery and brachial plexus. Superiorly, it is attached to the base of the skull, and inferiorly it enters the thorax to blend with the anterior longitudinal ligament of the vertebral column. The retropharyngeal space lies between the prevertebral fascia and the pharynx, extending down into the thorax.

Carotid sheath

The carotid sheath is a condensation of the fascia surrounding the common and internal carotid arteries, the internal jugular vein, the deep cervical chain of nodes, and the vagus nerve. It extends from the base of the skull to the root of the neck.

Posterior triangle of the neck

The inferior belly of omohyoid divides the posterior triangle into a large occipital triangle and a small supraclavicular triangle (Fig. 7.46).

The margins and contents of the posterior triangle are detailed in Figures 7.47 and 7.48, respectively.

Figure 7.49 outlines the muscles on the lateral aspect of the neck.

Infection in fascial planes of the neck

Abscess formation behind the prevertebral fascia can extend laterally in the neck, forming a swelling posterior to the sternocleidomastoid muscle. If it pierces the fascia anteriorly it enters the retropharyngeal space and can narrow the pharynx, causing difficulties in swallowing (dysphagia) and speaking (dysarthria) before spreading into the superior mediastinum anterior to the pericardium.

Fig. 7.46 Posterior triangle of the neck.

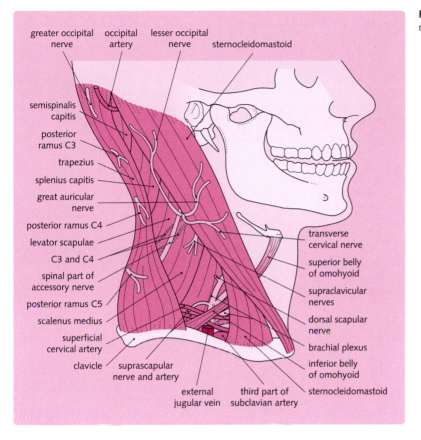

Labels on figure:
- greater occipital nerve
- occipital artery
- lesser occipital nerve
- sternocleidomastoid
- semispinalis capitis
- posterior ramus C3
- trapezius
- splenius capitis
- great auricular nerve
- posterior ramus C4
- levator scapulae
- C3 and C4
- spinal part of accessory nerve
- posterior ramus C5
- scalenus medius
- superficial cervical artery
- clavicle
- suprascapular nerve and artery
- external jugular vein
- third part of subclavian artery
- transverse cervical nerve
- superior belly of omohyoid
- supraclavicular nerves
- dorsal scapular nerve
- brachial plexus
- inferior belly of omohyoid
- sternocleidomastoid

Fig. 7.47 Margins of the posterior triangle

Margin	Components
Anterior	Posterior border of sternocleidomastoid
Posterior	Anterior border of trapezius
Inferior	Middle third of clavicle
Roof	Skin, superficial fascia, platysma, investing layer of deep fascia
Floor	Prevertebral fascia over prevertebral muscle

Fig. 7.48 Contents of the posterior triangle

Structure	Origin
Third part of subclavian artery	Enters anterior inferior angle of triangle
Superficial cervical artery	Branch of thyrocervical trunk of subclavian artery
Suprascapular artery	Branch of thyrocervical trunk
Brachial plexus	Roots of plexus enter posterior triangle by emerging between scalenus anterior and medius; trunks and divisions also lie in posterior triangle before entering the axilla
Accessory nerve	Spinal part of accessory nerve enters posterior triangle by emerging from deep to posterior border of sternocleidomastoid
Cervical plexus	The four cutaneous branches emerge from posterior border of sternocleidomastoid

Congenital torticollis

A fibrous tumour that develops in sternocleidomastoid before birth shortens the muscle, turning the head to one side. This awkward position requires a delivery by C-section.

Fig. 7.49 Major muscles of the lateral aspect of the neck

Name of muscle (nerve supply)	Origin	Insertion	Action
Platysma (VII nerve)	Inferior border of mandible; skin and subcutaneous tissues of lower part of the face	Fascia covering superior parts of pectoralis major and deltoid muscles	Used to express sadness and fright by pulling angles of mouth down
Sternocleidomastoid [XI nerve (spinal part), C2, C3]	Anterior surface of manubrium of sternum; medial third of clavicle	Mastoid process of temporal bone and superior nuchal line	Individually each muscle laterally flexes neck and rotates it so face is turned upwards toward opposite side; both muscles act together to flex neck
Trapezius [XI nerve (spinal part), C2, C3]	Superior nuchal line; external occipital protuberance; ligamentum nuchae; spinous processes of C7–T12 vertebrae	Lateral third of clavicle; acromion; spine of scapula	Elevates, retracts, and rotates scapula

Fig. 7.50 Branches of the cervical plexus.

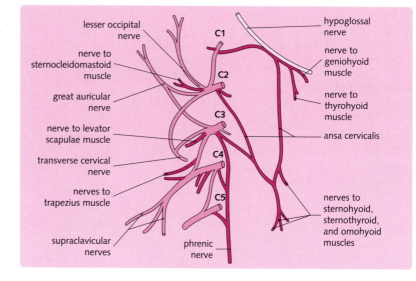

Cervical plexus

The cervical plexus (Fig. 7.50) is formed by the anterior rami of C1–C4 spinal nerves in the substance of the prevertebral muscles. It is covered by the prevertebral fascia and is related to the internal jugular vein in the carotid sheath.

External jugular vein

The external jugular vein is formed by the posterior auricular vein and the posterior division of the retromandibular vein behind the angle of the mandible. It crosses sternocleidomastoid and pierces the deep fascia just above the clavicle in the posterior triangle to enter the subclavian vein.

Anterior triangle of the neck

The anterior triangle is formed by the anterior border of sternocleidomastoid muscle, the midline of the neck, and the inferior border of the mandible. It is subdivided by the anterior and posterior bellies of digastric and the superior belly of omohyoid into the digastric (submandibular), carotid, and muscular

Fig. 7.51 Contents of the anterior triangle of the neck

Triangle	Main contents
Carotid	External carotid artery; larynx and pharynx, and internal and external laryngeal nerves
Muscular	Sternothyroid and sternohyoid muscles, superior belly of omohyoid; thyroid gland, trachea, and oesophagus
Digastric (submandibular)	Submandibular gland and lymph nodes; facial artery and vein; external carotid artery; internal carotid artery, internal jugular vein, glossopharyngeal (IX), vagus (X), and hypoglossal (XII) nerves
Submental	Submental lymph nodes

triangles. The boundaries and contents of these triangles are shown in Figures 7.51 and 7.52. More detail on the muscles is in Figure 7.53.

Vessels of the anterior triangle

Common carotid artery

The left common carotid artery arises from the aortic arch, the right from the brachiocephalic trunk. Both ascend in the neck deep to the sternocleidomastoid muscle from behind the sternoclavicular joint. At the upper border of the thyroid cartilage (level of C3) the arteries divide into the external and internal carotids (Fig. 7.54).

At the terminal part of the common carotid artery (the origin of the internal carotid artery) there is a dilatation, the carotid sinus. This contains baroreceptors that respond to changes in arterial pressure.

The carotid body is embedded in the tunica adventitia of the artery. It contains chemoreceptors that monitor blood carbon dioxide levels.

Both the carotid sinus and the carotid body are innervated by the carotid sinus branch of the glossopharyngeal nerve.

The common carotid pulse can be palpated at the upper border of the thyroid cartilage (C3, C4 vertebral levels), anterior to the sternocleidomastoid muscle.

External carotid artery

This commences at the upper border of the thyroid cartilage and ascends to enter the parotid. Its branches are:

- Ascending pharyngeal (to the pharynx).
- Superior thyroid (to the superior pole of the thyroid).
- Lingual (passes to the tongue with an upwards loop).
- Facial (loops over the submandibular gland to pass to the face).
- Occipital.
- Posterior auricular.
- Superficial temporal.
- Maxillary.

Internal carotid artery

This artery commences at the upper border of the thyroid cartilage and ascends in the carotid sheath to the carotid canal in the base of the skull. It supplies the cerebral hemispheres and the orbital contents.

It has no branches in the neck, unlike the external carotid.

Internal jugular vein

This vein commences at the end of the sigmoid sinus, leaving the cranial cavity through the jugular foramen. It descends through the neck in the carotid sheath, at first posterior then lateral to the carotid artery. It unites with the subclavian vein to form the brachiocephalic vein behind the sternoclavicular joint.

The vein has dilatations at its upper and lower ends—the superior and inferior bulbs.

Tributaries include the inferior petrosal sinus and the facial, pharyngeal, lingual and superior and middle thyroid veins.

Deep cervical nodes

These nodes form a chain along the internal jugular vein in the carotid sheath. They drain the entire head and neck. Efferent vessels join to form the jugular lymph trunk, which in turn drains into the

Central line

The internal jugular vein may be cannulated to measure blood pressure or administer drugs. Palpate the common carotid artery and aim a needle towards the apex of a triangle formed by the sternal and clavicular heads of sternocleidomastoid, angled at 30° in an inferolateral direction.

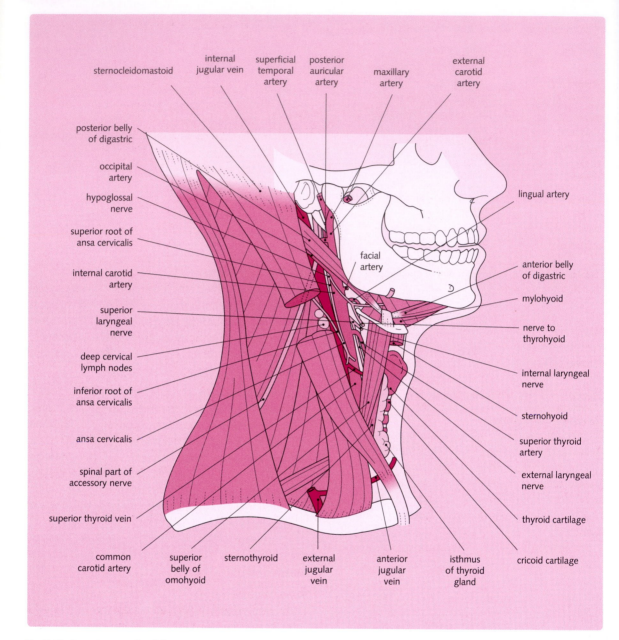

Fig. 7.52 Anterior triangle of the neck.

thoracic duct, right lymph duct, or subclavian trunk (see Fig. 7.15).

Nerves of the triangles of the neck

All the following nerves (except the accessory nerve) are found in the anterior triangle:

Glossopharyngeal nerve (IX)
This nerve emerges from the jugular foramen between the carotid arteries and passes lateral to stylopharyngeus, which it supplies. It gives a branch to the carotid body then passes between the superior and middle constrictors to supply sensory and taste fibres to the posterior third of the tongue and oropharynx.

Vagus nerve (X)
The vagus exits the skull through the jugular foramen, where its superior and inferior sensory ganglia lie. Below the superior ganglion the cranial part of the

Fig. 7.53 Suprahyoid and infrahyoid muscles. (Adapted from *Anatomy as a Basis for Clinical Medicine*, by E C B Hall-Craggs, Williams & Wilkins.)

Suprahyoid muscles			
Name of muscle (nerve supply)	Origin	Insertion	Action
Posterior belly of digastric (VII nerve)	Mastoid process	Intermediate tendon bound to hyoid bone	Depresses mandible and elevates hyoid bone
Anterior belly of digastric (inferior alveolar V_3 nerve)	Lower border of mandible near midline	Intermediate tendon bound to hyoid bone	Depresses mandible and elevates hyoid bone
Stylohyoid (VII nerve)	Styloid process of temporal bone	Body of hyoid bone	Elevates hyoid bone
Mylohyoid (inferior alveolar V_3 nerve)	Mylohyoid line on medial surface of mandible	Body of hyoid bone and mylohyoid raphe	Elevates floor of mouth and hyoid bone, and depresses mandible
Geniohyoid (C1 through XII nerve)	Inferior mental spine	Body of hyoid bone	Elevates hyoid bone and depresses mandible
Infrahyoid muscles			
Name of muscle (nerve supply)	Origin	Insertion	Action
Sternohyoid (ansa cervicalis C1–C3)	Manubrium sterni and clavicle	Body of hyoid bone	Depresses hyoid bone
Sternothyroid (ansa cervicalis C1–C3)	Manubrium sterni	Oblique line on lamina of thyroid cartilage	Depresses larynx
Thyrohyoid (C1 through XII nerve)	Oblique line on lamina of thyroid cartilage	Body of hyoid bone	Depresses hyoid bone and elevates larynx
Omohyoid–inferior belly (ansa cervicalis C1–C3)	Upper margin of scapula	Intermediate tendon bound to clavicle and first rib	Depresses hyoid bone
Omohyoid–superior belly (ansa cervicalis C1–C3)	Body of hyoid bone	Intermediate tendon bound to clavicle and first rib	Depresses hyoid bone

CN XI is the nerve of twos: it has two roots, passes through two foraminae and its spinal root supplies two muscles.

accessory nerve joins the vagus, to be distributed on pharyngeal and recurrent laryngeal nerves (Fig. 7.55). The vagus descends in the neck in the carotid sheath between the internal carotid artery and internal jugular vein. At the root of the neck it passes anterior to the first part of the subclavian artery to enter the thorax.

Accessory nerve (XI)

The spinal part of the accessory nerve arises from the upper five or six cervical segments and ascends to enter the skull via the foramen magnum. It joins the cranial root from the medulla oblongata and they exit the skull via the jugular foramen.

The cranial root joins the vagus; the spinal root supplies sternocleidomastoid and trapezius – it enters the posterior triangle one-third down the posterior border of sternocleidomastoid and leaves it one-third way up the anterior border of trapezius.

Hypoglossal nerve (XII)

This emerges from the hypoglossal canal then descends in the neck between the internal carotid artery and internal jugular vein. At the lower border of digastric the nerve loops around the occipital artery, passing lateral to internal and external carotid arteries

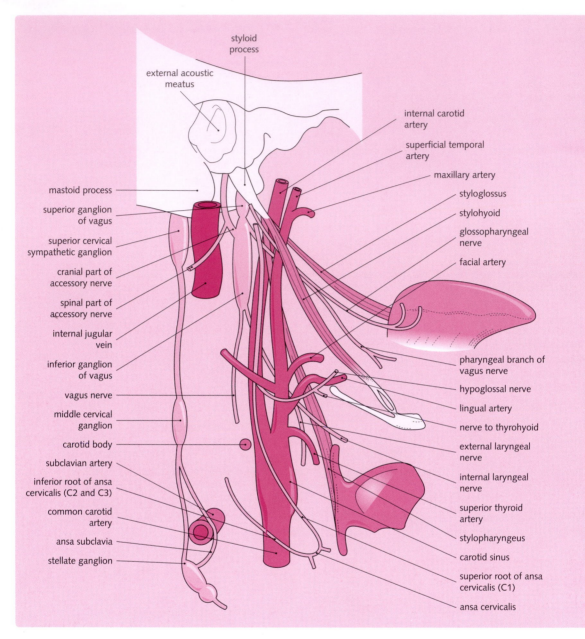

Fig. 7.54 The common carotid artery and the lower cranial nerves. (Adapted from *Clinical Anatomy For Medical Students*, 4th edn, by R S Snell. Little Brown & Co.)

to enter the submandibular region. It is motor to tongue muscles.

The nerve is joined by fibres of C1. Some of these are given off in the superior root of the ansa cervicalis, others pass to thyrohyoid and geniohyoid.

Ansa cervicalis

This nerve loop is formed from a superior root of C1 fibres travelling along the XII nerve and an inferior root from C2 and C3. It supplies omohyoid, sternohyoid and sternothyroid.

Sympathetic trunk

The trunk lies deep in the neck, between the carotid sheath and prevertebral fascia. It has superior, middle and inferior ganglia. The inferior ganglion usually fuses with the first thoracic ganglion to form the stellate ganglion. Postganglionic fibres form plexuses around

Fig. 7.55 Branches of the vagus nerve

Branch	Course and distribution
Meningeal branch	Dura mater of posterior cranial fossa
Auricular branch	Medial surface of auricle, external auditory meatus, and adjacent tympanic membrane
Pharyngeal branch	Contains motor fibres from XI nerve (cranial part); combines with pharyngeal branches of IX nerve (sensory fibres) to form pharyngeal plexus, which supplies all pharyngeal muscles except stylopharyngeus (IX) and all soft-palate muscles except tensor veli palatini (V_3)
Superior laryngeal nerve divides into internal and external laryngeal nerves	Internal laryngeal nerve is sensory to piriform fossa and mucosa of larynx above vocal folds; external laryngeal nerve is motor to cricothyroid muscle
Cardiac branches	Assist in forming cardiac plexus in thorax
Right recurrent laryngeal nerve	Arises from X nerve as it crosses subclavian artery; hooks backwards and upwards behind artery and ascends in a groove between trachea and oesophagus; supplies all laryngeal muscles (except cricothyroid) and laryngeal mucosa below vocal folds, trachea, and oesophagus
Left recurrent laryngeal nerve	Arises from X nerve as it crosses aortic arch; hooks beneath arch behind ligamentum arteriosum and passes into neck between trachea and oesophagus; has a similar distribution to right nerve

All sympathetic fibres to the head and neck are carried on blood vessel plexuses.

the major arteries to supply the structures of the head and neck. The trunks also give off cardiac branches.

MIDLINE STRUCTURES OF THE FACE AND NECK

Pharynx

The pharynx is a C-shaped fibromuscular tube lying behind the nasal cavity (nasopharynx), oral cavity (oropharynx), and larynx (laryngopharynx). It extends from the base of the skull to the inferior border of the cricoid cartilage (C6 vertebral level), where it is continuous with the oesophagus. There are three layers in the pharyngeal wall:

- The muscular layer is formed by the pharyngeal constrictors and longitudinal muscles (Figs 7.56 and 7.57). The constrictors sit inside each other like a series of cups.

Horner's syndrome

A cervical sympathetic trunk lesion results in ipsilateral papillary constriction, ptosis (eyelid drooping due to levator palpabrae superioris paralysis), facial and neck vasodilation, and lack of sweating. This is due to an interrupted sympathetic nerve supply and can be caused by an apical lung tumour invading the sympathetic chain at the neck of the first rib.

- The pharyngobasilar fascia separates the mucosa and the muscle layer. It blends with the periosteum of the base of the skull.
- The mucous membrane (Fig. 7.58).

Nasopharynx

The nasopharynx lies behind the nasal cavity above the soft palate. During swallowing, the soft palate elevates and the pharyngeal wall is pulled forward to form a seal, preventing food entering the nasopharynx. The pharyngeal tonsil (adenoid) lies in the posterior wall. The auditory tubes open at tubal elevations in the lateral wall – these also contain tonsillar tissue (the

Fig. 7.56 Muscles of the pharynx

Name of muscle (nerve supply)	Origin	Insertion	Action
Superior constrictor (pharyngeal plexus)	Medial pterygoid plate, pterygoid hamulus, pterygomandibular raphe, mylohyoid line of mandible	Pharyngeal tubercle of occipital bone, midline pharyngeal raphe	Assists in separating oro- and nasopharynx and propels food bolus downward
Middle constrictor (pharyngeal plexus)	Stylohyoid ligament, lesser and greater cornua of hyoid bone	Pharyngeal raphe	Propels food bolus downward
Inferior constrictor (pharyngeal plexus)			
Thyropharyngeus	Lamina of thyroid cartilage	Pharyngeal raphe	Propels food bolus downward
Cricopharyngeus	Cricoid cartilage	Contralateral cricopharyngeus	Upper oesophageal sphincter
Palatopharyngeus (pharyngeal plexus)	Palatine aponeurosis Horizontal plate of palatine bone	Thyroid cartilage	Elevates pharyngeal wall and pulls palatopharyngeal folds medially
Salpingopharyngeus (pharyngeal plexus)	Auditory tube	Merges with palatopharyngeus	Elevates pharynx and larynx
Stylopharyngeus (IX)	Styloid process of temporal bone	Thyroid cartilage	Elevates larynx during swallowing

Fig. 7.57 Muscles of the pharynx.

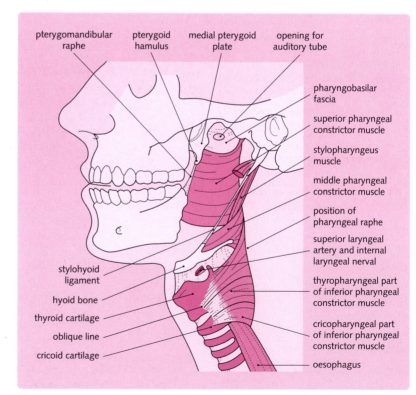

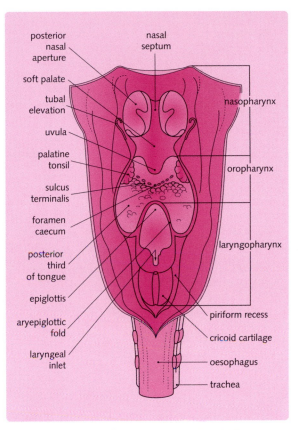

Fig. 7.58 Mucous membrane and the interior of the pharynx.

Pharyngeal pouch

Pharyngeal mucosa can bulge between the thyropharyngeus and cricopharyngeal muscles to form a pharyngeal pouch (Killian's dehiscence). As it enlarges, it pushes the oesophagus to one side, resulting in severe dysphagia (difficulty swallowing) and the possibility of foodstuffs being regurgitated into the lungs, causing infection. Treatment is surgical.

tubal tonsils). The tubal recess is a small depression in the lateral wall behind the tubal elevation. Anteriorly the nasopharynx is continuous with the nasal cavity through choanae and bordered by the soft palate, inferiorly.

Oropharynx

The oropharynx lies between the soft palate and the upper border of the epiglottis, behind the oral cavity. The palatine tonsils lie in its lateral walls. The posterior third of the tongue forms the anterior

wall of the oropharynx – it has an irregular surface owing to the presence of the underlying lingual tonsils.

The mucosa is reflected from the base of the tongue onto the epiglottis to form a median and two lateral glossoepiglottic folds with two pouches – valleculae – lying in between them.

Laryngopharynx

The laryngopharynx lies behind the laryngeal opening and the posterior surface of the larynx.

The piriform fossae are grooves on either side of the laryngeal inlet that direct food from the back of the tongue to the oesophagus.

Vessels of the pharynx

Blood supply is from branches of the ascending pharyngeal, ascending palatine, facial, maxillary and lingual arteries.

Veins drain via the pharyngeal venous plexus to the internal jugular vein.

Lymphatics drain into the deep cervical nodes either directly or indirectly via the retropharyngeal or paratracheal nodes.

Nerve supply of the pharynx

The motor nerve supply to the pharynx is the cranial part of XI via X and the pharyngeal plexus.

The sensory nerve supply is as follows:

- nasopharynx—maxillary nerve (V_2);
- oropharynx—IX nerve;
- laryngopharynx—internal laryngeal nerve (X).

Nose

The nose consists of:

- The external nose—this has a bony (nasal bones, frontal process of the maxilla) and cartilaginous skeleton, separated by the nasal septum.
- The nasal cavities—these communicate with the exterior via the nares or nostrils, and with the nasopharynx via the choanae.

Nasal cavity

The walls of the nasal cavity are listed in Figure 7.59. The openings in the lateral wall are listed in Figure 7.60. The nerve and blood supply of the lateral wall are illustrated in Figure 7.61.

Fig. 7.59 Walls of the nasal cavity

Surface	Components
Floor	Palatine process of maxilla, horizontal process of palatine bone— i.e. the hard palate
Roof	Nasal, frontal, sphenoid, and ethmoid bones; above lies the anterior cranial fossa and the sphenoidal sinus
Lateral wall	Maxillary, palatine, sphenoid, lacrimal, and ethmoid bones and the inferior concha; the superior and middle conchae are projections of the ethmoid bone; the superior, middle and inferior meatus Lie beneath their respective conchae; sphenoethmoidal recess lies above the superior concha
Medial wall (nasal septum)	The perpendicular plate of the ethmoid, the vomer and the septal cartilage

Fig. 7.60 Openings in the lateral wall of the nose

Region of lateral wall	Features and openings
Sphenoethmoidal recess	Sphenoidal sinus
Superior meatus	Posterior ethmoidal air cells
Middle meatus	The hiatus semilunaris lies below the middle concha; the frontal sinus, anterior ethmoidal cells, and maxillary sinus open into the hiatus; the bulla ethmoidalis is formed by the underlying middle ethmoidal cells which open onto it
Inferior meatus	Nasolacrimal duct

Paranasal sinuses

The paranasal sinuses lie around the nasal cavity, in the bones of the face and skull.

- Maxillary – lying laterally within the maxilla.
- Ethmoidal – lying medially within the ethmoid.
- Frontal – lying directly behind the forehead in the frontal bone.
- Sphenoidal – lying posterosuperiorly within the sphenoid. It is a direct relation of the pituitary and allows surgical access to it.

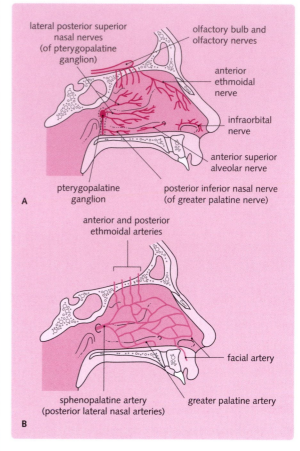

Fig. 7.61 Nerve (A) and blood (B) supplies of the lateral wall of the nose.

Mucous membrane of the nose

The vestibule lies just inside the anterior nares and is lined by hairy skin. The remainder of the nasal cavity is lined by ciliated columnar epithelium. There is a rich vascular plexus in the submucosa, together with numerous serous and mucous glands.

Dust from the inspired air is removed by the nasal hairs and the mucus of the nasal cavity. The air is also warmed by the vascular plexus and moistened before it enters the lower airway.

The roof and superior part of the lateral wall contain olfactory epithelium, which receives the distal processes of the olfactory nerve cells. These fibres play a role in both smell and taste sensations.

The sphenopalatine artery anastomoses with the septal branch of the superior labial artery around the vestibule of the nose.

Fig. 7.62 Communications of the pterygopalatine fossa

Surface	Communicates with
Lateral	Infratemporal fossa
Medial	Nasal cavity via the sphenopalatine foramen; hard palate via palatine canal
Anterior	Orbit via the inferior orbital fissure
Posterosuperior	Middle cranial fossa via the foramen rotundum and pterygoid canal
Posteromedial	Nasopharynx via palatovaginal canal

Pterygopalatine fossa

The pterygopalatine fossa is a small pyramidal space lying inferior to the apex of the orbit. It contains the terminal branches of the maxillary artery, the maxillary nerve, the nerve of the pterygoid canal, and the pterygopalatine ganglion. The communications of the fossa are listed in Figure 7.62.

Pterygopalatine ganglion

The pterygopalatine ganglion is a parasympathetic ganglion lying in the pterygopalatine fossa, just lateral to the sphenopalatine foramen. It is suspended from the maxillary nerve (V_2).

Preganglionic parasympathetic fibres from the superior salivary nucleus of the facial nerve enter the greater petrosal nerve. This joins the deep petrosal (sympathetic) nerve to form the nerve of the pterygoid canal, which joins the ganglion. Here, the parasympathetic fibres synapse and sympathetic fibres (from the deep petrosal branch of the carotid plexus) pass uninterrupted through the ganglion. Fibres of common sensation enter the ganglion via ganglionic branches of the maxillary nerve.

The branches of the ganglion are shown in Figure 7.63.

Fig. 7.63 Branches of the pterygopalatine ganglion

Branch	Course and distribution
Nasopalatine nerve	Passes through the sphenopalatine foramen to supply the nasal septum and incisive gum of the hard palate
Lateral posterior superior nasal nerve	Exits via the sphenopalatine foramen to supply the lateral wall of the nose
Greater palatine nerve	Passes through the greater palatine canal and foramen to supply the mucosa of the palate and the lateral wall of the nose
Lesser palatine nerve	Exits through the lesser palatine foramina to supply the soft palate and the mucosa over the palatine tonsil
Pharyngeal nerve	Passes via the palatovaginal canal to supply the nasopharynx
Lacrimal fibres	Parasympathetic fibres to the lacrimal gland join the zygomaticotemporal nerve of V_2 then the lacrimal nerve before supplying the gland

The pterygopalatine ganglion supplies the lacrimal gland, nasal cavity, nasopharynx, paranasal air sinuses and palate, so is 'The Ganglion of Hayfever'.

Branches of the maxillary nerve in the pterygopalatine fossa

- Infraorbital nerve—carries secretomotor fibres to the lacrimal gland.
- Zygomatic nerve—divides into zygomaticotemporal and zygomaticofacial branches.
- Posterior superior alveolar nerve.

Oral cavity

The oral cavity is divided into two parts:

The vestibule lies between the lips and cheeks externally and the gums and teeth internally.

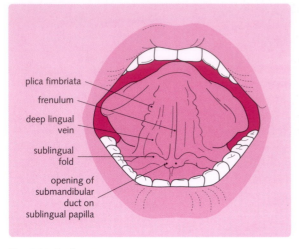

Fig. 7.64 Oral cavity.

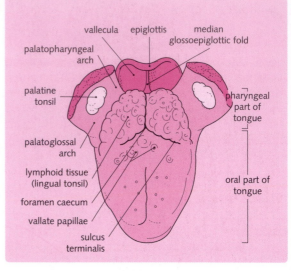

Fig. 7.65 Tongue.

The oral cavity proper is bounded by the teeth and gums anteriorly and laterally. The palate forms the roof; the floor is formed by the anterior two thirds of the tongue and the floor of the mouth. A midline fold of mucosa—the frenulum—lies beneath the tongue (Fig. 7.64).

The parotid, submandibular, sublingual and numerous minor salivary glands open into the oral cavity.

Nerve supply is as follows:

- Roof—greater and lesser palatine and nasopalatine nerves.
- Floor—lingual nerve.
- Cheek—buccal nerve (from V_3).

Folds of mucosa over the palatoglossus and palatopharyngeus muscle posteriorly form the palatoglossal and palatopharyngeal arches.

Lips

The lips seal the oral cavity and assist in speech. They are covered by mucosa internally and by skin externally. The orbicularis oris muscle, the superior and inferior labial vessels and nerves, and numerous minor salivary glands lie in the substance of the lips.

Tongue

The tongue is a mobile muscular organ covered by mucous membrane. The anterior two thirds lie in the mouth, the posterior third in the oropharynx (Fig. 7.65). A fibrous median septum runs from anterior to posterior.

The intrinsic muscles of the tongue are listed in Figure 7.66. They create an intermuscular cleft between mylohyoid externally and the muscles of the tongue internally, containing several structures.

Mucous membrane of the tongue

The sulcus terminalis divides the tongue into the anterior two thirds and the posterior third. It is V-shaped, the foramen caecum lying at its apex. It is the remnant of the upper end of the thyroglossal duct. Between 10 and 12 vallate papillae lie anterior to the sulcus.

The mucosa of the anterior two thirds of the tongue is relatively smooth, and it has numerous filiform and fungiform papillae on the dorsal surface. Lateral folds of mucosa, the plica fimbriata, are seen on the ventral surface of the tongue.

The irregular surface of the posterior third of the tongue is caused by the underlying lingual tonsils.

Blood and nerve supply to the tongue

Vessels of the tongue comprise the lingual arteries and veins.

Lymphatic drainage is to the deep cervical, the submandibular, and the submental nodes. The nerve supply to the tongue is shown in Figure 7.67.

Remember, the XII nerve is motor to all the muscles of the tongue except palatoglossus (pharyngeal plexus).

Fig. 7.66 Muscles of the tongue

Intrinsic muscles			
Name of muscle (nerve supply)	**Origin**	**Insertion**	**Action**
Longitudinal (XII nerve)	Mucous membrane	Mucous membrane	Shortens tongue
Transverse (XII nerve)	Mucous membrane and median septum	Mucous membrane	Narrows tongue
Vertical (XII nerve)	Mucous membrane	Mucous membrane	Lowers tongue
Extrinsic muscles			
Name of muscle (nerve supply)	**Origin**	**Insertion**	**Action**
Palatoglossus (pharyngeal plexus)	Palatine aponeurosis	Lateral aspect of tongue	Pulls tongue upward and backward and narrows oropharyngeal isthmus
Genioglossus (XII nerve)	Superior mental spine (genial tubercle) of mandible	Merges with other tongue muscles	Draws tongue forward and pulls tip backward
Hyoglossus (XII nerve)	Body and greater cornu of hyoid bone	Merges with other tongue muscles	Depresses tongue
Styloglossus (XII nerve)	Styloid process of temporal bone	Merges with other tongue muscles	Draws tongue upward and backward

Fig. 7.67 Nerve supply to the tongue

	Posterior third	**Anterior two thirds**
General sensory	Glossopharyngeal nerve (IX)	Lingual nerve (V$_3$)
Taste	Glossopharyngeal nerve (IX) (also vallate papillae)	Chorda tympani (VII) (via the lingual nerve)

Tongue carcinoma

Carcinoma of the tongue may spread via the lymphatics to both sides of the neck (lymphatics cross the midline), dramatically worsening its prognosis.

Floor of the mouth and submandibular region

This region lies between the mandible and hyoid bone. It contains the following:

- Muscles—digastric, mylohyoid, hyoglossus, geniohyoid, genioglossus, and styloglossus.
- Salivary glands—submandibular and sublingual.
- Nerves—lingual, glossopharyngeal, and hypoglossal; submandibular ganglion.
- Blood vessels—facial and lingual.
- Lymph nodes—submandibular.

Lingual nerve

From the mandibular third-molar region, the lingual nerve passes across styloglossus to the lateral surface of hyoglossus and across the submandibular duct, branching to supply the mucosa of the tongue.

Hypoglossal nerve

The hypoglossal nerve runs forward below the deep part of the submandibular gland, the submandibular duct, and the lingual nerve. It supplies all the muscles of the tongue except palatoglossus.

Submandibular gland

This consists of two parts—a large superficial part and a small deep part—that are continuous around the posterior border of mylohyoid. The deep part of the gland lies in the intramuscular cleft.

Blood supply is from the facial and lingual arteries. Nerve supply is from the submandibular ganglion, a parasympathetic ganglion with the following features:

- Preganglionic parasympathetic fibres from the facial (VII) nerve pass to the ganglion via the nervus intermedius, the chorda tympani, and the lingual nerve.
- Sympathetic and sensory fibres from the superior cervical ganglion and the lingual nerve pass through the ganglion.
- Postganglionic parasympathetic secretomotor fibres pass to the submandibular and sublingual glands via the lingual nerve or directly.

The submandibular ducts open onto the sublingual papillae on either side of the frenulum of the tongue.

Sublingual gland

The sublingual gland lies superficially under the sublingual fold extending back from the sublingual papilla under the tongue. Numerous short ducts open onto the fold. The lingual nerve and submandibular duct lie medially. It is supplied by the submandibular ganglion.

Palate and tonsils

The palate forms the roof of the mouth and the floor of the nose. It is divided into two components:

- The hard palate is composed of the palatine process of the maxilla and the horizontal process of the palatine bone. It is covered by mucous membrane.
- The soft palate is a mobile fibromuscular fold lying posteriorly. It is composed of muscles (Fig. 7.68) and the palatine aponeurosis—the expanded tendon of tensor veli palatini.

Blood supply to the palate is from the greater and lesser palatine arteries. Nerve supply is from the pterygopalatine ganglion.

The palatine tonsils are masses of lymphoid tissue lying in the tonsillar fossae between the palatoglossal and palatopharyngeal arches, covered by mucous membrane. The surface is pitted by many openings that lead to the tonsillar crypts. Lymphatics drain to the deep cervical nodes.

The four sets of tonsils (tubal, pharyngeal, lingual and palatine) form a ring of lymphoid tissue around the oropharynx – Waldeyer's ring.

Fig. 7.68 Muscles of the soft palate			
Name of muscle (nerve supply)	**Origin**	**Insertion**	**Action**
Tensor veli palatini (nerve to medial pterygoid V_3)	Spine of sphenoid, auditory tube, scaphoid fossa of pterygoid process	With muscle of other side, forms palatine aponeurosis	Tenses soft palate
Levator veli palatini (pharyngeal plexus)	Petrous part of temporal bone, auditory tube	Palatine aponeurosis	Elevates soft palate
Musculus uvulae (pharyngeal plexus)	Posterior border of hard palate	Mucous membrane of uvula	Elevates uvula
Palatopharyngeus (pharyngeal plexus)	Palatine aponeurosis horizontal plate of palatine bone	Posterior border of thyroid cartilage	Elevates pharyngeal wall and pulls palatopharyngeal folds medially and depresses soft palate
Palatoglossus (pharyngeal plexus)	Palatine aponeurosis	Lateral aspect of tongue	Pulls tongue upward and backward and narrows oropharyngeal isthmus and depresses soft palate

Larynx

The larynx is continuous with the laryngopharynx superiorly and with the trachea inferiorly at the level of C6. It acts as a sphincter, separating the lower respiratory system from the alimentary system, and is responsible for voice production.

The laryngeal cartilages are shown in Figure 7.69. The laryngeal membranes link these cartilages together, and join the larynx to the hyoid bone and the trachea (Fig. 7.70). The membranes thicken in places to form ligaments.

Mucous membrane of the larynx

The mucosa is tucked under the vestibular ligament to form the laryngeal ventricle between the vestibular ('false vocal') and vocal folds. Above the vocal fold the mucosa is supplied by the internal laryngeal nerve and the superior laryngeal artery. Below the vocal fold it is supplied by the recurrent laryngeal nerve and the inferior laryngeal artery (from the inferior thyroid artery).

Laryngeal cavity

The laryngeal inlet allows communication between the pharynx and the larynx. It is bounded by the epiglottis and the aryepiglottic and interarytenoid folds (Fig. 7.71).

The inlet leads to the vestibule, which extends to the vestibular folds. The laryngeal ventricle lies between the vestibular and vocal folds. The rima glottis is the space between the vocal folds. The infraglottic cavity lies below the vocal folds and is continuous with the trachea.

Intrinsic muscles of the larynx

The intrinsic muscles of the larynx are described in Figure 7.72. All intrinsic muscles are paired except the transverse arytenoid muscle. They can alter the tension and length of the vocal folds and the size and shape of the rima glottis (see Fig. 7.73).

Joints of the larynx

The synovial cricothyroid joint is formed by the inferior cornu (horn) of the thyroid cartilage articulating with the facet of the cricoid cartilage, allowing one cartilage to tilt backward and forwards on the other. This alters the vocal fold tension and length.

The synovial cricoarytenoid joint has a lax capsule. This allows rotation and gliding movements of the arytenoid cartilages upon the cricoid cartilage. These movements widen or narrow a V-shaped rima glottis.

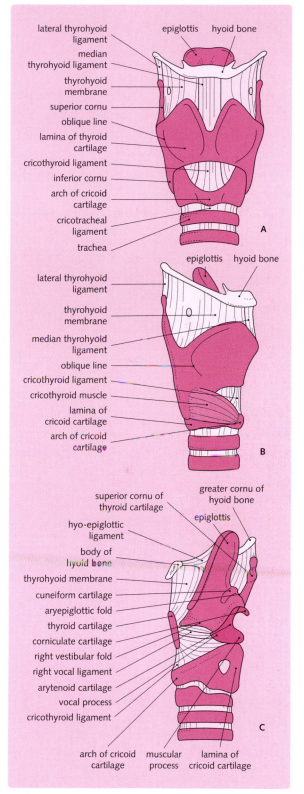

Fig. 7.69 Laryngeal cartilages from the front (A), from the right (B), and from the left without the left lamina of thyroid cartilage (C).

All intrinsic muscles are supplied by the recurrent laryngeal nerve except for the cricothyroid muscle, which is supplied by the external laryngeal nerve.

Fig. 7.70 Laryngeal membranes

Membrane	Attachments
Thyrohyoid	Runs between the thyroid cartilage and hyoid bone; has a midline thickening and two lateral thickenings, the median thyrohyoid ligament and lateral thyrohyoid ligaments, respectively
Quadrangular	Runs between the epiglottis and the arytenoid cartilage; its lower free border is the vestibular ligament
Cricothyroid	Joins the cricoid, thyroid, and arytenoid cartilages; its upper free border is the vocal ligament; there is also a midline thickening, the median cricothyroid ligament
Cricotracheal	Runs from the cricoid cartilage to the trachea

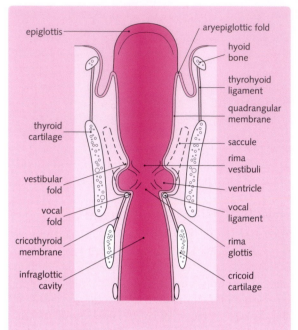

Fig. 7.71 Coronal section of the laryngeal cavity. (Adapted from *Gray's Anatomy* 38th edn, edited by L H Bannister et al. Harcourt Brace and Co.)

Fig. 7.72 Intrinsic muscles of the larynx

Muscle (nerve supply)	Origin	Insertion	Action
Cricothyroid (external laryngeal nerve)	Cricoid cartilage arch	Inferior border of thyroid cartilage and inferior cornu	Lengthens and tenses vocal cords by tilting cricoid and thus arytenoid cartilages
Posterior cricoarytenoid (recurrent laryngeal nerve)	Cricoid cartilage lamina	Arytenoid cartilage muscular process	Abducts vocal cords by laterally rotating arytenoid cartilages on cricoid cartilage
Lateral cricoarytenoid (recurrent laryngeal nerve)	Cricoid cartilage arch	Arytenoid cartilage muscular process	Adducts vocal cords by medially rotating arytenoid cartilages on cricoid cartilage
Thyroarytenoid (recurrent laryngeal nerve)	Posterior surface of thyroid cartilage	Arytenoid cartilage muscular process	Shortens vocal cord
Transverse arytenoid (recurrent laryngeal nerve)	Body of arytenoid cartilage	Body of contralateral arytenoid cartilage	Closes rima glottis by adducting arytenoid cartilages
Oblique arytenoid (recurrent laryngeal nerve)	Muscular process of arytenoid cartilage	Apex of contralateral arytenoid cartilage	Closes rima glottis by drawing arytenoid cartilages together
Vocalis (recurrent laryngeal nerve)	Vocal process of arytenoid cartilage	Vocal ligament	Maintains/increases tension in anterior part of vocal ligament; relaxes posterior part of vocal ligament

Tracheostomy (tracheotomy) and cricothyroidotomy

These are two techniques for creating a surgical airway. A tracheostomy is performed in an operating theatre and is more permanent: the skin of the neck is incised and the strap muscles moved to one side, the thyroid isthmus is moved inferiorly or clamped and divided if necessary – an incision is then made though the 2nd to 4th tracheal cartilages and a tracheostomy tube inserted.

A cricothyroidotomy is a short-term, emergency procedure performed by passing a needle through the cricothyroid membrane directly below the thyroid prominence. This is useful when there is a blockage at the rima glottidis, as the needle passes below this level.

Rotation of the arytenoids can open the rima glottis into a diamond shape or narrow it.

Trachea

The trachea commences at the level of C6 vertebra and is continuous with the larynx above. It ends at the sternal angle (T4 vertebral level) by dividing into the right and left main bronchi. Its walls are reinforced by C-shaped hyaline cartilages anteriorly.

Thyroid gland

The thyroid gland is an endocrine organ, lying in between trachea and infrahyoid strap muscles and covered by its capsule and the pretracheal fascia. It has a narrow isthmus (overlying tracheal rings 2–4)

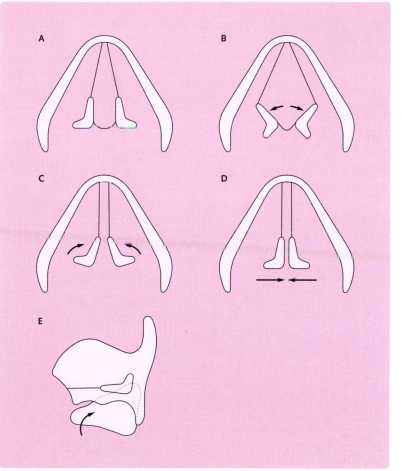

Fig. 7.73 Movements of the vocal folds, arytenoid and cricoid cartilages.

(A) Vocal cord position during quiet respiration, i.e. at rest.
(B) Vocal cord abduction by posterior cricoarytenoid muscles.
(C) Vocal cord adduction by lateral cricoarytenoid muscles.
(D) Vocal cord adduction by transverse arytenoid muscle.
(E) Increase in vocal cord tension by cricoid cartilage tilting through cricothyroid muscle contraction and drawing arytenoid cartilages posteriorly. (Adapted from *Gray's Anatomy* 38th edn, edited by L H Bannister et al. Pearson Professional Ltd.)

connecting two lobes (which extend up to the middle of the thyroid cartilage) (Fig. 7.74). It produces the hormones thyroxine and calcitonin.

Blood supply to the thyroid gland

The superior thyroid artery (the external carotid artery's first branch) has the external laryngeal nerve running with it. The artery branches at the upper pole of the gland to supply it. The inferior thyroid artery (arising from the thyrocervical trunk of the subclavian artery) has the recurrent laryngeal nerve running with it. The four arteries (two each side) anastomose posteriorly.

The thyroid ima artery is present in only 3% of individuals, arising from either the brachiocephalic trunk or the aortic arch and entering the lower part of the isthmus.

Fig. 7.74 Anterior view of the thyroid gland. The left side of the figure shows the arterial supply, and the right side shows the venous drainage. Inset shows thyroid gland anatomy.

The superior and middle thyroid veins join the internal jugular vein. The inferior thyroid veins join and empty into the left brachiocephalic vein.

Parathyroid glands

The parathyroid glands are four small glands (two each side) embedded in the posterior border of the thyroid gland. They are important in the regulation of calcium metabolism and may be damaged during thyroid surgery.

Blood supply to the parathyroid glands

The upper and lower parathyroid glands are supplied by the inferior thyroid artery. Small veins join the thyroid veins.

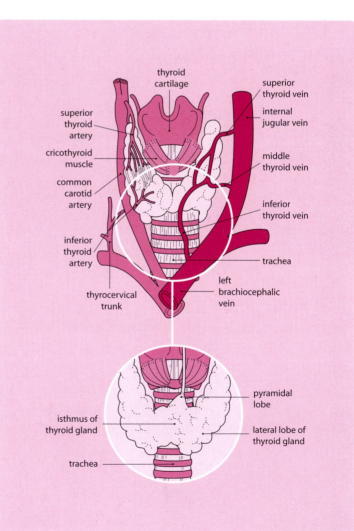

Thyroglossal cysts, goitre, thyroidectomy

The thyroid develops as a down growth from the back of the tongue – attached by a narrow tube called the thyroglossal duct. This usually disappears; however, it may remain and a cyst may form in it – these can be distinguished from midline sebaceous cyst (or goitre) by asking a patient to swallow or stick out the tongue, which will pull the cyst upwards.

An enlargement of the thyroid is referred to as a goitre and may compress structures adjacent to the thyroid. A thyroidectomy (removal of the thyroid) may be total (e.g. for carcinoma) or subtotal (e.g. in the treatment of hyperthyroidism), where the posterior part of the gland is preserved. Due to the close relationship between the inferior thyroid arteries and the recurrent laryngeal nerve, these are tied rather than cut during a thyroidectomy – damage to the nerve results in a hoarse voice.

RADIOLOGICAL ANATOMY

Imaging of the skull

Radiological imaging of the cranium is normally only for evaluation of the bones of the skull because the soft tissue such as the brain is not seen on plain films. However, because the skull is spherical in shape several different views are needed to assess and locate a fracture because the bones become superimposed upon each other.

Normal radiographic anatomy of an AP skull X-ray

In Figure 7.75 on an AP view of the skull, the anatomical landmarks to look for are the: frontal sinus (1), lesser wing of the sphenoid (18) below which is the superior orbit fissure (15). Medial to this

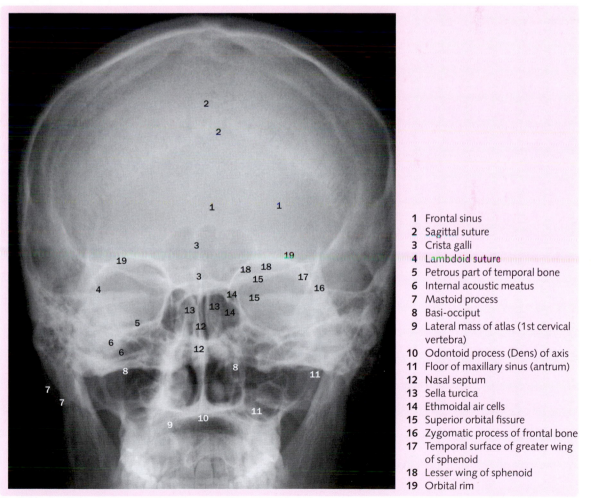

1 Frontal sinus
2 Sagittal suture
3 Crista galli
4 Lambdoid suture
5 Petrous part of temporal bone
6 Internal acoustic meatus
7 Mastoid process
8 Basi-occiput
9 Lateral mass of atlas (1st cervical vertebra)
10 Odontoid process (Dens) of axis
11 Floor of maxillary sinus (antrum)
12 Nasal septum
13 Sella turcica
14 Ethmoidal air cells
15 Superior orbital fissure
16 Zygomatic process of frontal bone
17 Temporal surface of greater wing of sphenoid
18 Lesser wing of sphenoid
19 Orbital rim

Fig. 7.75 Occipitofrontal view of skull.

are the ethmoidal air cells (14). Within the sphere of the orbit, the dense white shadow is the petrous part of the temporal bone (5). Below the orbit is the maxillary sinus (11). In the midline the dens (10) of the axis is seen with the lateral masses of the atlas (9) on either side of it.

Normal radiographic anatomy of a lateral skull X-ray

In Figure 7.76 on a lateral view of the skull, the anatomical landmarks to look for are the coronal suture (2) follow it inferiorly to find the sphenoidal sinus (9), positioned inferoanterior to the sella turcica (5) or pituitary fossa. Posteriorly identify the lambdoid suture (15) and follow it inferiorly to the mastoid air cells (17). Anteriorly on this lateral view, the paranasal sinuses are visible (from superior to inferior), the frontal (8), ethmoidal (10) and maxillary (13).

ENT

Sinusitis is inflammation of the sinuses, usually frontal or maxillary. A dull pain is felt over the affected sinus with tenderness of the overlying skin (referred pain due to same nerve supplying skin and sinus mucosa) and nasal discharge (a runny nose). If ethmoid or sphenoidal sinus is affected a deep pain is usually at the root of the nose.

How to examine a skull X-ray methodically

Examine the following features in sequence:

- Check the patient details of the X-ray, and the technical quality, i.e. the projection (is it AP?) and orientation (left from right).

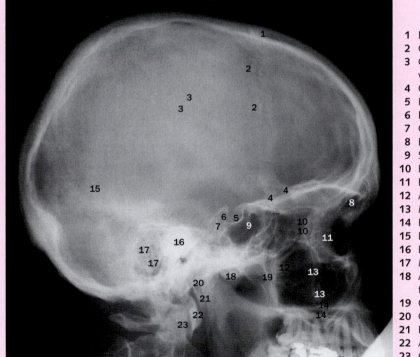

Fig. 7.76 Lateral view of skull.

1. Diploë
2. Coronal suture
3. Grooves for middle meningeal vessels
4. Greater wing of sphenoid
5. Pituitary fossa (sella turcica)
6. Dorsum sellae
7. Clivus
8. Frontal sinus
9. Sphenoid sinus
10. Ethmoidal air cells
11. Frontal process of zygoma
12. Arch of zygoma
13. Maxillary process of maxilla
14. Palatine process
15. Lambdoid process
16. External acoustic meatus
17. Mastoid air cells
18. Articular tubercle for temporomandibular joint
19. Coronoid process of mandible
20. Condyle of mandible
21. Ramus of mandible
22. Anterior arch of atlas
23. Odontoid process (Dens) of axis

- Examine the cortex of each bone. Look at the outline for any breaks in continuity and thickening, thinning or alterations in a normally smooth cortex.
- Check the sutures and that no fracture line is crossing them.
- Check any natural curves of skull, e.g. the orbital rim, and that no fracture line crosses it.
- Check sinuses for radiolucency (an opacity could indicate fluid and sinusitis).
- Finally, if you have found one abnormality, e.g. a fracture, keep looking because there may be more.

Radiology

As an individual ages the pineal gland within the brain undergoes calcification. This is sometimes seen on X-ray, giving a midline landmark but is of no clinical significance.

REGIONS AND COMPONENTS OF THE BACK

The back consists of the vertebral column, the spinal cord, the roots of the spinal nerves and associated muscles.

The vertebral column extends from the skull to the coccyx. It supports the weight of the body above the pelvic girdle. There is limited movement between adjacent vertebrae, but the total movement of the entire column is considerable.

There are 33 vertebrae arranged in five regions (seven cervical, twelve thoracic, five lumbar, five sacral, and four coccygeal). The sacral and coccygeal vertebrae fuse to form the sacrum and coccyx, respectively (see Fig. 8.2).

SURFACE ANATOMY AND SUPERFICIAL STRUCTURES

Visible and palpable features of the back are shown in Figure 8.1.

Cutaneous innervation of the back

The skin and muscles of the back are supplied segmentally by the posterior rami of the 31 pairs of spinal nerves. All posterior rami of the spinal nerves, except the first cervical nerve, divide into a medial

Back pain

Three factors combine to cause back pain. The nucleus pulposus dehydrates with age, weakened ligaments due to poor posture and lifting with a flexed vertebral column (which places strain on the muscles). As a protective mechanism, the back muscles go into spasm following injury or inflammation in the back, creating a muscular splint but causing pain and inhibiting movement.

and lateral branch. The posterior ramus of the 1st (suboccipital) cervical nerve supplies the deep muscles of the back of the neck (in the suboccipital region) and it does not supply the skin.

THE VERTEBRAL COLUMN

Skeleton of the vertebral column

The vertebral column consists of 33 vertebrae lying in five regions (Fig. 8.2). Individual vertebrae articulate with each other via intervertebral discs and articular facet (zygapophyseal) joints.

The vertebral column supports the weight of the upper body. The weight is transferred to the lower limb via the pelvic girdle. The column also transmits and protects the spinal cord.

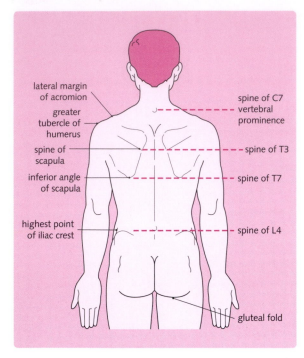

Fig. 8.1 Surface features of the back.

Abnormal curvatures

Scoliosis is an abnormal lateral curvature of the vertebral column, a true scoliosis also incorporating some element of rotation. This is usually idiopathic, but may also be congenital, neuropathic or due to muscular dystrophy.

Kyphosis is an abnormal increase in the thoracic curvature, resulting in a 'hunchback'. It can be due to wedge fractures in osteoporosis.

Lordosis is an abnormal increase in the lumbar curvature, accompanied by anterior rotation of the pelvis. It can be due to pregnancy or obesity, where the centre of gravity shifts anteriorly.

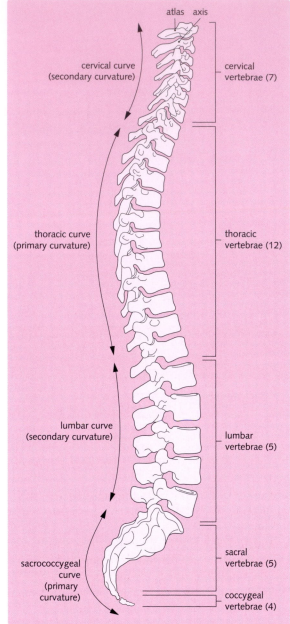

Fig. 8.2 Lateral view of the vertebral column.

There are four curvatures of the vertebral column in adults. The cervical and lumbar curvatures (secondary curvatures) are concave posteriorly; the thoracic and sacrococcygeal curvatures (primary curvatures) are concave anteriorly. The primary curvatures develop during the fetal period, whereas the secondary curvatures begin to appear before birth, but they become obvious only during infancy.

Features of individual vertebrae

The cervical, thoracic and lumbar vertebrae, together with the sacrum and coccyx, are discussed in Chapters 3 (**p. 60**), 4 (**p. 87**), 5 (**p. 118**) and 7 (**p. 181**).

Figure 8.3 illustrates the features of typical vertebra:

- A vertebral body – the weight-bearing part of the vertebra, which increases in size going down the vertebral column.

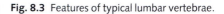

Fig. 8.3 Features of typical lumbar vertebrae.

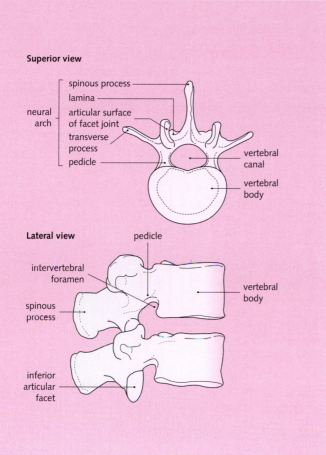

- A vertebral foramen, forming the vertebral canal running down the vertebral column for the spinal cord.
- A neural arch (Fig. 8.3), forming the lateral and posterior walls of the vertebral canal and consisting of two pedicles and two laminae. A single spinous process projects posteriorly from the junction of the laminae and transverse processes extend posterolaterally from the junctions of the pedicles and laminae, one on each side. Superior and inferior articular processes also project posteriorly from the junctions of the pedicles and laminae.
- The pedicles are notched superiorly and inferiorly, forming an intervertebral foramen between two vertebrae which transmits spinal nerves and vessels.

Joints of the vertebral column

The craniovertebral joints are discussed in Chapter 7.

Vertebral fractures and dislocations

These usually result from sudden forceful flexion–compression injuries, most commonly causing a compression fracture of a vertebral body. If a violent anterior movement also occurs, this can result in an anterior dislocation of the vertebra, dislocating or fracturing the articular facets and impinging on the spinal cord.

Intevertebral discs

These are the joints between the bodies of adjacent vertebrae (Fig. 8.4). They are secondary cartilaginous joints and absorb compressive forces.

The disc is composed of:

- The annulus fibrosus – an outer ring made up of concentric layers of fibrous tissue.
- The nucleus pulposus – a gelatinous core.

Joints of the vertebral arches

These are between the articular processes on the vertebral arches and are called facet (zygapophyseal) joints. They are plane synovial joints and their orientation affects the movements that can take place at the different vertebral levels.

Ligaments of the vertebral column

These are described in Figure 8.5.

Movement of the vertebral column

Flexion, extension, lateral flexion and rotation are possible, due to the shape of the joints between vertebrae (see Fig. 8.6). Movements of the atlanto-occipital and atlanto-axial joints are discussed in Chapter 7.

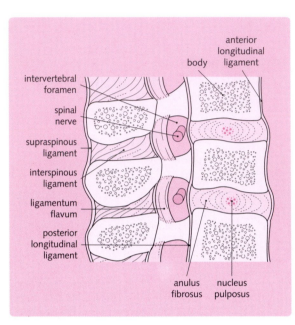

Fig. 8.4 Sagittal section of vertebrae showing the intervertebral discs and ligaments of the vertebral column.

> **Prolapsed disc**
>
> As individuals age, the nuclei pulposi lose their water content, becoming less turgid and thinner due to the compression forces upon the vertebral column, and this change can herniate through a worn annulus fibrosus. This is commonly called a slipped disc and occurs most frequently in the lumbar region. Herniation of the nucleus pulposus posterolaterally can compress the L5 and S1 nerve roots (sciatica) or the S1 alone (lumbago). This causes lower back pain that radiates down the back of the lower limb.

Fig. 8.5 Ligaments of the vertebral column	
Ligament	**Action**
Anterior longitudinal	Strong band covering the anterior part of the vertebral bodies and the intervertebral discs running from the anterior tubercle of C1 vertebra to the sacrum; maintains stability of the intervertebral discs and prevents hyperextension of the vertebral column
Posterior longitudinal	Is attached to the posterior aspect of the intervertebral discs and posterior edges of the vertebral bodies from C2 vertebra to the sacrum; prevents hyperflexion of the vertebral column and posterior protrusion of the discs
Supraspinous	Accessory ligament uniting the tips of the spinous processes
Interspinous	Accessory ligaments uniting the spinous processes
Ligamentum flavum	Unites adjacent laminae; helps to preserve the curvature of the vertebral column and support the joints between the vertebral arches

Fig. 8.6 Movements of the vertebral column

Vertebral region	Movements and accommodating factors	Limited movements and factors
Cervical	Flexion, extension, and lateral flexion occur because the intervertebral discs are thick compared to the vertebral bodies, facet joint capsules are loose, and the facet joints of C3 to C7 are horizontal, ovoid-shaped, and large	Lateral rotation is limited due to the shape of the articular processes of the facet joints of C3 to C7
Thoracic	Rotation and lateral flexion occur due to the oblique, nearly vertical shape of the facet joints and laminae	Flexion and extension are inhibited by facet joint shape, long spinous processes, the ribs, sternum, and thin intervertebral discs
Lumbar	Flexion, extension, and lateral flexion occur due to large intervertebral discs, and the shape of the facet joints	Rotation is prevented by the interlocking articular processes of the facet joints

---

Whiplash

This is the name given to a hyperextension of the vertebral column, which may stretch or tear the anterior longitudinal ligament – commonly occurring in rear-end car impacts.

Muscles of the vertebral column

An individual's body weight, for the greater part, is anterior to their vertebral column. To support this and move the vertebral column, there is a strong mass of muscle that runs longitudinally on the posterior aspect of the vertebrae. There are three main groups of back muscles:

- The superficial extrinsic muscles associated with the upper limb – trapezius, latissimus dorsi, levator scapulae and rhomboideus minor and major (see Chapter 2).
- The intermediate extrinsic muscles, these provide accessory respiratory movements by attaching vertebrae to ribs – serratus posterior and levatores costarum.
- The deep intrinsic muscles of the back (see Figs 8.7 and 8.8) – vertical superficial muscles (erector spinae), oblique intermediate muscles (transversospinalis), and deepest muscles (interspinales and intertransversarii).

Blood supply to the vertebral column

Spinal arteries supplying the vertebral column and spinal cord are branches of:

- Vertebral and ascending cervical arteries of the neck.
- Posterior intercostal arteries in the thoracic region.
- Subcostal and lumbar arteries in the abdomen.
- Iliolumbar and lateral sacral arteries in the sacrum.

The spinal artery branches enter the intervertebral foramina and divide into radicular arteries. These supply the anterior and posterior roots of the spinal nerves and the spinal cord.

Spinal veins form plexuses inside (internal vertebral venous plexus – in extradural fat) and outside (external vertebral venous plexus) the vertebral canal. Neither plexus has valves.

Back of the neck

At the back of the neck is a complex arrangement of muscles that connect the skull to the spine and pectoral girdle.

Metastasis via vertebral veins

Blood may return from the pelvis and abdomen to the heart via the vertebral venous plexuses and the azygos veins to the superior vena cava. Abdominal and pelvic tumours may metastasize to the vertebrae in this way.

Fig. 8.7 Deep intrinsic muscles of the back

Muscle	Origin	Insertion	Action
Deep layer			
Interspinales	Spinous process	Adjacent spinous process	Extension and rotation of vertebral column
Intertransversii	Transverse process	Adjacent transverse process	Lateral flexion and stabilize vertebral column
Transversospinalis (intermediate layer)			
Rotatores	Transverse process	Lamina of vertebra above	Stabilize vertebrae
Multifidus	Sacrum, ilium, thoracic transverse processes, cervical articular processes	2nd to 4th spinous process above	Stabilize vertebrae
Semispinalis	Transverse processes C4 to T12	Spinous processes above and occipital bone	Rotate column, extend head, cervical and thoracic regions
Erector spinae (superficial layer)			
Iliocostalis	Sacrum, iliac crest, lumbar spinous processes	Angles of ribs, cervical and thoracic transverse processes, mastoid process	Erector spinae muscles extend column and head, control flexion by relaxation of their fibres, lateral flexion
Longissimus	Sacrum, iliac crest, lumbar spinous processes	Angles of ribs, cervical and thoracic transverse processes, mastoid process	
Spinalis	Spinous processes	Spinous processes	
Splenius	T1–T6 spinous processes	Mastoid process	

Ligamentum nuchae

The ligamentum nuchae is a strong triangular fibroelastic ligament attaching superiorly to the external occipital protuberance and the cervical vertebrae spinous processes, essentially a continuation of the supraspinous ligament. It provides muscular attachments for trapezius and rhomboid minor.

Suboccipital region

This region is inferior to the occipital bone of the cranial base, covered by the deep intrinsic semispinalis capitis muscle and containing four muscles (Fig. 8.9). Within this region is the suboccipital triangle – bounded by three muscles (Fig. 8.10), which contains the C1 (suboccipital) nerve and the vertebral artery before it enters the skull through the foramen magnum.

THE SPINAL CORD AND MENINGES

The spinal cord lies in the vertebral canal. It commences just below the foramen magnum and it ends opposite L2 vertebra at the conus medullaris in adults (Fig. 8.11). In children the spinal cord can end as low as the L4 vertebra. Note that because of this, vertebral and spinal levels do not correspond and nerve rootlets become increasingly long at lower spinal cord levels: lumbar and sacral rootlets form the cauda equina below the conus medullaris.

A cervical enlargement extends from the C4 to T1 spinal cord segments. Ventral rami from these segments form the brachial plexus. A lumbosacral enlargement extends from the L2 to S3 spinal cord segments. Ventral rami from these segments form the lumbar and sacral plexuses.

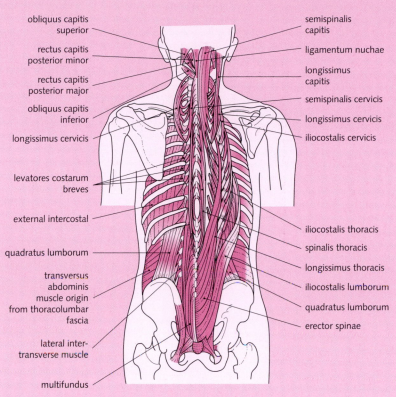

Fig. 8.8 Deep intrinsic muscles of the back. The right side shows the erector spinae components. Note that longissimus cervicus has been moved laterally and semispinalis captis has been removed. (Adapted from *Gray's Anatomy*, 38th edn, edited by L H Bannister et al. Pearson Professional Ltd.)

obliquus capitis superior

rectus capitis posterior minor

rectus capitis posterior major

obliquus capitis inferior

longissimus cervicis

levatores costarum breves

external intercostal

quadratus lumborum

transversus abdominis muscle origin from thoracolumbar fascia

lateral inter-transverse muscle

multifundus

semispinalis capitis

ligamentum nuchae

longissimus capitis

semispinalis cervicis

longissimus cervicis

iliocostalis cervicis

iliocostalis thoracis

spinalis thoracis

longissimus thoracis

iliocostalis lumborum

quadratus lumborum

erector spinae

Fig. 8.9 Muscles of the suboccipital region

Muscle (nerve supply)	Origin	Insertion	Action
Rectus capitis posterior minor (suboccipital nerve)	Posterior tubercle of atlas (C1)	Inferior nuchal line	Extend head
Rectus capitis posterior major (suboccipital nerve)	Spinous process of axis (C2)	Inferior nuchal line	Extend and rotate head
Obliquus capitis inferior (suboccipital nerve)	Spinous process of axis (C2)	Transverse process of atlas (C1)	Rotate altas and hence head
Obliquus capitis superior (suboccipital nerve)	Transverse process of atlas (C1)	Occipital bone	Lateral flexion

There are 31 pairs of spinal nerves, each composed of a dorsal and a ventral root (see Fig. 1.9).

Spinal meninges and cerebrospinal fluid

The meninges and the cerebrospinal fluid (CSF) surround and protect the spinal cord.

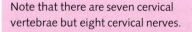

Note that there are seven cervical vertebrae but eight cervical nerves.

Fig. 8.10 The suboccipital region and contents. The right side shows the contents and the left side shows the boundaries of the suboccipital triangle. (Adapted from *Gray's Anatomy*, 38th edn, edited by L H Bannister et al. Pearson Professional Ltd.)

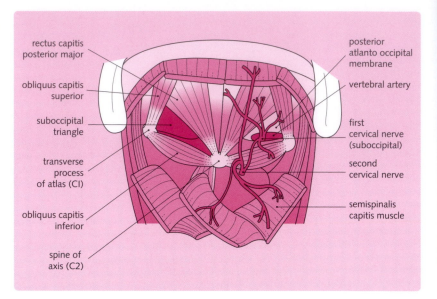

rectus capitis posterior major

obliquus capitis superior

suboccipital triangle

transverse process of atlas (CI)

obliquus capitis inferior

spine of axis (C2)

posterior atlanto occipital membrane

vertebral artery

first cervical nerve (suboccipital)

second cervical nerve

semispinalis capitis muscle

Dura mater

The dura mater is tough fibrous membrane continuous with the dura of the brain. It is separated from the vertebral periosteum by the epidural (extradural) space, which contains fat, connective tissue and the internal vertebral venous plexus. It is attached to the foramen magnum superiorly and to the coccyx inferiorly by the filum terminale. The dura mater extends into, and adheres to the intervertebral foramina. It forms a sleeve around the spinal nerve roots and eventually blends with the epineurium of the spinal nerves.

Arachnoid mater

The arachnoid mater is a delicate avascular membrane that encloses the subarachnoid space. It may be separated from the dura by a potential space – the subdural space. Like the dura it covers the spinal nerve roots and spinal ganglia.

Subarachnoid space

The subarachnoid space lies between the arachnoid and the pia mater, and it contains the spinal cord, nerve roots, ganglia and CSF.

Pia mater

The pia mater is a finely vascular membrane that is closely adherent to the spinal cord. It covers the roots of the spinal nerves and the spinal ganglia. Below the conus medullaris the pia continues as the filum terminale. It pierces the dural sac at the S2 vertebral level to attach to the coccyx. The pia mater extends laterally as the denticulate ligament, which passes out laterally to attach to the dural sac's inner surface.

Blood supply to the spinal cord

Anterior and posterior spinal arteries arise in the cranial cavity from the vertebral arteries or the inferior cerebellar artery. Anterior and posterior radicular branches of the spinal arteries reinforce the blood supply, the largest (the arteria radicularis magna) is variably located in the lower thoracic or upper lumbar regions.

Internal vertebral venous plexuses lie on the surface of the cord. They communicate with the cranial veins and the venous sinuses of the skull and with the external vertebral plexuses.

The spinal cord has no lymphatic vessels.

Remember the adult spinal cord ends at the L2 vertebral level. The dural sac ends at the S2 vertebral level.

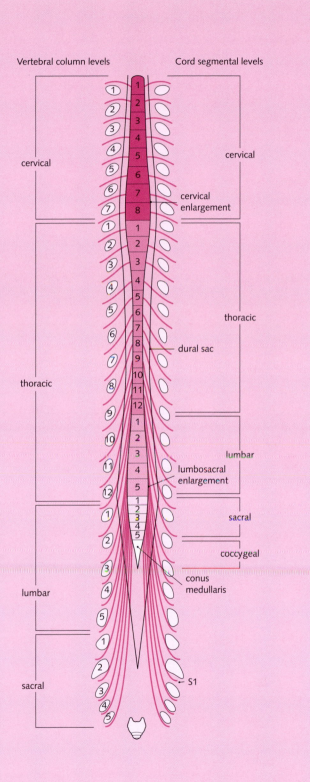

Fig. 8.11 Spinal cord, showing vertebral and segmental levels. (Adapted from *Anatomy as a Basis for Clinical Medicine*, by E C B Hall-Craggs. Courtesy of Williams & Wilkins.)

Vertebral column levels

Cord segmental levels

cervical

cervical

cervical enlargement

thoracic

dural sac

thoracic

lumbar

lumbosacral enlargement

sacral

coccygeal

conus medullaris

lumbar

S1

sacral

Lumbar puncture

By inserting a needle into the lumbar cistern below L2, a sample of CSF may be obtained without damaging the cord. This is done at the intervertebral space either directly below or above L4 (found by a line between the highest point of the iliac crests), with the patient lying on their side with back flexed to open up spaces between vertebrae. A hollow needle is passed slightly off-centre through skin, supraspinous ligament, infraspinous ligament, ligamentum flavum and dura (the latter two giving perceptible 'gives' as the needle passes through them) into the cistern. This is done to take samples of CSF for analysis (e.g. for meningitis) or to inject contrast agents or antibiotics. Lumbar puncture should not be attempted in raised intracranial pressure as the sudden drop can cause the cerebellum and brainstem to fatally herniate through the foramen magnum.

Anaesthesia

In epidural anaesthesia, an anaesthetic agent is injected into the epi(extra)dural space, affecting lumbar and sacral nerve roots: the procedure is as above except that the dura is not penetrated and the patient must not lie on their side (this would not result in unilateral anaesthesia).

In spinal anaesthesia, the anaesthetic agent is passed into the subarachnoid space for a more profound and longer-lasting anaesthesia.

In caudal anaesthesia, the needle is passed into the extradural space via the sacral hiatus.

Aortic aneurysm

An aortic aneurysm can compress a segmental artery that gives rise to a spinal branch. This impairs blood supply to that spinal segment level and results in loss of sensation and voluntary movement below this level.

SELF ASSESSMENT

Multiple-choice Questions (MCQs)

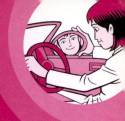

Indicate whether each answer is true or false.

Chapter 1 Basic concepts of anatomy

1. **Concerning the anatomical position:**
   a. The body is vertical with the vertebral column positioned anteriorly.
   b. The lower limbs are together in contact with each other.
   c. The palms of the hand face medially.
   d. The feet point laterally.
   e. The head faces anteriorly with the eyes looking upwards.

2. **Concerning anatomical planes and terms of position:**
   a. The horizontal plane runs perpendicular to the median sagittal plane of the body.
   b. A parasagittal plane is perpendicular to the median sagittal plane.
   c. A coronal plane is parallel to the median sagittal plane.
   d. Inferior describes a structure as being below another.
   e. Deep describes a structure as being closer to the body surface.

3. **Regarding terms of movement:**
   a. Adduction is a movement away from the median plane.
   b. Flexion is a movement in a sagittal plane that decreases the angle of a joint.
   c. Circumduction is a movement combination of flexion and abduction.
   d. Abduction of the thumb is when the thumb moves anteriorly away from the palm.
   e. Extension of the thumb is when the thumb moves laterally away from the palm abduction/adduction.

4. **Regarding the skin:**
   a. It has metabolic functions.
   b. It is composed of three layers.
   c. It is involved in thermoregulation due to presence of sebaceous glands.
   d. Its dermis contains a rich network of collagen that allows skin to stretch.
   e. The hypodermis acts as a waterproof barrier.

5. **Concerning bone:**
   a. Long bones contain yellow marrow that is involved in red blood cell synthesis.
   b. It is surrounded by an acellular periosteum (no cells present in it).
   c. It has an outer spongy layer that resists external forces.
   d. With ageing the cortices thicken and trabeculae increase in number.
   e. The metaphysis lies between the diaphysis and the epiphysis.

6. **Regarding joints:**
   a. Synovial joints lack a fibrous capsule.
   b. They receive their nerve supply from a nerve that innervates a muscle, which moves that joint.
   c. Ligaments prevent excessive joint movement.
   d. Only ligaments and muscles stabilize joints.
   e. There are four types of joint.

7. **Concerning muscle:**
   a. A fixator is a muscle responsible for preventing unwanted movements in an intermediate joint.
   b. Muscle fibres running oblique to the pull of a muscle allow a greater range of mobility.
   c. Smaller motor units are recruited (activated) for powerful muscle contractions.
   d. For a fixed muscle volume shorter muscle fibres produce a greater contractile force.
   e. An aponeurosis is a flattened tendon.

8. **Concerning the cardiovascular and lymphatic systems:**
   a. The left side of the heart pumps deoxygenated blood.
   b. All veins contain valves to prevent the backflow of blood.
   c. An arteriovenous shunt is a communication between two vessels under parasympathetic control.
   d. The lymphatic system removes excess tissue fluid only.
   e. Movement of fluid through lymphatic vessels is aided by muscle contraction.

9. **Concerning the gastrointestinal system:**
   a. The process of digestion begins in the stomach.
   b. The products of digestion are absorbed in the large intestine.
   c. Pancreatic enzymes and bile enter the duodenum.
   d. The area available for absorption of the products of digestion is increased by folding of the mucosa.
   e. The portal circulation transports carbohydrates, proteins and fats.

10. **Concerning the respiratory system:**
    a. Its upper part (nasal and oral cavities, pharynx and larynx) conditions the air, e.g. humidifying it.
    b. The walls of the bronchioles contain plates of cartilage.

c. The alveoli are where gaseous exchange occurs.
d. The only function of the respiratory system is gaseous exchange.
e. The trachea divides into two bronchi.

11. **Concerning the urinary system:**
   a. The glomerulus sits within Bowman's capsule and is the site of blood filtration.
   b. The basic unit of the kidney is the glomerulus.
   c. The nephron plays no role in formation of urine.
   d. Selective reabsorption occurs in the bladder.
   e. The ureters and bladder are lined by urothelium.

Chapter 2 The upper limb

12. **Regarding the surface anatomy of the upper limb:**
   a. The inferior angle of the scapula lies opposite the T7 vertebra.
   b. The corocoid process is palpated in the deltopectoral triangle.
   c. The anterior axillary fold contains the pectoralis minor muscle.
   d. The brachial artery is palpated in the cubital fossa lateral to the biceps brachii tendon.
   e. The olecranon process is palpated anteriorly through the cubital fossa.

13. **Regarding the muscles of the upper limb:**
   a. The latissimus dorsi muscle is supplied by the long thoracic nerve.
   b. The pectoralis minor muscle divides the axillary artery into three parts.
   c. The subscapularis muscle is the only muscle supplied by the lower subscapular nerve.
   d. Damage to the long thoracic nerve during breast surgery causes winging of the scapula.
   e. The infraspinatus muscle initiates abduction of the arm.

14. **Concerning the quadrangular and triangular spaces and triangular interval in the axillary region:**
   a. The triangular space transmits a branch of the subscapular artery.
   b. The quadrangular space is bounded by the humerus, long head of biceps brachii, teres major and minor muscles.
   c. The triangular interval contains the profunda brachii artery.
   d. The quadrangular space transmits a nerve branch of the posterior cord of the brachial plexus.
   e. The triangular interval is bounded by teres major, lateral and long heads of triceps brachii muscles.

15. **Concerning the joints of the upper limb:**
   a. In the adult they are all synovial joints (except the interosseus membrane if included as a joint).
   b. The shoulder joint is completely surrounded by the rotator cuff muscles.
   c. In the elbow joint the ulna articulates with the capitulum of the humerus.

d. Pronation and supination occur at the proximal radioulnar joint.
e. The sternoclavicular joint has an intra-articular disc.

16. **Concerning the axilla:**
   a. It contains lymph nodes that drain the upper limb only.
   b. The axillary artery commences at the inner border of the first rib.
   c. The axillary vein lies within the axillary sheath.
   d. It is bounded laterally by the intertubercular sulcus, and coracobrachialis and biceps brachii muscles.
   e. The cords of the brachial plexus are found in the axilla.

17. **Regarding the brachial plexus:**
   a. It is formed by the anterior rami of C5–C8 and T1 spinal nerves.
   b. The anterior division of the middle trunk joins the lower trunk.
   c. The thoracodorsal, upper and lower subscapular nerves arise from the posterior cord.
   d. The medial and lateral cords form the ulnar nerve.
   e. The radial nerve supplies muscles in the arm, forearm and hand.

18. **Regarding the vessels of the upper limb:**
   a. The axillary artery becomes the brachial artery at the inferior border of teres major.
   b. The brachial artery is deep throughout most of its course in the arm.
   c. The radial artery may be palpated in the anatomical snuffbox.
   d. The ulnar artery runs lateral to the ulnar nerve in the wrist region.
   e. The common interosseous artery arises from the ulnar artery just before it enters the hand.

19. **Concerning the cubital fossa:**
   a. The supinator and brachialis muscles form the floor of the fossa.
   b. The brachial artery usually divides in the fossa into radial and ulnar arteries.
   c. The biceps brachii tendon is found medial to the brachial artery.
   d. The radial nerve divides into its deep and superficial branches in the fossa.
   e. The median nerve lies lateral to the brachial artery.

20. **Regarding the nerves of the upper limb:**
   a. The ulnar nerve supplies cutaneous innervation to the medial border of the forearm.
   b. The median nerve supplies all the muscles of the thenar eminence.
   c. The median and ulnar nerves supply flexor digitorum superficialis.
   d. The median and radial nerves supply flexor digitorum profundus muscles.
   e. The ulnar nerve is motor to all the interossei and lumbrical muscles of the hand.

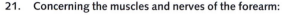

21. Concerning the muscles and nerves of the forearm:

a. The supinator muscle is supplied by the main trunk of the radial nerve.
b. The median nerve and ulnar artery pass distally in the forearm superficial to flexor digitorum superficialis.
c. The median nerve passes into the forearm between the origins of the pronator teres.
d. The ulnar nerve enters the forearm between the heads of flexor carpi ulnaris muscle.
e. The extensor carpi radialis longus muscle adducts and flexes the wrist.

22. Concerning the intrinsic muscles of the hand:

a. The dorsal interosseous muscles adduct the digits.
b. The adductor pollicis muscle has two heads that insert into the base of the proximal phalanx.
c. The radial artery enters the palm between the two heads of adductor pollicis to form the superficial palmar arch.
d. The opponens pollicis muscle inserts into the base of the proximal phalanx.
e. The lumbrical muscles arise from the tendons of flexor digitorum superficialis.

23. Radiographic anatomy of the upper limb:

a. On X-ray the bone cortex appears to be thinner in the carpal bones than in the humerus.
b. The bone cortex is smooth throughout the length of the bone.
c. On an X-ray film only the cortex is seen.
d. In osteoporosis the bones appear darker on an X-ray.
e. A scaphoid fracture is always visible at the first X-ray.

24. Clinical aspects of the upper limb:

a. In a fracture of the clavicle the commonest site is between the outer and middle thirds.
b. The median cubital vein is commonly used to take blood.
c. A Colles fracture is a fracture of the lower end of the ulnar.
d. After a fall on the outstreched hand tenderness over the anatomical snuffbox is likely to be due to a fracture of the scaphoid.
e. Thickening of the palmar aponeurosis is called Dupuytren's contracture.

Chapter 3 The thorax

25. Concerning the thoracic wall:

a. The manubrium only articulates with the clavicles, sternum, first and second costal cartilages.
b. The body of the sternum articulates with the second to seventh costal cartilages.
c. A typical rib articulates with the same numerical vertebral body and the vertebral body below.

d. The eleventh and twelfth ribs do not articulate with the ribs above to form the costal margin and therefore have no costal cartilage on their tips.
e. The weakest part of the rib is the neck.

26. Regarding the thoracic wall and intercostal spaces:

a. The neurovascular bundle runs between the deepest two muscle layers.
b. The intercostal nerves are the anterior rami of the thoracic spinal nerves.
c. Motor innervation to the intercostal muscles is from the phrenic nerves.
d. The intercostal arteries all arise from the aorta.
e. Insertion of a needle into the intercostal space should be at the inferior border of the upper rib.

27. The diaphragm:

a. Has a motor nerve supply from the phrenic and intercostal nerves.
b. Transmits the aorta at the level of T12 vertebra.
c. Transmits the oesophagus through the central tendon.
d. Is pierced by the greater, lesser and least splanchnic nerves.
e. Is the main muscle used in quiet respiration.

28. The pericardium:

a. Is divided into serous and fibrous layers.
b. Lies in the middle mediastinum.
c. The fibrous layer is attached to the central tendon of the diaphragm, sternum and great vessels.
d. The nerve supply to the fibrous and parietal serous layers is by the phrenic nerve.
e. The reflection of the serous pericardium around the pulmonary veins forms the oblique sinus.

29. Regarding the heart:

a. The right ventricular wall is thicker than the left ventricular wall.
b. The fossa ovalis lies in the interatrial wall.
c. The apex of the heart normally lies in the 7th left intercostal space.
d. The atrioventricular node is the normal cardiac pacemaker.
e. The mitral valve lies in the right atrioventricular orifice.

30. Concerning the blood supply of the heart:

a. The coronary arteries are the first branches of the aorta.
b. The anterior cardiac veins drain into the coronary sinus.
c. The great cardiac vein runs in the interventricular groove with the anterior interventricular artery.
d. If the posterior interventricular artery arises from the circumflex artery, the heart is said to have right dominance.
e. The cardiac veins drain into the right atrium (excluding the venae cordis minimae).

31. **Regarding the thoracic aorta:**
    a. The ascending aorta has no branches.
    b. The aortic arch is attached to the right pulmonary artery via the ligamentum arteriosum.
    c. The descending aorta commences at the level of the sternal angle.
    d. The descending aorta gives branches to the pericardium, oesophagus and bronchi.
    e. The aorta leaves the thorax by passing through the central tendon of the diaphragm at the level of T12 vertebra.

32. **Concerning thoracic nerves:**
    a. The phrenic nerve passes posterior to the lung hilum.
    b. The phrenic nerve arises from posterior rami of C3–C5 spinal nerves.
    c. The vagus nerves contribute to the formation of the cardiac, pulmonary and oesophageal plexuses.
    d. Both right and left vagi leave the thorax with the oesophagus.
    e. The thoracic sympathetic ganglia supply both thoracic and abdominal structures.

33. **Regarding the oesophagus:**
    a. Is a continuation of the laryngopharynx at the level of C6 vertebra.
    b. Passes inferiorly anterior to the trachea.
    c. Has constrictions caused by the cricopharyngeus muscle, aorta, left main bronchus and diaphragm.
    d. Its lowest part has a blood supply from direct oesophageal branches of the descending aorta.
    e. Exits the thorax by piercing the diaphragm with oesophageal arterial and venous branches of the left gastric vessels.

34. **Concerning the lungs:**
    a. The right main bronchus is shorter and wider and more vertical than the right.
    b. The right lung has two lobes, and the left lung has three lobes.
    c. Bronchopulmonary segments are the functional units of the lungs.
    d. The apex of the lung lies above the clavicle.
    e. The visceral pleura has a rich somatic innervation and is very sensitive to pain.

35. **Regarding the mechanics of the respiration:**
    a. In quiet inspiration the diaphragm contracts, increasing the vertical diameter of the thorax.
    b. In adult males thoracic movement is greater than diaphragmatic movement.
    c. In forced inspiration, the twelfth rib is fixed by quadratus lumborum muscle, allowing a more forceful diaphragmatic contraction.
    d. In quiet expiration, the intercostal muscles contract.
    e. In forced expiration the abdominal wall muscles contract, pushing abdominal viscera and the diaphragm upwards.

36. **Radiographic anatomy of the thorax:**
    a. On a PA chest X-ray the aortic knuckle is seen on the right hand side of the trachea.
    b. On a PA chest X-ray the left hemidiaphragm is higher than the right hemidiaphragm.
    c. On a lateral chest X-ray the left atrium forms the posterior border of the heart.
    d. The superior vena cava forms a curved shadow on a PA chest X-ray.
    e. No muscle shadow is seen on a PA chest X-ray.

37. **Clinical aspects of the thorax:**
    a. In breast carcinoma, skin dimpling is caused by shortening of the suspensory ligaments.
    b. The mediastinal contents are pulled to the left in a left sided tension pneumothorax.
    c. Pericarditis can cause shoulder pain.
    d. The anterior interventricular artery is most commonly affected in ischaemic heart disease.
    e. Tracheobronchial node enlargement in bronchial carcinoma causes compression of the right recurrent laryngeal nerve and paralysis of the laryngeal muscles.

Chapter 4 The Abdomen

38. **Concerning the surface anatomy of the abdomen:**
    a. The liver lies mostly behind the ribcage.
    b. The fundus of the gall bladder is marked by the linea semilunaris intersecting the transpyloric plane.
    c. The spleen lies deep to the right ninth, tenth and eleventh ribs.
    d. The head of the pancreas lies in the transpyloric plane.
    e. The right kidney is lower than the left.

39. **Regarding the anterolateral abdominal wall:**
    a. Nerves run in a plane between internal and external oblique muscles.
    b. The aponeurosis of transversus abdominis lies against the posterior aspect of the rectus abdominis along its length.
    c. The inferior epigastric artery enters the rectus sheath and runs deep to the rectus abdominis muscle.
    d. The ilioinguinal nerve (L1) forms part of the nerve supply to all anterolateral abdominal wall muscles except external oblique.
    e. Both internal oblique and transversus abdominis arise from the thoracolumbar fascia.

40. **Concerning the peritoneum and the peritoneal cavity:**
    a. The parietal layer lines the anterior and posterior abdominal walls, inferior surface of the diaphragm, and the pelvic cavity.
    b. A retroperitoneal organ is suspended by a mesentery.
    c. Fluid may accumulate in the hepatorenal pouch when a patient is supine.

d. The greater sac is divided into two compartments by the transverse mesocolon.
e. The epiploic foramen is bounded anteriorly by the portal vein, and posteriorly by the inferior vena cava.

41. The stomach:

a. Is derived from the foregut.
b. The stomach is an intraperitoneal structure.
c. Part of the stomach may pass into the thoracic cavity in a hiatus hernia.
d. Has a blood supply mainly derived from the coeliac trunk.
e. The stomach is connected to the transverse colon by the lesser omentum.

42. Regarding the small intestine:

a. The pancreatic ducts open into the 4th part of the duodenum.
b. Lymph from the duodenum drains into the coeliac and superior mesenteric nodes.
c. The jejunum has shorter vasa recta than the ileum.
d. The pancreas and duodenum are direct relations.
e. The small intestine is supplied by the vagus nerve and sympathetic fibres of T9 and T10 spinal cord levels.

43. Concerning the colon:

a. It is retroperitoneal throughout its course.
b. It is supplied by the superior mesenteric artery only as far as the hepatic flexure.
c. Appendices epiploicae and taeniae coli are distinguishing features of the large intestine.
d. The vermiform appendix opens into the caecum.
e. All the arteries of the large intestine are end arteries.

44. Regarding the liver:

a. It is completely covered by peritoneum except over its anterior surface.
b. Deoxygenated blood leaves the liver via the porta hepatis.
c. The bare area of the liver lies in direct contact with the stomach.
d. The division into left, quadrate and caudate lobes is based on function.
e. The falciform ligament attaches the liver to the anterior abdominal wall.

45. Concerning the gall bladder:

a. The bile duct is formed by the union of the cystic duct with the common hepatic duct.
b. The bile duct runs in free margin of the lesser omentum.
c. The gall bladder is usually supplied by a branch of the left hepatic artery.
d. The fundus of the gall bladder lies at the tip of the ninth costal cartilage.
e. A gallstone may be the cause of jaundice.

46. Regarding the posterior abdominal wall:

a. Thoracolumbar fascia attaches to the bodies of lumbar vertebrae.

b. The kidneys are surrounded by fatty tissue.
c. The left kidney has a longer vein than the right.
d. The ureters lie on quadratus lumborum muscle.
e. The suprarenal glands are supplied by three branches of the superior mesenteric artery.

47. Regarding the abdominal blood vessels:

a. The abdominal aorta ends at the level of L4 vertebra by dividing into the common iliac arteries.
b. The superior mesenteric artery arises from the aorta at the level of L2 vertebra.
c. The inferior mesenteric artery supplies the derivatives of the hindgut.
d. The inferior mesenteric vein joins the inferior vena cava at the level of L4.
e. Haematemesis can be a consequence of liver cirrhosis.

48. Concerning the nerves of the abdomen:

a. The lumbar plexus is formed by the anterior rami of L1–L4 spinal nerves.
b. The femoral nerve and obturator nerve lie medial to psoas major.
c. The iliohypogastric and ilioinguinal nerves arise from L1 spinal nerve.
d. Sympathetic fibres pass along branches of the lumbar plexus to gut tube structures.
e. Pelvic splanchnic nerves innervate the descending colon.

Chapter 5 The Pelvis and Perineum

49. Concerning the bony pelvis:

a. The greater or false pelvis lies below the pelvic brim.
b. The sacrum is attached to the rest of the pelvis via two synovial joints.
c. The pubic tubercle lies in the midline.
d. In an erect individual, the anterior inferior iliac spines and pubic symphysis lie in the same vertical plane.
e. The female pubic arch is wider than the male pubic arch.

50. Concerning the rectum:

a. It commences where the sigmoid mesocolon ends.
b. The superior and middle rectal arteries supply the rectum.
c. The rectum has taeniae coli.
d. The rectovesical pouch in females separates the rectum from the bladder.
e. The middle third of the rectum is covered at the sides by peritoneum.

51. Concerning the pelvic ureters and bladder:

a. The ureters turn anteriorly towards the bladder at the level of the ischial spine.
b. The base of the bladder is related to internal sexual organs in both sexes.

c. In the female the uterine artery passes inferior to the ureter.
d. Detrusor muscle has a sympathetic nerve supply.
e. The trigone is a smooth area of mucosa lying between urethral and ureteric orifices.

52. **Regarding the pelvic viscera:**

a. The bladder is covered by peritoneum on its superior surface.
b. The broad ligament of the uterus contains the uterine tubes and ovarian vessels.
c. If an enlarged smooth prostate is palpated, it can be a sign of malignant disease.
d. The ovary is supplied by a branch of the internal iliac artery.
e. The posterior fornix of the vagina is deeper than the anterior fornix.

53. **Concerning the pelvic vessels:**

a. The walls of the pelvis are supplied by the internal iliac artery.
b. The internal pudendal artery leaves the pelvis through the lesser sciatic foramen.
c. The obturator artery is crossed laterally by the ureter.
d. The superior vesical artery is continuous with the medial umbilical ligament.
e. The prostate has venous drainage to the portal venous system.

54. **Concerning the nerves of the pelvis:**

a. The sacral plexus is formed by the S1–S5 anterior rami only.
b. The two sacral sympathetic trunks unite at the ganglion impar.
c. The pelvic splanchnic nerves carry sympathetic nerve fibres.
d. The pudendal nerve roots are S2, S3 and S4.
e. The right and left hypogastric plexuses receive a right and left hypogastric nerve, respectively.

55. **Regarding the perineum:**

a. It can be divided into an anterior (urogenital) triangle and a posterior (anal) triangle.
b. The line dividing anal and urogenital triangles runs between the two ischial tuberosities.
c. The structures of the perineum are supplied by the obturator artery and nerve.
d. The urogenital triangle contains the perineal membrane, which lies above the pelvic floor.
e. The ischioanal fossa are filled with venous plexuses which enlarge to form haemorrhoids.

56. **Concerning the anal canal:**

a. It is supplied entirely by the autonomic nervous system.
b. It commences at the anorectal junction.
c. At the pectinate line, the epithelium becomes stratified squamous.
d. The anal sphincter consists of four parts.
e. Haemorrhoids are formed by dilatations of rectal venous plexuses.

57. **Regarding the external genitalia:**

a. The penis is formed by two cylinders of erectile tissue.
b. The penis receives its blood supply from the internal pudendal artery.
c. The greater vestibular glands open directly into the vagina.
d. In a pudendal nerve block, the ischial spine is palpated by a finger within the vagina
e. Either side of the vagina there are two erectile masses that form the bulb of the vestibule.

Chapter 6 The lower limb

58. **Concerning the surface anatomy of the lower limb:**

a. The lesser trochanter is palpable in the hip region.
b. The iliotibial tract is on the medial surface of the thigh.
c. The muscles of the anterior compartment of the leg lie anteromedial to the tibia.
d. The great saphenous vein passes anterior to the medial malleolus.
e. The skin of the great toe (hallux) is supplied by the dermatome of L5.

59. **Concerning the gluteal region:**

a. The close fit of the femoral head in the acetabulum contributes to the stability of the hip joint.
b. Abduction of the hip is performed by all three gluteus muscles.
c. All the structures that pass from the greater sciatic foramen to supply the gluteal region and lower limb lie inferior to the piriformis muscle.
d. Cutaneous innervation is supplied by the gluteal branches of the posterior rami of lumbar and sacral nerves.
e. The pudendal nerve exits the pelvis through the greater sciatic foramen and re-enters through the lesser sciatic foramen.

60. **Regarding the femoral triangle:**

a. The femoral vein, artery and nerve lie in the femoral sheath.
b. The femoral nerve lies most laterally in the femoral triangle.
c. The medial border of the femoral triangle is formed by the medial border of the adductor magnus muscle.
d. The femoral canal is bounded proximally by the inguinal ligament, lacunar ligament, pectinate line (of pubis) and femoral vein.
e. The floor of the femoral triangle is formed by the iliopsoas, pectineus, adductor longus and brevis muscles.

61. **Regarding the vessels of the lower limb:**

a. The femoral artery is a direct continuation of the internal iliac artery as it passes below the inguinal ligament.

b. The profunda femoris artery supplies the muscles of the medial and posterior compartments of the thigh.
c. The great saphenous vein drains into the femoral vein.
d. The profunda femoris vein drains into the great saphenous vein.
e. In increased venous return the femoral vein can expand into the femoral canal.

62. **Concerning nerves of the lower limb:**
   a. The ilioinguinal nerve supplies the skin over the femoral triangle.
   b. The lateral cutaneous nerve passes medial to the posterior superior iliac spine.
   c. The obturator nerve has a branch to the pectineus muscle.
   d. The posterior femoral cutaneous nerve has nerve root values of S2–S3.
   e. The tibial division of the sciatic nerve supplies all the muscles of the posterior compartment of the thigh.

63. **Concerning movements of the hip joint:**
   a. The gluteus medius and minimus muscles resist excessive adduction.
   b. Extension is limited by the pubofemoral and iliofemoral ligaments.
   c. The axis of rotation passes through the femoral head and femoral medial condyle.
   d. The ischiofemoral ligament is stretched by lateral rotation.
   e. The anteroposterior axis of abduction–adduction passes through the femoral neck.

64. **Regarding the popliteal fossa:**
   a. The popliteal artery is the deepest structure of the popliteal fossa.
   b. The popliteal artery has no branches in the popliteal fossa.
   c. The small saphenous vein joins the popliteal vein in the popliteal fossa.
   d. The upper boundaries of the fossa are formed by the semimembranosus and biceps femoris muscles only.
   e. The popliteus muscle locks the knee joint.

65. **Concerning the knee joint:**
   a. The knee joint is an articulation between the femur, tibia and fibula.
   b. Only flexion and extension movements are possible at the knee joint.
   c. The cavity of the knee joint communicates with the suprapatella bursa.
   d. The anterior cruciate ligament prevents posterior displacement of the femur when tibia is fixed.
   e. Inflammation of the prepatella bursa is known as clergyman's knee.

66. **Regarding the leg:**
   a. All peroneal muscles are supplied by the superficial peroneal nerve.
   b. The extensor digitorum longus muscle inserts into the medial four digits.

c. The inferior extensor retinaculum is Y-shaped.
d. No movement occurs at the inferior tibiofibular joint.
e. The interosseous membrane has no defects within it, i.e. a hiatus.

67. **Concerning the nerves of the lower limb:**
   a. The tibial nerve ends by dividing into the medial and lateral plantar nerves.
   b. The saphenous nerve passes behind the medial malleolus to supply the medial side of the foot.
   c. Compression of the deep peroneal nerve causes sensory loss in the first interdigital cleft of the foot.
   d. The tibial nerve supplies the muscles of the anterior compartment of the leg.
   e. The sural nerve is cutaneous only.

68. **Concerning the dorsum of the foot:**
   a. The dorsalis pedis artery is a continuation of the anterior tibial artery in the foot.
   b. The extensor digitorum longus tendons are joined by lumbrical and interossei muscle tendons to form an extensor expansion.
   c. Extensor hallucis brevis muscle inserts into the proximal phalanx of the great toe.
   d. The dorsal venous arch drains laterally into the small saphenous vein.
   e. The extensor digitorum brevis is supplied by the superficial peroneal nerve.

69. **Concerning the foot:**
   a. The four lumbricals are supplied by the lateral plantar nerve.
   b. Flexor digitorum brevis inserts into the distal phalanges of the lateral four digits.
   c. The adductor hallucis muscle moves the hallux away from the second digit.
   d. The skin of the foot sole is innervated by the medial and lateral plantar nerve only.
   e. The spring ligament is also known as the calcaneonavicular ligament.

70. **Clinical aspects of the lower limb:**
   a. Varicose veins are due to incompetent valves that allow venous flow from deep to superficial veins.
   b. The femoral pulse is palpated at the midpoint of the inguinal ligament.
   c. A femoral neck fracture causes the axis of rotation to lie along the shaft of the femur.
   d. On X-ray of a femoral neck fracture, Shenton's line is lost.
   e. On X-ray loss of the joint space is a feature of osteoarthritis.

Chapter 7 The Head and Neck

71. **Concerning the skull:**
   a. The sagittal suture is formed by the parietal bones articulating with the frontal bone.

b. The bregma is where the lambdoid suture joins the sagittal suture.

c. The lambda is where the coronal suture joins the lambdoid suture.

d. The pterion is formed by the sphenoid, temporal, frontal and parietal bones.

e. The anterior fontanelle closes in the first 6 months of life.

72. **Regarding the skull foramina:**

a. The jugular foramen transmits deoxygenated blood from the brain.

b. The internal acoustic meatus transmits the vestibulocochlear nerve only.

c. The optic canal conveys a blood vessel that gives a branch to the forehead.

d. The maxillary nerve (V_3) passes through the foramen rotundum.

e. The internal carotid artery enters the skull through the foramen lacerum.

73. **Concerning the face and scalp:**

a. The buccal branch of the facial nerve is sensory to the buccal mucosa.

b. Buccinator is a muscle of facial expression.

c. The trigeminal nerve is sensory to the entire scalp region.

d. The facial vein is formed by the union of the supraorbital and supratrochlear veins.

e. The arterial supply to the face and scalp is from branches of the external carotid artery only.

74. **Concerning the cranial cavity:**

a. The optic chiasma lies adjacent to the pituitary fossa.

b. The superior sagittal sinus runs in the inferior border of the falx cerebri.

c. The falx cerebelli separates the two cerebral hemispheres.

d. The sigmoid venous sinus becomes the internal jugular vein at the jugular foramen.

e. The circulus arteriosus connects the internal and external carotid arteries.

75. **Regarding the cranial nerves:**

a. Cranial nerves V, VII and X are the only ones to give cutaneous innervation.

b. The cranial part of the accessory nerve is sensory to the mucosa of the pharynx.

c. The trigeminal nerve gives a motor supply to the muscles of mastication.

d. Preganglionic parasympathetic fibres come from cranial nerves III, V and VII.

e. The constrictors of the pharynx are supplied by the glossopharyngeal nerve.

76. **Concerning the orbit:**

a. Superior oblique muscle is supplied by the infratrochlear nerve.

b. Inferior oblique and superior rectus, acting together, displace the pupil upwards.

c. If the abducent nerve is damaged the pupil is displaced laterally.

d. Inferior rectus moves the pupil downward and medially.

e. If the oculomotor nerve is damaged the pupil is constricted.

77. **Concerning the orbit:**

a. The nasolacrimal duct empties into the middle meatus of the nasal cavity.

b. The parasympathetic fibres that supply the lacrimal gland synapse in the pterygopalatine ganglion.

c. The roof of the orbit is formed by the frontal bone.

d. The inferior orbital fissure communicates with the pterygopalatine fossa.

e. The long ciliary branch of the nasociliary nerve carries sympathetic fibres.

78. **Regarding the salivary glands:**

a. The external carotid artery and the retromandibular vein lie in the substance of the parotid gland.

b. The parotid gland duct opens in the oral cavity opposite the second premolar tooth.

c. The facial nerve gives off its five terminal branches before it enters the parotid gland.

d. The submandibular gland has superficial and deep parts.

e. The lingual nerve carries parasympathetic fibres to the sublingual and submandibular glands.

79. **Regarding the temporal and infratemporal fossae:**

a. The coronoid process of the mandible forms part of the temporomandibular joint.

b. None of the muscles of mastication are used to open the jaw wide.

c. The pterygoid venous plexus communicates with veins inside the skull.

d. The temporomandibular joint is strengthened by the lateral temporomandibular ligament.

e. Preganglionic parasympathetic fibres to the optic ganglion are carried in part of their course by the glossopharyngeal (IX) nerve.

80. **In the neck region:**

a. Neck muscles that lie outside the prevertebral fascia are innervated by cervical nerves only

b. The accessory nerve supplies the trapezius muscle.

c. There are three sympathetic ganglia in the neck.

d. The pretracheal space extends inferiorly into the thorax.

e. The phrenic nerve arises from cervical roots C3, 4 and 5.

81. **Concerning the neck:**

a. The sympathetic trunk lies within the carotid sheath.

b. The cervical plexus is formed by the anterior rami of C1–C4 spinal nerves.

c. A typical cervical vertebra has a triangular vertebral foramen.

d. The internal carotid artery has only two branches in the neck.

e. The external jugular vein is formed by the continuation of the facial vein.

82. **Concerning the neck region:**
   a. The spinal part of the accessory nerve ascends through the foramen magnum
   b. The carotid sinus is innervated by a branch of the glossopharyngeal nerve.
   c. The brachial plexus roots emerge between the scalenus medius and scalenus posterior muscles.
   d. The internal jugular vein lies posterior to the internal carotid immediately below the skull.
   e. All lymph from the head and neck drains into nodes within the carotid sheath.

83. **Regarding the neck:**
   a. The common carotid artery divides at the upper border of the thyroid cartilage.
   b. The common carotid artery lies adjacent to sternocleidomastoid.
   c. The tendinous sling of omohyoid attaches to the hyoid bone.
   d. The external laryngeal nerve is sensory to the mucosa above the vocal folds.
   e. The superior root of the ansa cervicalis is a branch of the hypoglossal nerve.

84. **Regarding the pharynx:**
   a. The pharyngeal plexus supplies all the muscles of the pharynx.
   b. The pharynx ends at the level of the vocal folds.
   c. Lymphoid tissue surrounds the opening of the auditory tube in the nasopharynx.
   d. During swallowing, the soft palate is elevated.
   e. The inferior constrictor may be divided into two parts.

85. **Concerning the pharynx:**
   a. The posterior third of the tongue forms the anterior wall of the oropharynx.
   b. The oropharynx receives a sensory innervation through the glossopharyngeal nerve.
   c. The pharyngobasilar fascia separates pharyngeal mucosa and muscle.
   d. The tubal recess lies anterior to the tubal elevation.
   e. The epiglottic valleculae are formed by reflections of mucous membrane from the posterior third of the tongue.

86. **Regarding the nose:**
   a. The nasal septum is completely cartilaginous.
   b. The maxillary air sinus opens out into the middle meatus.
   c. The sphenoethmoidal recess has the sphenoid sinus opening into it.
   d. The entire nasal cavity is lined by olfactory mucosa.
   e. The sphenoid sinus lies directly below the pituitary fossa.

87. **Regarding the nasal cavity and the pterygopalatine fossa:**
   a. The cribriform plate of the ethmoid bone forms part of the roof of the nasal cavity.

   b. Three conchae divide the lateral nasal wall into three meatus.
   c. The pterygopalatine fossa communicates with the middle cranial fossa.
   d. The nerve of the pterygoid canal is formed by the deep petrosal nerve and the greater petrosal nerve.
   e. The pterygopalatine ganglion gives a sensory branch that supplies the nasopharynx.

88. **Concerning the bones of the skull and face:**
   a. The sphenoid bone forms a boundary (or boundaries) of the superior orbital fissure.
   b. The maxilla takes part in formation of the hard palate.
   c. The temporal bone attaches sternocleidomastoid.
   d. The temporal bone transmits CN VII (facial nerve) and CN VIII (vestibulocochlear nerve).
   e. The coronoid process articulates with the mandibular fossa of the temporal bone.

89. **Concerning the oral cavity:**
   a. The submandibular gland opens into the vestibule of the mouth.
   b. Taste sensation from the posterior one-third of the tongue passes along the chorda tympani nerve.
   c. The tubal tonsils form part of the ring of lymphoid tissue around the pharynx.
   d. Damage to the hypoglossal nerve results in a tongue that deviates to the affected side.
   e. The sensory supply of the walls of the oral cavity comes entirely from branches of the mandibular (V_3) nerve.

90. **Concerning the oral cavity:**
   a. The intrinsic muscles of the tongue are all supplied by the hypoglossal nerve.
   b. The hard palate is formed by the horizontal process of the palatine bones alone.
   c. The lymphatic supply to the tongue drains into the deep cervical lymph nodes.
   d. There are between 10 and 12 vallate papillae.
   e. The palatine tonsil lies between the palatoglossal and palatopharyngeal arches.

91. **Concerning the floor of the mouth and the soft palate:**
   a. The submandibular gland is supplied by the facial and lingual arteries.
   b. The palatine tonsils lie at the back of the mouth and are related to two muscles of the soft palate.
   c. The sublingual gland is supplied by the lingual nerve.
   d. Tensor veli palatini is supplied by the pharyngeal plexus.
   e. The pharyngeal plexus is formed by the glossopharyngeal and vagus nerves.

92. **Concerning the larynx:**
   a. A needle passing through the cricothyroid membrane would enter the ventricle.
   b. The cricothyroid muscle is supplied by the internal laryngeal nerve.

c. The epiglottis is composed of elastic cartilage.
d. The vocal folds are formed by the free borders of the cricothyroid membrane.
e. The arytenoid cartilages articulate with the thyroid cartilage.

93. **Concerning the intrinsic muscles of the larynx:**
    a. The recurrent laryngeal nerve supplies all the muscles except cricothyroid and is sensory to the mucosa below the vocal folds.
    b. The tilting of the cricoid and arytenoids by cricothyroid muscle abducts the vocal folds.
    c. Both transverse arytenoid and oblique arytenoid muscles adduct the vocal folds.
    d. The vocalis muscle relaxes the vocal ligament.
    e. The transverse arytenoid muscle is the only unpaired intrinsic muscle of the larynx.

94. **Regarding the larynx:**
    a. The thyrohyoid membrane is pierced by the external laryngeal nerve.
    b. The inferior border of the quadrangular membrane forms the vestibular ligament.
    c. The laryngeal inlet is bounded by the thyroid cartilage, aryepiglottic and interarytenoid folds.
    d. The cricoarytenoid joint has a lax capsule.
    e. In swallowing, the larynx is pulled upwards.

95. **Regarding the thyroid gland:**
    a. It lies anterior to the trachea and part of the larynx.
    b. It is drained by two pairs of veins.
    c. The superior and inferior thyroid arteries are both branches of the external carotid.
    d. The inferior thyroid artery is closely associated with the recurrent laryngeal nerve.
    e. An enlargement of the thyroid is known as a goitre.

Chapter 8 The Back

96. **Concerning the back:**
    a. The highest point of the iliac crest lies at the level of the spinous process of L4 vertebra.
    b. Back muscles and skin are supplied by the posterior rami of spinal nerves.

c. There are 33 vertebrae.
d. Thoracic and sacrococcygeal curvatures are concave anteriorly.
e. The C7 vertebra's spine is the highest easily palpable spinous process.

97. **Concerning the vertebral column:**
    a. There are eight cervical vertebrae.
    b. The laminae of vertebrae face posteriorly.
    c. The bodies of vertebrae become smaller passing down the spinal column.
    d. Intervertebral foraminae transmit the spinal cord.
    e. An intervertebral joint is a secondary cartilaginous joint.

98. **Regarding the vertebral column:**
    a. The anterior longitudinal ligament unites vertebral laminae.
    b. The vertebral arteries give branches that supply the entire length of the spinal cord.
    c. Flexion, extension and lateral rotation occur in the cervical region.
    d. The shape of facet joints is the main factor that determines the movements between vertebrae.
    e. There is free rotation in the lumbar region.

99. **Concerning the spinal cord:**
    a. The spinal cord commences below the foramen magnum, and it ends at the level of vertebra L2 in adults.
    b. The cervical enlargement supplies the cervical plexus.
    c. In epidural anaesthesia the needle punctures dura.
    d. The largest radicular artery usually occurs in the lower thoracic or upper lumbar region.
    e. There are 31 pairs of spinal nerves.

100. **Concerning the meninges:**
    a. The epidural space is between the dura mater and the vertebral periosteum.
    b. The dural sac ends at the same level as the spinal cord.
    c. The arachnoid mater is separated from the dura mater by the potential subarachnoid space.
    d. The cauda equina lies within the lumbar cistern.
    e. The pia mater continues below the conus medullaris as the filum terminale.

Short-answer Questions (SAQs)

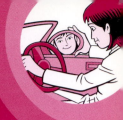

1. Briefly, describe the descriptive anatomical terms used in anatomy and clinical practice.

2. Describe the components of a spinal nerve.

3. Write short notes that describe the boundaries and contents of the axilla.

4. Draw a diagram to illustrate the components of the brachial plexus and list the branches with their distribution.

5. Describe the carpal tunnel, including contents and a syndrome that affects it.

6. Write short notes on the diaphragm.

7. List the muscles and their actions involved in respiration.

8. Write short notes on the blood supply of the heart.

9. Briefly describe the surface anatomy of the abdomen.

10. Briefly describe the inguinal canal, explaining the difference between direct and indirect inguinal hernias.

11. Illustrate the components of the rectus sheath.

12. List the main branches of the abdominal aorta, including the levels they arise at and the structures they supply.

13. Describe the main areas of portosytemic anastomosis and their clinical significance.

14. Explain the lymphatic drainage of the pelvis.

15. Describe the femoral triangle.

16. Summarize the venous drainage of the lower limb and a clinical condition that can affect these veins.

17. Using a diagram show the possible movements of the vocal folds, the muscles responsible for them and indicate the innervation of those muscles.

18. Given an account of the parasympathetic ganglia of the head.

19. Describe the thyroid gland and its blood supply.

20. Describe the arrangement of the spinal meninges, including a note on lumbar puncture.

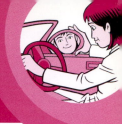

Extended Matching Questions (EMQs)

For each scenario described below, choose the *single* most correct response from the list of options. *Each option may be used once, more than once or not at all.*

1. Concerning the nervous system:

A. Central nervous system
B. Cranial nerves
C. Motor nerves
D. Parasympathetic nerves
E. Peripheral nervous system
F. Sensory nerves
G. Spinal nerves
H. Sympathetic nerves
I. Sacral nerves
J. Thoracic nerves

1. Nerves that contain preganglionic fibres, which synapse in ganglia associated with organs. ☐
2. Nerves that innervate structures of the head and neck. ☐
3. Term that applies to the structures that comprise the brain and spinal cord. ☐
4. Nerves that have cell bodies in the anterior horn of the spinal cord. ☐
5. Nerves arise from the thoracic and upper lumbar segments of the spinal cord only. ☐

2. Nerve injuries affecting limb movements:

A. Axillary nerve
B. Common peroneal nerve
C. Femoral nerve
D. Long thoracic nerve
E. Median nerve
F. Radial nerve
G. Sciatic nerve
H. Tibial nerve
I. Thoracodorsal nerve
J. Ulnar nerve

1. A 40-year-old man presents to A&E with a traumatic injury to his left arm. An X-ray reveals a midshaft fracture of the humerus. On examination, you find he cannot extend his wrist. ☐
2. A 45-year-old woman has a left mastectomy and removal of her left axillary lymph nodes. After the operation, she complains that she cannot wash or comb her hair with her left hand. Examination reveals winging of the left scapula. ☐

3. A 35-year-old woman is involved in a road traffic accident. Examination reveals that she is unable to dorsiflex her right foot (clinically known as foot drop). An X-ray demonstrates a fracture of the neck of the fibula. ☐
4. A 20-year-old man presents with a left shoulder dislocation after playing rugby. As part of your assessment, you test his sensation of the upper arm and find that he has anaesthesia (no sensation) over the upper lateral aspect of his arm. ☐
5. A 25-year-old man is involved in a fight at a nightclub. He presents with a puncture wound to the anterior aspect of his right wrist. Examination reveals paraesthesia (numbness) in the lateral three and a half digits and weak abduction of the pollicis (thumb). ☐

3. Osteology of the limbs:

A. Adductor tubercle
B. Lateral condyle
C. Lateral epicondyle
D. Linea aspera
E. Lunate
F. Medial condyle
G. Medial epicondyle
H. Neck of femur
I. Scaphoid
J. Shaft of femur

1. A fracture of this bone causes anatomical snuffbox tenderness and can cause necrosis of its proximal part. ☐
2. Its larger surface area allows rotation and locking of the knee joint during knee extension. ☐
3. Fracture of this bone causes a change in its axis of rotation and lateral rotation of the leg with the foot pointing outwards. ☐
4. The insertion of the hamstring part of adductor magnus. ☐
5. Fracture of this structure can cause weakness in the interossei muscles, adductor pollicis, hypothenar eminence and anaesthesia (no sensation) in the medial one and a half digits. ☐

4. Concerning the surface markings of the thorax:

A. Angle of Louis
B. Azygos vein
C. Brachiocephalic trunk
D. Brachiocephalic vein
E. Common carotid artery
F. Right atrium
G. Subclavian artery
H. Superior vena cava
I. Trachea (carina)
J. Ventricular apex

1. A structure that begins at the level of right first costal cartilage.
2. The surface landmark used to determine the level of the second costal cartilage.
3. A structure that joins the superior vena cava at the level of the right second costal cartilage.
4. A structure found in the left fifth intercostal space.
5. A structure that bifurcates at the level of the sternoclavicular joint

5. Concerning the anatomy of the heart:

A. Atrioventricular (coronary) groove
B. Atrioventricular node
C. Chordae tendineae
D. Interventricular groove
E. Left atrium
F. Left atrioventricular bundle branch
G. Moderator band
H. Right atrium
I. Right atrioventricular bundle branch
J. Sinoatrial node

1. On an anteroposterior chest X-ray, this heart structure is adjacent to the middle lobe of the right lung.
2. The location of the right coronary artery, part of the left coronary and its circumflex branch.
3. The term that is used for the area of the heart that controls its inherent rhythmicity.
4. The structure that conducts electrical activity in the interventricular septum and has two branches.
5. The structure that attaches the papillary muscles to the cusps of the atrioventricular valve.

6. Intracranial haemorrhage:

A. Extradural haemorrhage
B. Subdural haemorrhage
C. Subarachnoid haemorrhage
D. Subaponeurotic haematoma
E. Endocranium
F. Subarachnoid space
G. Arachnoid
H. Cavernous sinus
I. Dural venous sinuses
J. Circle of Willis

1. Can be caused by fracture of the pterion.
2. Term used to describe bleeding into the CSF.
3. A subdural haemorrhage occurs between this layer and the dura.
4. A subarachnoid haemorrhage may be due to rupture of vessels connected to this structure.
5. Site to which infection from the face may spread via the ophthalmic veins.

7. Nerve palsy and the eye:

A. Oculomotor nerve CNIII
B. Trochlear nerve CNIV
C. Trigeminal nerve CNV
D. Abducent nerve CNVI
E. Ptosis
F. Dilated pupil
G. Constricted pupil
H. Horner's syndrome
I. Divergent squint
J. Convergent squint

1. The cranial nerve most vulnerable to damage due to its long intracranial course.
2. Damage to this nerve causes ptosis with a dilated pupil.
3. The sign other than ptosis that is observed in Horner's syndrome
4. The result of damage to the abducent nerve (CNVI)
5. The only nerve listed above to provide general sensory innervation to the eyeball.

8. Inguinal hernia:

A. Indirect inguinal hernia
B. Direct inguinal hernia
C. Inguinal triangle
D. Processus vaginalis
E. Deep inguinal ring
F. Superficial inguinal ring
G. Inferior epigastric artery
H. Inguinal ligament
I. Spermatic cord

J. Abdominal wall weakness

1. This type of hernia is more common in older men.

2. The structure that lies medial to the neck of an indirect inguinal hernia.

3. The structure that an indirect inguinal hernia may pass through before entering the scrotum.

4. The structure through which a direct inguinal hernia enters the inguinal canal.

5. An indirect inguinal hernia always lies inside this structure.

9. Autonomic supply of abdomen and pelvis:

A. Sympathetic
B. Parasympathetic
C. Thoracic and lumbar splanchnic nerves
D. Pelvic splanchnic nerves
E. Sympathetic trunks
F. Vagal trunks
G. Coeliac plexus
H. Ganglion impar
I. Superior hypogastric plexus
J. Inferior hypogastric plexus

1. Type of innervation provided by greater splanchnic nerves.

2. Autonomic plexus supplying the stomach with sympathetic innervation.

3. Origin of parasympathetic innervation for the bladder.

4. Origin of parasympathetic innervation for foregut structures.

5. The structure formed in the pelvis by the hypogastric nerves.

10. Spinal meninges and lumbar puncture:

A. L2
B. L3
C. L4
D. Pia mater
E. Arachnoid mater
F. Dura mater
G. Subarachnoid space
H. Extradural space
I. Conus medullaris
J. Cauda equina

1. The lumbar cistern typically commences at the level of this vertebra in adults.

2. A lumbar puncture needle is inserted directly above or below this vertebra.

3. The lumbar cistern contains CSF and what structure?

4. What separates dura from vertebral periosteum and may be used in anaesthesia?

5. Which is the last layer of the meninges to be penetrated when sampling CSF?

Chapter 1 Basic concepts of anatomy

1. a. False the body is vertical with the head and face directed forwards.
    b. False the lower limbs are together with the feet slightly apart.
    c. False the palms are turned forwards (anterior).
    d. False the feet point anteriorly.
    e. False the head and eyes are directed forwards, looking into the distance.

2. a. True   this plane is at 90° to the median sagittal plane.
    b. False the parasagittal plane runs parallel to the median sagittal plane.
    c. False the coronal plane is at 90° to the median sagittal plane.
    d. True   this term is used in contrasting positions, e.g. the leg is inferior to the thigh.
    e. False it describes a structure, as further away from the body surface, e.g. bone is deep to muscle.

3. a. False adduction is toward the median sagittal plane.
    b. True   flexion is in the sagittal plane but it reduces the angle of a joint.
    c. False circumduction is a combination of flexion, extension, abduction and adduction.
    d. True   remember that thumb movements are at right angles to the rest of the digits.
    e. True   remember that thumb movements are at right angles to the rest of the digits.

4. a. True   vitamin D synthesis occurs in the skin.
    b. True   there are three layers, the epidermis, dermis and hypodermis.
    c. False sweat glands in dermis and dermal–hyodermal border aid thermoregulation.

d. False dermal collagen resists stretching. A genetic mutation in its synthesis (e.g. Ehlers–Danlos) causes very elastic skin.
    e. False the epidermis is waterproof; the hypodermis acts as a shock-absorbing layer.

5. a. False this occurs in red marrow found in the medullary cavity of the long bones of children. Yellow bone marrow is found in the long bones of adults.
    b. False this connective tissue membrane with an inner cellular layer that surrounds the bone.
    c. False the spongy (cancellous) layer lies deep to the outer compact bone layer.
    d. False the cortices are thinner and trabeculae decrease in number. This predisposes bone to fracturing.
    e. True   this growing portion of bone lies between the epiphysis and the diaphysis.

6. a. False this joint type has a fibrous capsule that covers articulating bone surfaces.
    b. True   this is the definition of Hilton's law.
    c. True   ligaments are pulled tight in excessive joint movements.
    d. False ligaments, muscles and bony contours all contribute to joint stability.
    e. True   primary, and secondary cartilaginous, fibrous and synovial joints.

7. a. False fixators are two opposing muscles that fix a joint.
    b. False this muscle exerts a greater force but with reduced mobility.
    c. False larger motor units are recruited for powerful contraction since they innervate larger muscles.
    d. True   force generated is related to the cross sectional area of muscles fibres.

e. True   an aponeurosis unites one muscle to another or muscle to bone.

8.
a. False   the right side pumps deoxygenated blood to lungs; left side pumps oxygenated blood to rest of body.

b. False   some veins lack valves, e.g. pelvic, head and neck veins.

c. False   these communications have a sphincter regulated by sympathetic nerve control.

d. False   functions include removal of excess tissue fluid, fat transportation and an immunological role against infection.

e. True   movement is by muscle contraction, pulsation of an adjacent artery, negative intrathoracic pressure and pressure gradient within vessel itself.

9.
a. False   the process of digestion begins in the mouth with mastication and salivary gland enzyme secretion.

b. False   the products of digestion are absorbed in the small intestine.

c. True   pancreatic enzymes and bile enter the second part of the duodenum to continue digestion.

d. True   an increased surface area is due to plicae circularis (folds), villi (finger-like projections) and microvilli.

e. False   the portal circulation transports carbohydrates and proteins. Fat enters the lymphatic system.

10.
a. True   humidification is by blood vessels in the nasal cavity and trapping of foreign material is by nasal hair and mucous secretion.

b. False   bronchioles lack cartilage. The bronchi have cartilaginous walls.

c. True   the alveoli are the site of gaseous exchange.

d. False   respiratory system functions include gaseous exchange, metabolism of proteins, blood reservoir, phonation and olfaction.

e. True   the trachea bifurcates at the carina to form two principal bronchi.

11.
a. True   See Fig. 1.15. Blood pressure within the glomerulus causes filtration of blood.

b. False   the nephron is the basic unit of the kidney. See Fig. 1.15.

c. False   selective reabsorption and secretion occur along the length of the nephron unit.

d. False   the function of the bladder is to store urine until such time it can be voided.

e. True   urothelium allows the ureters and bladder to stretch, thus allowing the latter to accommodate large amounts of urine.

Chapter 2   The upper limb

12.
a. True   the inferior angle of the scapula lies opposite the T7 vertebra.

b. True   the corocoid process is palpated in the deltopectoral triangle.

c. False   the anterior axillary fold contains the pectoralis major muscle.

d. False   the brachial artery is palpated in the cubital fossa medial to the biceps brachii tendon.

e. False   the olecranon process is palpated posteriorly.

13.
a. False   latissimus dorsi is supplied by the thoracodorsal nerve.

b. True   first part is medial, second part behind, and the third part lateral to the muscle.

c. False   teres major also receives nerve supply from the lower subscapular nerve.

d. True   long thoracic nerve damage paralyses serratus anterior. It is difficult to raise the arm above the head and the winging of the scapula is seen by pushing arm against wall.

e. False   supraspinatus initiates the first 15° of abduction.

14.
a. True   the circumflex scapular branch passes through the triangular space.

b. False is bounded by the humerus, long head of triceps brachii, teres major and minor muscles.

c. True the interval also contains the radial nerve.

d. True the axillary nerve and posterior circumflex artery passes through the space.

e. True see Fig. 2.10.

15. a. True the synovial joints have a fibrous capsule lined by a synovial membrane.

b. False the rotator cuff muscles are deficient inferiorly.

c. False the trochlea notch of the ulnar articulates with the trochlea of the humerus.

d. True the radial head rotates in the anular ligament at the proximal radioulnar joint.

e. True an articular disc 'sits' in the cavity of the sternoclavicular joint dividing it into two.

16. a. False axillary lymph nodes drain the upper limb, breast and thoracic wall.

b. False it is the continuation of the subclavian artery and commences at the outer border of the first rib.

c. False the vein lies outside the sheath so it can expand on increased venous return.

d. True the sulcus lies anteriorly on the humerus; the muscles are shoulder joint flexors.

e. True trunks are found in the posterior triangle of the neck; the divisions are behind the clavicle.

17. a. True anterior rami of the C5–C8 and T1 spinal nerves.

b. False posterior divisions of upper and lower trunks join the middle trunk; anterior division of middle trunk joins the upper trunk.

c. True see Fig. 2.15.

d. False the ulnar nerve arises from the medial cord.

e. False the radial nerve supplies some arm and forearm muscles. It gives only sensory innervation to the hand.

18. a. True the axillary artery finishes at the inferior border of teres major.

b. False the brachial artery can be palpated easily under biceps brachii medially.

c. True the radial artery passes through the snuffbox before passing between the first dorsal interosseous heads.

d. True they pass superficial to the flexor retinaculum to reach the hand.

e. False the common interosseous artery arises from the ulnar artery proximally in the forearm.

19. a. True supinator supinates the forearm; brachialis flexes the elbow.

b. True however sometimes it may divide in the arm and a superficial ulnar artery arises.

c. False the biceps brachii tendon is lateral to the brachial artery.

d. True the radial nerve divides anterior to the lateral epicondyle.

e. False the median nerve lies medially to the brachial artery.

20. a. False the cutaneous innervation of the medial forearm border is by a branch of medial cord of brachial plexus.

b. True a recurrent (muscular) branch of the median nerve supplies the thenar eminence.

c. False median nerve supplies flexor digitorum superficialis.

d. False median nerve supplies the muscle laterally; ulnar nerve supplies the muscle medially.

e. False the ulnar nerve supplies all intrinsic hand muscles except lateral two lumbricals.

21. a. False its posterior interosseous branch supplies the supinator muscle as it pierces it to pass to the posterior forearm compartment.

b. False the median nerve and the ulnar artery pass distally deep to flexor digitorum profundus.

c. True pronator teres forms the medial border of the cubital fossa.

d. True the ulnar nerve passes deep between the two heads of the flexor carpi ulnaris muscle.

e. False the action of the muscle is abduction and extension of the wrist.

22. a. False dorsal interossei abduct the digits towards the middle digit.

b. True see Fig. 2.33. From between the two heads the radial artery passes to form the deep palmar arch.

c. False it passes between the two adductor pollicis muscle heads and forms the deep palmar arch.

d. False the muscle inserts into the first metacarpal bone.

e. False the lumbrical muscles arise from the tendons of flexor digitorum profundus.

23. a. True the bone cortex appears to be thicker in the long bones than in the short bones.

b. False the smooth surface of the cortex is interrupted by tendon insertion and entry of nutrient arteries into bone.

c. False the trabeculae can be seen as thin white lines in areas of bone, which bear external forces.

d. True osteoporotic bones appear darker due to loss of bone density.

e. False this fracture is not always evident and a repeat X-ray 10 days later confirms its presence.

24. a. True this is the thinnest part of the clavicle.

b. True the median cubital vein lies in the cubital fossa.

c. False the fracture causes the normally distal radial styloid process to lie at the same level as the ulnar styloid process.

d. True a fractured scaphoid may present as tenderness over the snuffbox, but it could also be due to a Colles fracture.

e. True the thickening normally affects the 4th and 5th digits and is relieved by cutting the contracture.

Chapter 3 The thorax

25. a. True but only the upper part of the second costal cartilage articulates with the manubrium.

b. True second to seventh costal cartilages articulate with the sternal body.

c. False there are upper and lower articular facets on the rib head separated by a crest articulating with vertebral body above and same numerical rib.

d. False these ribs do have costal cartilages.

e. False the weakest part is anterior to the rib angle. Trauma can cause a fracture which may lead to a pneumothorax.

26. a. True the neurovascular bundle runs between the innermost and internal intercostal muscles.

b. True intercostal nerves give rise to collateral, lateral cutaneous and anterior cutaneous branches.

c. False the phrenic nerve does not supply the intercostal muscles.

d. False the anterior intercostal arteries arise from the internal thoracic artery.

e. False needle insertion is equidistant between the ribs to avoid damage to the intercostal neurovascular bundle.

27. a. False the phrenic nerve arises from C3–C5 spinal segments and is motor to the diaphragm.

b. True the aorta passes behind the diaphragm at the T12 vertebra, with the azygos, accessory azygos and thoracic duct.

c. False the oesophagus passes through the muscle at T10 vertebral level.

d. True   the splanchnic nerves pierce the crurae of the diaphragm.

e. True   it is the main muscle of quiet respiration.

28.
a. True   the serous layer is within the fibrous layer.

b. True   it lies in the middle mediastinum only.

c. True   it is connected to the sternum by weak sternopericardial ligaments.

d. True   the visceral serous layer is sensitive to stretch only with autonomic innervation.

e. True   this serous reflection forms the oblique sinus. Reflection around great vessels forms the transverse sinus.

29.
a. False   the left ventricular wall is thicker since it has to pump against a high systemic blood pressure.

b. True   this is the remnant of the foramen ovale in the fetal heart, an atrial communication.

c. False   the apex is formed by the left ventricle and lies normally in the 5th left intercostal space in the mid clavicular line.

d. False   the sinoatrial node is the pacemaker and is influenced by sympathetic and vagus nerves.

e. False   this valve consists of two cusps and separates the left atrium and ventricle.

30.
a. True   arise from left and right aortic sinuses.

b. False   they drain directly into the right atrium.

c. True   the great cardiac vein ends in the coronary sinus.

d. False   the heart has left dominance when the posterior interventricular artery arises from the circumflex artery (branch of left coronary artery)

e. True   the venae cordis minimae empty into the heart chambers directly.

31.
a. False   coronary arteries arise from the ascending aorta.

b. False   the ligamentum arteriosum links the pulmonary trunk and aortic arch.

c. True   the sternal angle is at the level of T4 vertebral level.

d. True   the descending aorta runs to the left of the vertebral column. These branches are small.

e. False   it leaves the thorax behind the diaphragm.

32.
a. False   the phrenic nerve passes anteriorly and the vagus nerve passes posteriorly to the lung hilum.

b. False   the nerve is formed by the anterior rami and is the sole motor supply to the diaphragm.

c. True   the vagus nerve contributes parasympathetic fibres to these plexuses. Sympathetic trunk postganglionic fibres also contribute.

d. True   the nerves form the oesophageal plexus and pass through the diaphragm at the level of T10 vertebra.

e. True   the thoracic sympathetic ganglia supply abdominal structures, e.g. stomach or liver, through splanchnic nerves.

33.
a. True   the oesophagus is a continuation of the laryngopharynx at the C6 vertebral level.

b. False   the oesophagus is a posterior relation to the trachea.

c. True   the cricopharyngeus muscle forms an upper oesophageal sphincter.

d. False   the left gastric artery has oesophageal branches that supply the lower oesophagus.

e. True   the oesophagus pierces the diaphragmic muscle at T10 vertebral level.

34.
a. True   the right main bronchus is prone to inhaled foreign objects lodging in it.

b. False   the right has three lobes separated by oblique and horizontal fissures; the left has two lobes separated by a horizontal fissure.

c. True   there are ten segments in each lung.

d. True   the apex lies 1 cm above the clavicle.

e. False   it has autonomic nerve supply and is insensitive to pain.

35.   a. True   as the diaphragm contracts it lowers, thus increasing the vertical diameter.
      b. False   in adult males diaphragmatic movement is greater than thoracic. This is opposite for females.
      c. True   scalene muscles elevate ribs, intercostal muscles contract forcefully and erector spinae arch back, contributing to inspiration.
      d. False   the intercostal muscles relax and expiration is entirely due to lung elastic recoil.
      e. True   the muscle reinforces the elastic recoil.

36.   a. False   the aortic knuckle is seen on the left hand side of the trachea.
      b. False   the liver pushes the right hemidiaphragm superiorly and is higher.
      c. True   the left atrium forms the posterior border.
      d. True   the superior vena cava forms a curved shadow on PA X-ray.
      e. False   the pectoralis major muscle forms a shadow which is seen on PA chest X-ray.

37.   a. True   shortening of the suspensory ligaments causes peau d'orange or skin dimpling.
      b. False   the mediastinal contents are pushed to the opposite side by a tension pneumothorax.
      c. True   referred pain to the C4 dermatome via the phrenic nerve (C3–C5).
      d. True   the anterior interventricular artery is known as the widow's artery.
      e. False   the left recurrent laryngeal nerve is compressed and the majority of the left laryngeal musculature is paralysed.

Chapter 4 The abdomen

38.   a. True   it dips slightly below the costal margin in the midline.
      b. True   transpyloric plane intersects the linea semilunaris at the ninth costal cartilage and gall bladder fundus.

      c. False   it lies deep to the left ninth to eleventh ribs.
      d. False   the pancreatic head lies to the right of the L2 vertebral level.
      e. True   it is pushed down by the liver.

39.   a. False   the nerves run between transversus abdominis and internal oblique.
      b. False   below the arcuate line, it passes in front of transversus abdominis.
      c. True   the artery runs superiorly and anastomoses with the superior epigastric artery.
      d. True   the external oblique is supplied by T7–T12 nerves only.
      e. True   external oblique arises from the lower eight ribs.

40.   a. True   it is attached to these walls by extraperitoneal tissue.
      b. False   a retroperitoneal organ lies against the posterior abdominal wall.
      c. True   it is the lowest part of the peritoneal cavity in this position.
      d. True   the superior compartment lies above the mesocolon, the inferior compartment below.
      e. True   the foramen is a communication between the lesser and greater sacs.

41.   a. True   the oesophagus, liver, and gall bladder are also foregut derivatives.
      b. True   it is separated from the posterior abdominal wall by the omental bursa.
      c. True   it passes up through the oesophageal opening in the diaphragm due to a weakened right crus.
      d. True   left gastric artery from coeliac trunk; right gastric artery from the common hepatic artery.
      e. False   the lesser omentum connects the stomach to the liver.

42.   a. False   they open into the 2nd part at the major and minor duodenal papillae.

b. True   remember that lymphatic supply follows the arterial supply.

c. False   the jejunum has longer vasa recta.

d. True   the pancreas may be eroded by a duodenal ulcer.

e. True   the vagal input increases secretion and peristaltic activity; sympathetic input decreases these activities.

43.
a. False   the transverse colon has a mesentery (the transverse mesocolon).

b. False   this artery supplies as far as the splenic (left colic) flexure.

c. True   they may be used by a surgeon to distinguish bits of bowel.

d. True   roughly 2 cm inferior to the ileocaecal orifice.

e. False   they anastomose along the marginal artery of the colon.

44.
a. False   posteriorly on the liver there is the bare area, which lacks peritoneum.

b. False   deoxygenated blood passes directly to the inferior vena cava via hepatic veins.

c. False   it lies against the diaphragm.

d. False   it is an anatomical division: their blood supply and drainage is different.

e. True   it is the remnant of the embryonic ventral mesentery.

45.
a. True   left and right hepatic ducts form the common hepatic duct, which joins the cystic duct.

b. True   it forms a 'portal triad' with the portal vein and hepatic artery.

c. False   the right hepatic artery usually gives rise to the cystic artery.

d. True   it is marked by the transpyloric plane intersecting the linea semilunaris.

e. True   biliary obstruction results in reabsorption of bile pigments.

46.
a. False   it attaches to their spinous and transverse processes.

b. True   perinephric fat—this may disappear in extreme weight loss, causing the kidneys to drop down.

c. True   it must pass in front of the aorta.

d. False   psoas muscle.

e. False   they are supplied by three branches but none from the superior mesenteric artery.

47.
a. True   the common iliac arteries then divide to supply the pelvis and lower limb.

b. False   the superior mesenteric artery arises at the L1 vertebral level from the aorta.

c. True   the artery supplies the descending and sigmoid colon and the rectum superiorly.

d. False   all venous drainage of the gut goes to the hepatic portal vein.

e. True   portal hypertension can cause oesophageal varices, which may rupture.

48.
a. True   the plexus is formed within the substance of the psoas major muscle.

b. False   the femoral nerve is lateral to the psoas major muscle.

c. True   the ilioinguinal nerve is a collateral branch of the iliohypogastric nerve.

d. False   postganglionic fibres run along arterial plexuses.

e. True   pelvic splanchnic nerves innervate the distal half of the transverse colon onwards.

Chapter 5 The pelvis and perineum

49.
a. False   the greater pelvis lies above the pelvic brim.

b. True   the shape of these joints restricts movement.

c. False   it lies just lateral to the pubic symphysis.

d. False   anterior superior iliac spine and pubic symphysis lie in the vertical plane.

e. True   this wide angle allows a fetal head to pass through it.

50.
a. True   the sigmoid mesocolon ends at the third sacral segment.

b. True   superior rectal artery is a branch of the inferior mesenteric artery and the middle rectal artery is a branch of the internal iliac artery.

c. False   it has a layer of longitudinal muscle, like the small intestine.

d. False   the rectovesical pouch is in the male.

e. False   it is covered only at the front.

51. a. True   they turn anteriorly to run along the pelvic floor.

b. True   ductus deferens and seminal vesicles in the male, vagina and cervix in female.

c. False   the uterine artery is superior to the ureter.

d. False   it has a parasympathetic supply, its action being to empty the bladder.

e. True   it is easily visible on viewing the internal structure of the bladder.

52. a. True   only the superior surface is covered by peritoneum.

b. True   the broad ligament is a double fold of peritoneum.

c. False   an enlarged craggy prostate is a sign of malignant disease, e.g. prostatic carcinoma.

d. False   the ovarian artery is a branch of the abdominal aorta.

e. True   the posterior fornix is closely related to the rectouterine pouch.

53. a. True   the external iliac artery mainly supplies the lower limb.

b. False   the internal pudendal artery leaves the pelvis through the greater sciatic foramen.

c. False   the obturator artery is crossed medially by the ureter.

d. True   it is a remnant of the obliterated fetal umbilical artery.

e. False   only the gut tube and associated structures drain into the portal system.

54. a. False   the plexus is formed by the anterior rami of L4, L5, and S1–S5

b. True   this lies in front of the coccyx.

c. False   the pelvic splanchnic nerves carry parasympathetic nerves.

d. True   remember: 'S2, 3, 4 keeps your guts off the floor'.

e. True   the hypogastric nerves arise from the superior hypogastric plexus.

55. a. True   the posterior triangle is larger than the anterior triangle.

b. True   it forms a boundary for each of these regions.

c. False   they are supplied by the pudendal nerve (S2, 3, 4) and internal pudendal artery

d. False   the perineal membrane lies below the pelvic floor.

e. False   they contain ischioanal fat pads.

56. a. False   the external sphincter is supplied by the pudendal nerve (inferior rectal branch).

b. True   the anorectal junction is where puborectalis forms a 'sling' around the rectum.

c. True   the epithelium changes from columnar epithelium just below the anal valves.

d. True   an internal sphincter and an external sphincter in three parts.

e. True   usually caused by straining at stool in chronic constipation.

57. a. False   three cylinders: two corpora cavernosa and a corpus spongiosum.

b. True   the artery divides to form the artery of the bulb, the deep artery, and the dorsal artery of the penis.

c. False   they open into the vestibule and are active during sexual arousal.

d. True   this is used to alleviate pain in childbirth.

e. True   it is the female equivalent of the male corpus spongiosum.

Chapter 6 The lower limb

58. a. False   the greater trochanter is palpable in the hip region.

b. False   the iliotibial tract is palpated on the lateral surface of the thigh.

c. False   the subcutaneous surface of the tibia is anteromedial. The muscles lie anterolaterally.

d. True   the small saphenous vein passes posterior to the lateral malleolus.

e. True   it is an important dermatome to know when testing the spinal cord roots in neurological examination.

59. a. True   the depth of the acetabulum is increased by an acetabular labrum, increasing stability further.

b. False   the gluteus medius and minimus muscles abduct (and also medially rotate) the femur at the hip joint. Gluteus maximus extends the hip and laterally rotates the femur.

c. False   the superior gluteal nerve (L4, L5 and S1) passes above the piriformis muscle.

d. True   gluteal (or clunial) nerves arise from the posterior cutaneous nerve of the thigh, L1–3 and S1–3 posterior rami.

e. True   the pudendal nerve exits via the greater sciatic foramen and enters the lesser sciatic foramen.

60. a. False   the femoral artery and vein are within the femoral sheath.

b. True   the femoral nerve is a lateral structure. Remember the mnemonic N-A-V-Y from lateral to medial.

c. False   the medial border of the adductor longus muscle forms the medial border of the femoral triangle.

d. True   the femoral canal begins superiorly at the femoral ring.

e. True   the adductor brevis muscle is seen in the gap between pectineus and adductor longus muscles.

61. a. False   the femoral artery is a direct continuation of the external iliac artery.

b. True   the four perforating branches of the profunda femoris artery supply adductor magnus and the hamstring muscles.

c. True   the great saphenous vein pierces the cribriform fascia of the saphenous opening before joining the femoral vein.

d. False   the profunda femoris vein joins the femoral vein just below the inguinal ligament.

e. True   the femoral canal contains a few lymphatic vessels and loose connective tissue.

62. a. True   the ilioinguinal nerve (L1) is a branch of the lumbar plexus. It also supplies scrotal (or labia majus) skin.

b. False   the lateral cutaneous nerve passes medial to the anterior superior iliac spine.

c. True   the pectineus muscle has a dual nerve supply from femoral and obturator nerves.

d. True   the posterior femoral cutaneous nerve supplies skin of posterior thigh and perineum.

e. False   the short head of biceps femoris is innervated by the common peroneal nerve of the sciatic nerve.

63. a. True   these muscles are abductors of the thigh. Note that adduction is restricted by the contralateral lower limb.

b. True   extension stretches the pubofemoral and iliofemoral ligaments.

c. True   the pull of iliopsoas about this axis causes medial rotation of the thigh.

d. False   the ischiofemoral ligament resists medial rotation.

e. False   the anteroposterior axis passes through the femoral head.

64. a. True   the femoral artery lies adjacent to the distal end of the femur and fractures may damage it.

b. False   the popliteal artery has genicular, muscular and sural branches.

c. True   the small saphenous vein pierces the popliteal fascia to join the popliteal vein.

d. False the superior boundary is biceps femoris (laterally) and semimembranosus and semitendinosus (medially).

e. False the popliteus muscle unlocks the knee joint by lateral rotation of the femur.

65. a. False the knee joint is an articulation between the femur and the tibia.

b. False popliteus laterally rotates the femur on the tibia. Rotation can occur in the flexed knee.

c. True   other bursae that communicate with the joint are popliteus and gastrocnemius bursae.

d. True   the anterior cruciate ligament attaches the lateral femoral condyle to the anterior part of the intercondylar area of tibia.

e. True   prepatella bursitis is called clergyman's knee. Housemaid's knee is infrapatella bursitis.

66. a. False the peroneus tertius muscle is supplied by the deep peroneal nerve.

b. False extensor digitorum longus inserts into the lateral four digits.

c. True   the inferior extensor retinaculum attaches to the calcaneus (laterally), medial malleolus and fascia.

d. True   the stability of this joint is reinforced by the tibiofibular ligaments and stabilizes the ankle joint.

e. False superiorly the anterior tibial artery passes through a hiatus in the membrane.

67. a. True   the tibial nerve divides just below the flexor retinaculum.

b. False the saphenous nerve, a terminal branch, of the femoral nerve, passes anterior to the medial malleolus.

c. True   the deep peroneal nerve supplies the skin of the first interdigital cleft (and anterior compartment of the leg).

d. False the tibial nerve supplies the posterior compartment.

e. True   the sural nerve supplies the skin on the posterior and lateral parts of the leg.

68. a. True   the dorsalis pedis artery can be palpated between the extensor hallucis and digitorum longus tendons.

b. True   the foot has an extensor expansion similar to the expansion found in the hand.

c. True   extensor hallucis brevis inserts into the proximal phalanx of the great toe (hallux).

d. True   the dorsal venous arch also drains medially into the great saphenous vein.

e. False extensor digitorum brevis is supplied by the deep peroneal nerve.

69. a. False the first medial lumbrical is supplied by the medial plantar nerve.

b. False it inserts into the middle phalanges of the lateral four digits.

c. False it moves the hallux towards the second digit.

d. False the saphenous, sural and calcaneal branches of the tibial nerve also innervate the skin (see Fig. 6.40).

e. True   the spring ligament helps to maintain the foot arches.

70. a. True   normally the venous valves allow venous flow from superficial to deep veins.

b. False it is palpated at the mid-inguinal point (half way between the anterior superior iliac spine and pubic symphysis.

c. True   this change in axis causes iliopsoas to become a lateral rotator of the femur.

d. True   Shenton's line is a smooth line traced along the femur shaft, neck and superior pubic ramus.

e. True   other features that would be present also are osteophytes, subchondral sclerosis and bone cysts.

Chapter 7 The head and neck

71. a. False the sagittal suture is formed by the articulation of the parietal bones alone.

b. False   the coronal suture joins the sagittal suture at the bregma.

c. False   the sagittal suture joins the lambdoid suture at the lambda.

d. True   the pterion overlies the anterior branches of middle meningeal artery.

e. False   it closes on average between 18–24 months.

72.
a. True   it transmits the internal jugular vein.

b. False   it also transmits the facial nerve and labyrinthine artery.

c. True   the ophthalmic artery.

d. True   it runs on into the pterygopalatine fossa.

e. False   it enters the carotid canal, then enters the top part of the foramen lacerum (the lower part being blocked off by fibrocartilage).

73.
a. False   the buccal branch of the facial nerve is motor to the facial muscles.

b. True   it is involved in mastication but innervated by the facial nerve.

c. False   the greater occipital and lesser occipital cervical nerves supply the scalp posteriorly.

d. True   the facial vein eventually empties into the internal jugular vein.

e. False   the internal carotid artery, through supraorbital and supratrochlear branches, also contributes to the supply.

74.
a. True   an enlargement of the pituitary gland here can cause bitemporal hemianopia.

b. False   the superior sagittal sinus runs in the superior border of the falx cerebri.

c. False   the falx cerebelli separates the cerebellar hemispheres.

d. True   the sigmoid sinus also receives the superior petrosal sinus.

e. False   the circulus arteriosus connects the internal carotid and vertebral arteries.

75.
a. True   VII and X are involved in supplying skin around the ear.

b. False   CN XI (cranial part) is motor to pharyngeal and laryngeal muscles via the vagus nerve.

c. True   the muscles are supplied by the mandibular branch of the trigeminal nerve.

d. False   III, VII and IX.

e. False   they are supplied by cranial IX fibres carried by X and the pharyngeal plexus.

76.
a. False   it is supplied by the trochlear nerve.

b. True   their medial and lateral movements cancel out.

c. False   lateral rectus is paralysed, so it is displaced medially.

d. True   true downwards movement occurs together with superior oblique.

e. False   the pupil is dilated due to unopposed sympathetic innervation.

77.
a. False   the nasolacrimal duct empties into the inferior meatus of the nasal cavity.

b. True   the greater petrosal branch of the facial nerve carries parasympathetic nerve fibres to the ganglion.

c. True   the orbital part of the frontal bone forms the roof of the orbit.

d. True   the inferior orbital fissure connects the orbit with the pterygopalatine fossa.

e. True   the long ciliary nerve carries sympathetic fibres to the dilator pupillae muscle of the eye.

78.
a. True   the vein is superficial to the artery, but both are deep to the facial nerve.

b. False   the parotid duct opens opposite the upper second molar tooth.

c. False   the facial nerve divides into its five terminal branches within the parotid gland.

d. True   the submandibular gland has superficial and deep parts, around mylohyoid.

e. True   both preganglionic to the submandibular ganglion and postganglionic fibres to the glands.

79.
a. False the condyloid process takes part in the joint; the coronoid attaches temporalis.
b. False the lateral pterygoid is used to pull the mandible forward in wide opening.
c. True it communicates with the dural venous sinuses.
d. True the temporomandibular ligament prevents posterior dislocation.
e. True carried by the tympanic branch.

80.
a. True the infrahyoid strap muscles are innervated by the ansa cervicalis (C1, 2 and 3 and fibres from CNXII hypoglossal).
b. True the accessory nerve appears in the posterior triangle from behind the posterior border of sternocleidomastoid.
c. True superior, middle and inferior ganglia. The inferior ganglion usually fuses with the first thoracic ganglion.
d. True it is a possible route for spread of infection.
e. True spinal cord transsection above C3 results in paralysis of the diaphragm.

81.
a. False it lies between the carotid sheath and the prevertebral fascia.
b. True the nerves form loops and off these loops arise the branches of the cervical plexus.
c. True it is proportionally larger to accommodate the cervical expansion of the spinal cord.
d. False the internal carotid artery has no branches in the neck.
e. False the external jugular is formed by the posterior auricular vein and the posterior division of the retromandibular vein.

82.
a. True it joins the cranial part inside the cranial cavity.
b. True the carotid sinus branch.
c. False the brachial plexus roots emerge between the scalenus anterior and scalenus medius muscles.
d. True it lies posteriorly then laterally.
e. True the deep cervical lymph nodes, which drain into the jugular lymph trunk.

83.
a. True the common carotid divides into external and internal carotid arteries.
b. True sternocleidomastoid covers over the carotid sheath.
c. False it attaches to the clavicle and first rib.
d. False the external laryngeal nerve is motor to cricothyroid muscle.
e. True the superior root comes from this nerve.

84.
a. False the glossopharyngeal nerve supplies stylopharyngeus.
b. False it ends at the level of the cricoid and start of the oesophagus (C6).
c. True the tubal tonsils.
d. True the soft palate forms a seal so that food cannot enter the nasopharynx.
e. True thyropharyngeus and cricopharyngeus.

85.
a. True the tongue surface has an irregular appearance due to the lingual tonsil.
b. True the vagus nerve provides the motor innervation.
c. True the fascia blends with the periosteum of the skull above.
d. False it lies behind.
e. True they are created by the glossoepiglottic folds and food may stick in them.

86.
a. False septal cartilage, perpendicular plate of the ethmoid bone and vomer bone form the nasal septum.
b. True it opens in the hiatus semilunaris; however, cannot be drained by gravity as the opening is too high on its medial wall.
c. True the sphenoid sinus lies below the pituitary fossa.
d. False olfactory mucosa exists only in the very uppermost part of the nasal cavity.
e. True this allows surgical access to the pituitary.

87.
a. True the olfactory nerves pass through to innervate olfactory mucosa.

b. True   three conchae separate the sphenoethmoidal recess into the superior meatus, middle meatus and inferior meatus.

c. True   pterygopalatine fossa communicates via the foramen rotundum and pterygoid canal with the middle cranial fossa.

d. True   the deep petrosal nerve carries sympathetic fibres; the greater petrosal nerve carries parasympathetic fibres.

e. True   the pharyngeal nerve, passing out through the palatovaginal canal.

88.
a. True   the fissure lies between lesser and greater wings.

b. True   the hard palate is formed by the maxilla and palatine bones.

c. True   to the mastoid process.

d. True   the internal acoustic meatus transmits both nerves. The stylomastoid foramen transmits the facial nerve.

e. False   the condyloid process articulates with the mandibular fossa of the temporal bone.

89.
a. False   it opens in the floor of the mouth.

b. False   the posterior one-third is innervated by the glossopharyngeal nerve.

c. True   this is called Waldeyer's ring.

d. True   the hypoglossal nerve innervates almost all tongue muscles.

e. False   the roof is innervated by branches of the maxillary (V_2) nerve.

90.
a. True   the hypoglossal nerve innervates all the muscles of the tongue except the extrinsic muscle palatoglossus.

b. False   the maxilla and palatine bones form the hard palate.

c. True   a carcinoma may spread to neck structures through the lymphatics.

d. True   the vallate papillae are on the oral part of the tongue.

e. True   the palatoglossus muscle forms the palatoglossal arch; the palatopharyngeus muscle forms the palatopharyngeal arch.

91.
a. True   the glandular branch of the facial and the sublingual branch of the lingual arteries both contribute.

b. True   palatoglossus and palatopharyngeus.

c. False   the sublingual gland receives a parasympathetic supply from the submandibular ganglion.

d. False   the medial pterygoid nerve supplies the tensor veli palatini muscle.

e. True   the glossopharyngeal supplies sensory fibres; the vagus nerve carries motor fibres from the accessory nerve.

92.
a. False   it would enter the infraglottic cavity, below the vocal folds.

b. False   the external laryngeal nerve supplies the cricothyroid muscle.

c. True   the epiglottis covers the laryngeal inlet as a food bolus passes towards the oesophagus.

d. True   they run from the vocal processes of the arytenoids to the back of the thyroid cartilage.

e. False   they articulate with the cricoid cartilage.

93.
a. True   in nerve damage the ipsilateral vocal fold is adducted and the voice is hoarse.

b. False   it tightens them.

c. True   this closes the rima glottidis.

d. False   vocalis tenses the vocal ligament anteriorly and relaxes it posteriorly.

e. True   the transverse arytenoid adducts the vocal ligaments, closing the rima glottis.

94.
a. False   the thyrohyoid membrane is pierced by the internal laryngeal nerve.

b. True   the vestibular ligament is superior to the vocal ligament, separated by a ventricle.

c. False   the laryngeal inlet is bounded by the epiglottis, aryepiglottic and interarytenoid folds.

d. True   this allows gliding and rotating movements.

e. True   this pushes the epiglottis down, closing the laryngeal inlet.

95.   a. True   the isthmus lies over tracheal rings 2–4.
    b. False   it is drained by three pairs – the superior, middle and inferior.
    c. False   the inferior is a branch of the thyrocervical trunk of the subclavian artery.
    d. True   the superior artery is closely associated with the external laryngeal nerve.
    e. True   a thyroidectomy can be performed to remove it.

Chapter 8   The back

96.   a. True   this is a useful landmark in lumbar puncture.
    b. True   except C1.
    c. True   eight cervical, twelve thoracic, five lumbar, five sacral, and four coccygeal vertebrae.
    d. True   the thoracic curvature results from the wedge shaped vertebral bodies.
    e. True   the C7 vertebral process is called the 'vertebra prominens'.

97.   a. False   there are seven cervical vertebrae (although eight cervical spinal nerves).
    b. True   they form part of the neural arch.
    c. False   they increase in size, as they have more weight to bear.
    d. False   they lie laterally, transmitting spinal nerves and vessels.
    e. True   each disc consists of anulus fibrous and nucleus pulposus.

98.   a. False   it lies on the anterior surfaces of vertebral bodies and IV discs.
    b. False   the blood supply is reinforced segmentally by spinal arteries.
    c. True   thick intervertebral discs, a lax capsule, and horizontal facets accommodate these movements.
    d. True   the interlocking of facet joints prevents rotation in the lumbar region.
    e. False   rotation is prevented in the lumbar region by interlocking articular facets.

99.   a. True   the spinal cord is shorter than the vertebral column, and it ends in the conus medullaris.
    b. False   it supplies the brachial plexus.
    c. False   the anaesthetic is delivered into the epidural space, not the subarachnoid.
    d. True   this is called the arteria radicularis magna.
    e. True   note that this is two less than the number of vertebrae.

100.   a. True   into this space anaesthetic agent can be introduced, producing an epidural block, e.g. in childbirth.
    b. False   it continues down to the level of S2, creating the lumbar cistern.
    c. False   the subdural space is between the dura mater and the subarachnoid mater.
    d. True   it is created by spinal nerve roots passing downwards to their respective intervertebral foraminae.
    e. True   the pia mater attaches to the coccyx via the filum terminale.

1. The anatomical position allows an accurate description of the body, especially the relationship of one structure to another. This standard position consists of (i) the head directed forwards, with eyes looking into the distance, (ii) the body upright, with legs together and feet directed anteriorly, and (iii) the palms of the hands facing forwards with the thumbs laterally.

   Anatomical planes are frequently used in medical imaging, e.g. CT scans and MRIs when cross-sectional images of the body are produced. Such cross-sectional planes include (i) the median sagittal plane, which is a vertical plane that passes through the midline of the body from anterior to posterior. Any plane parallel to this is known as a parasagittal plane; (ii) the coronal plane is a vertical plane that is at 90° to the median sagittal plane (dividing the body into anterior and posterior portions), and (iii) the horizontal plane transverses the body from anterior to posterior, dividing the body into superior and inferior parts. The terms of position are described in Fig. 1.3. These terms allow description of the relationships between body parts, e.g. the arm is proximal to the forearm or the skin is superficial to muscle.

   The terms of movement are described in Fig. 1.4. However, these terms of movement are different for the thumb (pollex) and the ankle. The thumb (pollex) is rotated 90° medially relative to the fingers and so abduction of the thumb occurs in the same plane as flexion of the fingers. The extension (dorsiflexion) of the ankle causes a reduction in the angle of the joint and flexion (plantar flexion) increases the angle.

2. In the peripheral nervous system there are 31 pairs of spinal nerves, including 8 cervical, 12 thoracic, 5 lumbar, 5 sacral and 1 coccygeal. The roots of the spinal nerves arise from the spinal cord, which terminates at the lower border of the first lumbar vertebra in the adult. Inferior to this the nerve roots form the cauda equina. Anterior and posterior nerve roots unite to form a spinal nerve. The spinal nerve then divides into anterior and posterior rami that supply the anterior and posterior parts of the body respectively. The anterior rami form the great nerve plexuses that supply the limbs, e.g. brachial plexus.

   The spinal nerve anterior root contains motor fibres that innervate skeletal muscle, as well as autonomic fibres, e.g. sympathetic fibres from T1 to L2 spinal cord levels and parasympathetic fibres from S2–S4 spinal cord levels that innervate viscera. The spinal nerve posterior root contains sensory fibres that carry information from the periphery to the spinal cord. Thus spinal nerves (and some cranial nerves) contain a mixture of motor, sensory and autonomic fibres.

   A motor fibre originates from a cell body in the anterior horn of the spinal cord, travels in the anterior root and synapses with the sarcolemma of muscle to form the neuromuscular junction.

   A sensory fibre carries an impulse from a receptor in the periphery, e.g. skin, viscera or muscle to the spinal cord. It enters through the posterior root; its cell body lies in the posterior root ganglion. The fibres may synapse in the posterior horn of the spinal cord before ascending higher centres, e.g. cerebellum or cerebral cortex.

   A sympathetic preganglionic fibre from the spinal cord synapses in a ganglion, i.e. either in the sympathetic chain (either side of the vertebral column) or in a prevertebral ganglion, e.g. coeliac ganglion. The sympathetic postganglionic fibre leaves the ganglion to enter a spinal nerve or innervate viscera. A parasympathetic preganglionic fibre in sacral spinal nerves (and some cranial nerves) synapses in ganglia closely associated with organs which they innervate through a postganglionic fibre.

3. The axilla is a pyramidal space between the arm and the thoracic wall that is bounded anteriorly and posteriorly by axillary folds.

   Superiorly, the axilla communicates via its apex with the posterior triangle of the neck, and it contains the neurovascular structures for the upper limb. The boundaries of the axilla are:

   - apex—the superior border of the scapula, the clavicle and the outer border of the first rib.
   - anterior wall—pectoralis major, pectoralis minor muscles, and clavipectoral fascia (these form the anterior axillary fold).
   - lateral wall—intertubercular groove.
   - posterior wall—teres major, latissimus dorsi, and subscapularis muscles (these form the posterior axillary fold).
   - medial wall—serratus anterior, upper four ribs, and intercostal muscles.
   - floor—axillary fascia and skin.

   The contents of the axilla are the axillary artery, axillary vein, lymph nodes, and the three cords of the brachial plexus. These structures enter or exit through the apex of the axilla. The axillary artery is a continuation of the subclavian artery from the outer border of the first rib, and it finishes at the lower border of the teres major muscle. The artery is divided into three parts by the pectoralis minor muscle. The first part is medial to the muscle and has one branch. The second part is behind the muscle and has two branches. The third part lies lateral to the muscle and has three branches. The axillary vein is formed by joining of the brachial veins and basilic vein at the lower border of teres major muscle, and it becomes the subclavian vein at the outer border of the first rib. The tributaries are the same as the arterial branches. The cords of the brachial plexus run with the axillary artery in the axillary sheath. The axillary sheath is derived from the prevertebral fascia of the deep cervical fascia of the neck. The cords divide into branches within the axilla that supply the upper limb. The axillary vein lies outside the axillary sheath and this allows it to expand in increased venous return.

Within the fatty tissue of the axilla are five groups of axillary lymph nodes. These lymph nodes drain the upper limb and the majority of the breast. The lymph nodes empty into a subclavian lymph trunk that empties into the thoracic duct on the left or the right lymphatic duct.

4. See Figs 2.14 and 2.15.

5. The carpal tunnel is an osseofibrous tunnel formed by the flexor retinaculum and the carpal bones of the hand. The flexor retinaculum is a strong thickening of deep fascia that serves to bind the long flexor tendons of the forearm against the carpal bones. It is attached to the pisiform bone and hook of hamate medially, and the trapezium and scaphoid bones laterally. The intrinsic muscles of the thenar and hypothenar eminences take origin from the flexor retinaculum.

Through the carpal tunnel pass the four tendons of flexor digitorum superficialis, the four tendons of flexor digitorum profundus, the tendon of flexor pollicis longus, and the median nerve. As the tendons of flexor digitorum superficialis enter the carpal tunnel, the index finger and little finger tendons lie deep to the middle finger and ring finger tendons. At the distal row of carpal bones, these four tendons all lie in the same plane. A synovial sheath surrounds all the tendons within the carpal tunnel. The median nerve is the most superficial structure in the carpal tunnel, and it supplies the thenar eminence, lateral two lumbrical muscles, and the skin of the lateral three and a half digits.

Compression of the median nerve in the carpal tunnel can occur, and this is known as carpal tunnel syndrome, a common clinical condition. This compression paralyses the thenar eminence muscles. Paralysis of the two lateral lumbrical muscles can be seen when the patient is asked to make a fist and the two lateral fingers lag behind the two medial digits. Paraesthesia (numbness) occurs over the lateral three and a half digits. The skin of the palm is unaffected due to the palmar cutaneous branch of the median nerve arising before the nerve enters the carpal tunnel and passing over the flexor retinaculum. The compression is relieved by division of the flexor retinaculum.

6. The diaphragm is a thin sheet of muscle that separates the thoracic and abdominal cavities. In profile, the diaphragm is an inverted 'J-shape' with two domes. The right dome is higher than the left. The diaphragm is the primary muscle of inspiration and on contraction it flattens. This action is seen in adult respiration; however, there is greater movement of the thoracic wall during inspiration in women and children.

The diaphragm arises from two crura. The right crus arises from the upper three lumbar vertebral bodies and intervening intervertebral discs, and fibres of the right crus form a sling around the oesophageal opening in the diaphragm. The left crus arises from the upper two lumbar bodies and intervening intervertebral disc. These crura pass superiorly into a central tendon. The tendinous fibres of the medial edge of the crura unite with each other in front of the T12 vertebra and form the median arcuate ligament (anterior to the aortic hiatus). The medial arcuate ligament is a thickening of psoas fascia, and the lateral arcuate ligament is a thickening of the quadratus lumborum fascia. Muscle fibres arise from the medial and lateral arcuate ligaments, the twelfth rib, and the costal margin and adjacent ribs as far as the seventh rib. The muscle fibres then pass upwards and insert into a central tendon.

There are three large openings in the diaphragm. An aortic opening is opposite T12 vertebra behind the median arcuate ligament. It transmits the aorta, azygos vein, hemiazygos vein, and thoracic duct. The oesophageal opening is opposite T10, and it is within the muscle of the diaphragm. It transmits the oesophagus, vagus nerves, and oesophageal branches of the left gastric vessels. The vena caval opening is opposite the T8 vertebra in the central tendon. It transmits the inferior vena cava and the right phrenic nerve. Other structures pass between the diaphragm and the body wall. Splanchnic nerves and the sympathetic trunk pass behind the diaphragm. Lymphatics and the superior epigastric vessels pass anteriorly to the diaphragm. The lower six intercostal neurovascular bundles pass laterally to diaphragm.

The motor nerve supply to the diaphragm is phrenic nerve (C3–C5). The sensory nerve supply is the phrenic nerve centrally and the lower five intercostal and subcostal nerves peripherally. The blood supply is from the musculophrenic branch and superior epigastric branch of the internal thoracic artery. It receives phrenic branches from the thoracic and abdominal aorta.

7. See Fig. 3.35.

8. The arterial supply of the heart is through the two coronary arteries, which arise from the ascending aorta. The left and right coronary arteries arise from the aortic sinuses and run for a variable distance in the coronary groove.

The right coronary artery in 60% of individuals supplies the sinoatrial node (the pacemaker of the heart) and in 90% of individuals supplies the atrioventricular node. The atrioventricular bundle, and its right and left branch, are supplied by this artery. Most commonly the right coronary artery gives rise to the posterior interventricular artery. This is known as right dominance. Dominance refers to the coronary artery from which the posterior interventricular artery arises.

The left coronary divides into a circumflex artery that continues to run in the left coronary groove and an anterior interventricular artery, which, as the name suggests, lies between right and left ventricles. It supplies the left branch of the atrioventricular bundle.

Venous drainage of the heart mostly enters the coronary sinus that lies in the coronary groove posteriorly. It receives tributaries from the great cardiac, middle cardiac and small cardiac veins that accompany the anterior interventricular, posterior interventricular and right marginal artery respectively. A small proportion of venous blood does not enter the coronary sinus and instead is returned in either the anterior cardiac veins directly into the right atrium or into any of the chambers of the heart via small veins known as venae cordis minimae.

Narrowing of the coronary arteries or their branches causes ischaemic heart disease (angina) and complete occlusion causes a myocardial infarction (heart attack). The narrowing can be 'bypassed' by surgically grafting the great saphenous vein or the internal thoracic artery onto the affected coronary artery.

9. To facilitate description of abdominal pain and/or swellings, the abdomen is divided into four quadrants by vertical and horizontal lines through the umbilicus. However, a more accurate division of the abdomen into nine regions is also used. These nine regions are formed by two vertical lines that correspond to the midclavicular lines, and two horizontal lines. One horizontal line corresponds to the transpyloric plane (L1 vertebral level, intersecting with the 9th costal cartilage) and the second runs between the tubercles of the iliac crests (intertubercular plane).

The inferior border of the liver extends from the right 10th costal cartilage in the midaxillary line to the left 5th rib in the midclavicular line. The upper border of the liver lies along the 5th ribs (and their costal cartilages) between the midclavicular lines. The right border of the liver runs from the 5th right rib to the 10th costal cartilage.

The fundus of the gall bladder lies deep to where the linea semilunaris intersects the right costal margin in the transpyloric plane in the midclavicular line. At this point the fundus lies behind the 9th right costal cartilage.

The spleen lies deep to the 9, 10 and 11th ribs on the left. It is not palpable unless it is enlarged, at which point the spleen extends inferiorly and anteriorly along the 10th rib to below the costal margin.

The hilum of the kidney lies in the transpyloric plane, 5 cm from the midline. The upper poles of the kidneys lie anterior to the 12th rib. The right kidney is lower than the left because of the presence of the liver, but they both lie roughly opposite the first three lumbar vertebrae.

The ureters begin at the hilum of the kidney in the transpyloric plane. They run inferiorly on the anterior surface of the psoas major muscle, in front of the tips of the lumbar vertebrae transverse processes (as seen on a urogram), to the sacroiliac joint to enter the pelvis.

10. The inguinal canal is an oblique slit, approximately 6 cm long. The canal runs parallel and just above the medial half of the inguinal ligament, commencing at the deep inguinal ring and ending at the superficial inguinal ring medially. In males the inguinal canal transmits the spermatic cord and ilioinguinal nerve. In females the round ligament and ilioinguinal nerve form the canal contents.

The anterior wall of the inguinal canal is formed by the external oblique aponeurosis. The inguinal ligament forms the floor, which is the lower free edge of the external oblique aponeurosis. The floor is reinforced medially by the lacunar ligament, which extends from the inguinal ligament to the pectinate line of the superior pubic ramus. The internal oblique and transversus abdominis muscles form the roof laterally. The posterior wall is formed by the transversalis fascia laterally and by the conjoint tendon medially.

The deep ring is an opening in the transversalis fascia bounded laterally by the arching fibres of transversus abdominis and the inguinal ligament and medially by the transversalis fascia. The superficial ring is a triangular slit in the external oblique aponeurosis. The fibres of the aponeurosis split into two crura. A medial crus attaches to the pubic crest and a lateral crus attaches to the pubic tubercle.

Structures that comprise the spermatic cord enter the inguinal canal at the deep inguinal ring. As they pass through the inguinal canal they gain three covering layers from the anterior abdominal wall. Only when these structures exit the canal at the superficial ring are they completely invested in the three layers. The ilioinguinal nerve lies outside the spermatic cord because it does not enter the canal at the deep inguinal ring. It enters the canal from the side as the nerve runs between the external oblique and internal oblique layers. However, it does leave the canal through the superficial ring.

An indirect hernia is where the hernia tracks through the inguinal canal within the spermatic cord, passing through the deep inguinal ring. In a direct hernia, the hernia does not pass through the deep inguinal ring, instead entering the inguinal canal through a weakness in the abdominal wall.

11. See Fig. 4.6.

12. The main branches of the abdominal aorta are;
Unpaired ventral branches:
- Coeliac trunk – arises at level of T12, supplies foregut structures (stomach, first one and a half parts of duodenum, liver, spleen, pancreas).
- Superior mesenteric artery – arises at level of L1, supplies midgut structures (distal duodenum, caecum, appendix, ascending colon, first half of transverse colon).
- Inferior mesenteric artery – arises at level of L3, supplies hindgut structures (distal half of transverse colon, descending and sigmoid colons, rectum, upper anal canal).

Paired lateral branches:
- Inferior phrenic arteries – arise at T12, pass to the diaphragm. Also give superior suprarenal branches.
- Middle suprarenal arteries – arise at T12, pass to the adrenal glands.

277

- Renal arteries – arise at L2, pass to the kidneys. The left is longer than the right and gives rise to inferior suprarenal and gonadal branches which are direct branches of the aorta on the right.
- Lumbar arteries – four pairs arising segmentally. Supply posterior abdominal wall including vertebrae and spinal cord.
- Common iliac arteries – terminal branches at L4. Supply pelvis and lower limb.

13. Areas of portosystemic anastomosis occur between tributaries of the portal vein (draining back to the liver) and tributaries of the systemic venous system (draining back to the heart). Portal hypertension can be caused by liver tumours or cirrhosis – this increases the pressure in the portal venous system (portal hypertension), causing increased blood flow through and enlargement of areas of portosystemic anastomosis.

   The first site of anastomosis is the lower end of the oesophagus between the left gastric vein and tributaries of the azygos – the increased blood flow causes oesophageal varices which may rupture causing haematemesis (vomiting of blood).

   Para-umbilical veins around the umbilicus are another site of anastomosis – visibly enlarged veins radiating out from the umbilicus are referred to as Caput Medusae.

   There is anastomosis between the superior (portal) and inferior (systemic) rectal veins – hypertension causes varicoses of the internal rectal venous plexuses, resulting in haemorrhoids (note that portal hypertension is not the most common cause of haemorrhoids).

   There are also anastomoses where gut viscera lie retroperitoneal (such as the ascending and descending colon and the bare area of the liver) but these do not give rise to significant clinical symptoms.

14. See Fig. 5.21.

15. The femoral triangle is formed in the thigh. Its boundaries are:
    - the inguinal ligament, superiorly.
    - the medial aspect of sartorius, laterally.
    - the medial aspect of adductor longus, medially.
    - iliopsoas, adductor longus and pectineus muscles form the floor.
    - the fascia lata and cribriform fascia form the roof.

   The femoral triangle contains, from lateral to medial, the femoral nerve, femoral artery, and the femoral vein. Medial to the femoral vein is the femoral canal. The femoral artery, femoral vein, and the femoral canal are enclosed within the femoral sheath. This sheath is derived from the transversalis fascia anteriorly, and from the iliopsoas fascia posteriorly.

   The femoral nerve is not enclosed by the femoral sheath because it lies outside the fascia, which forms the sheath. The femoral artery has a profunda femoris branch that arises at the apex of triangle, which then passes behind the adductor longus muscle. At the apex of the triangle, the femoral vessels pass into the adductor canal.

The femoral canal is bounded superiorly by the femoral ring. This is formed by the inguinal ligament, femoral vein, pectinate line and lacunar ligament. The canal contains loose connective tissue and lymphatics including a deep node. Because the canal is medial to the femoral vein it provides a dead space into which the vein can expand in increased venous return from the lower limb.

A femoral hernia is a condition in which an abdomen visceral content, e.g. usually intestine, enters the femoral canal through the femoral ring. It is more common in women because the femoral ring is larger.

16. Venous drainage of the lower limb can be divided into superficial and deep. These are connected to each other by perforator veins.

   The deep veins of the lower limb are known as venae comitantes. They accompany the arteries and thus have the same name as the artery, e.g. popliteal vein and artery.

   The superficial veins of the lower limb originate from the dorsal venous arch of the foot, which receives venous blood from the digits. The medial part of the arch drains into the great saphenous vein and the lateral part of the arch drains into the small saphenous vein. The small saphenous vein passes posterior to the lateral malleolus, running posteriorly and superiorly to pierce the deep fascia of the popliteal fossa to join the popliteal vein. Along its length, it communicates with the deep veins through perforator veins and drains the lateral part of the leg. The great saphenous vein receives venous blood from the medial part of the arch. It passes anterior to the medial malleolus before passing superiorly and medially. It curves posteriorly around the knee and then anteromedially in the thigh. The great saphenous vein passes through a defect in the fascia lata (deep fascia of the thigh) known as the saphenous opening, which is covered over by the cribriform fascia. The great saphenous vein joins the femoral vein; however, before this it receives tributaries, which drain the abdominal wall, external genitalia and thigh. These include the superficial epigastric, superficial circumflex iliac, superficial and deep external pudendal, anteromedial and posterolateral veins of the thigh.

   Varicose veins are due to incompetent valves within the perforating veins, with blood no longer passing from superficial to deep veins. The superficial veins become tortuous and dilated because blood can now flow from deep to superficial veins. If valve incompetence is at sapheno-femoral junction, it is known as a saphena varix.

17. See Fig. 7.73
   B – A lateral rotation of the vocal cords, producing a diamond-shaped rima glottidis is produced by the posterior cricoarytenoid muscle.
   C – Lateral cricothyroid produces a medial rotation of the arytenoids, opposing the movement by posterior cricoarytenoid.

D – Both the transverse and oblique arytenoid muscles adduct the vocal folds by drawing the two arytenoid cartilages together in a gliding motion.

The thyroarytenoid muscles shorten the vocal cords by tipping the cricoid (and thus arytenoid) cartilages downwards.

E – The cricothyroid muscle rotates the cricoid (and thus arytenoid) cartilages downwards, lengthening the vocal folds.

All the above muscles are innervated by the recurrent laryngeal nerve, except the cricothyroid muscle – this is innervated by the external laryngeal nerve.

---

18. Each of the parasympathetic ganglia in the head has three roots: a preganglionic parasympathetic root, which synapses in the ganglion, postganglionic sympathetic fibres, which are vasoconstrictor, and sensory fibres from one of the divisions of the trigeminal nerve.

The ciliary ganglion lies within the orbit. It receives preganglionic parasympathetic fibres from the inferior division of the occulomotor (III) nerve, sensory fibres from the nasociliary nerve (a division of the ophthalmic nerve V1) and postganglionic sympathetic fibres from the carotid plexus. It sends postganglionic parasympathetic fibres to the smooth muscle of constrictor pupillae, sensory fibres and vasomotor sympathetic fibres to the eyeball via short ciliary nerves. The long ciliary nerves are branches of the nasociliary nerve which carry sympathetic fibres to the dilator pupillae muscles of the eye.

The pterygopalatine ganglion lies within the pterygopalatine fossa, suspended from the maxillary nerve (V_2) which supplies it with sensory fibres. Preganglionic parasympathetic fibres are given off from the facial nerve (VII – nervus intermedius root) to form the greater petrosal nerve within the temporal bone. The greater petrosal nerve runs on the floor of the middle cranial fossa and joins with the deep petrosal nerve consisting of postganglionic sympathetic nerves from the carotid plexus. Together, these form the nerve of the pterygoid canal, which passes forward through the pterygoid canal into the pterygopalatine fossa. The ganglion gives branches to the lacrimal gland (parasympathetic secretomotor fibres via the zygomatic then lacrimal nerves) and also to glands in the nose, nasopharynx and palate via branches of the maxillary nerve. Because its branches supply the glands involved in an attack of hay fever, it is sometimes called the ganglion of hay fever.

The otic ganglion lies in the infratemporal fossa, just below the foramen ovale. Preganglionic parasympathetic fibres arise from the tympanic branch of the glossopharyngeal nerve (IX) – forming the tympanic plexus within the ear and subsequently as the lesser petrosal nerve it passes through a tiny foramen in the skull to the otic ganglion. Postganglionic sympathetic fibres are carried on blood vessel plexuses to the ganglion and it receives sensory fibres from the auriculotemporal nerve (V_3). Branches pass from the ganglion via the auriculotemporal nerve to give a secretomotor supply to the parotid gland.

The submandibular ganglion lies in the intramuscular cleft between mylohyoid muscle and the muscles of the tongue. Preganglionic parasympathetic fibres arise from the facial nerve (VII) nervus intermedius root, to form the chorda tympani nerve within the inner ear. This passes through the skull and into the infratemporal fossa, where it joins the lingual nerve (a branch of the mandibular nerve V_3). This passes down into the oral cavity and gives branches to the submandibular ganglion – the lingual nerve also providing sensory nerve fibres. Postganglionic sympathetic nerves are carried on the facial artery. Branches from the ganglion pass to the submandibular and sublingual glands via branches of the lingual nerve.

---

19. The thyroid gland is an endocrine organ that regulates rate of metabolism. The gland consists of two lateral lobes that are connected together by an isthmus. The isthmus lies in front of, and adheres to, the second to fourth tracheal cartilaginous rings. A small glandular projection often arises from the isthmus. This pyramidal lobe is to the left of the midline, and it is attached to the hyoid bone. It represents the development of the glandular tissue from the caudal end of the thyroglossal duct. The thyroid gland is enclosed within its own capsule and within the pretracheal fascia of the deep cervical fascia of the neck.

The blood supply arises from the superior and inferior thyroid arteries. The superior thyroid artery arises from the anterior aspect of the external carotid artery and enters the upper pole of the lateral lobe. With the superior thyroid artery runs the external laryngeal nerve, which supplies the cricothyroid muscle. The inferior thyroid artery arises from the thyrocervical trunk of the second part of the subclavian artery. The inferior thyroid artery enters the lower pole of the lateral lobe. The recurrent laryngeal nerve runs with the inferior thyroid artery and the nerve supplies all the intrinsic laryngeal muscles (except cricothyroid) and the mucosa below the vocal cords. These two thyroid arteries anastomose with each other on the posterior surface and supply the parathyroid glands that lie embedded in the thyroid tissue. The venous return consists of three pairs of veins, which are the superior, middle, and inferior thyroid veins. The superior and middle thyroid veins join the internal jugular vein, and the inferior thyroid veins join together and empty into the left brachiocephalic vein. In 3% of individuals a thyroid ima artery enters the isthmus after arising from either the brachiocephalic trunk or aortic arch.

The relationship of the thyroid arteries to laryngeal nerves is important to surgeons performing a complete or partial removal of the thyroid gland because the arteries need to be ligated. If the laryngeal nerves are damaged, the voice becomes weak and hoarse because the intrinsic muscles are paralysed.

---

20. There are three meningeal layers: pia, arachnoid and dura.

The dura is the outermost membrane, separated from vertebral periosteum by the extradural space.

The arachnoid is loosely adherent to the inner surface of the dura, a potential (subdural) space existing between the two. The space between the arachnoid and pia is filled with cerebrospinal fluid and is referred to as the subarachnoid space. In an adult, the spinal cord terminates at the level of L2 the most inferior part is known as the conus medullaris. The arachnoid and dura continue beyond the conus medullaris to S2 vertebral level, leaving a large CSF-filled space containing the remaining nerve roots (cauda equina) which is known as the lumbar cistern.

In a lumbar puncture, a needle is passed in between vertebrae and into this space (usually at the level of L4, marked by a line in between iliac crests), so a sample of CSF may be obtained without danger of damaging the spinal cord.

The pia is a thin membrane that closely adheres to the spinal cord and roots of the spinal nerves. It projects laterally as denticulate ligaments, attaching to the inner surface of the dural sac and it continues inferiorly below the conus meduallaris as the filum terminale, which attaches to the coccyx.

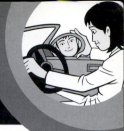

1.

1. D Parasympathetic nerves. Arise from the cranial and sacral portions of the central nervous system.

2. B Cranial nerves. There are 12 pairs of these nerves that supply the sense organs, muscles and skin of the head and neck.

3. A Central nervous system. Consists of aggregated nerve cell bodies (nuclei) and fibres that run together in tracts.

4. C Motor nerves. These innervate muscle cells via a synapse, which forms a motor end plate.

5. H Sympathetic nerves. These fibres synapse in a sympathetic ganglion and then enter a spinal nerve or innervate an organ.

2.

1. F Radial nerve. It runs in the spiral (radial) groove of the humerus. Damage at this level causes loss of function in the forearm extensors. The triceps brachii muscle is unaffected as its branches arise more proximally.

2. D Long thoracic nerve. Arises from the brachial plexus roots C5–C7. It crosses the lateral chest wall and supplies the serratus anterior muscle. This muscle rotates the scapula, allowing the arm to be raised above the head.

3. B Common peroneal nerve. It winds around the neck of the fibula and passes beneath the peroneus longus muscle to divide into superficial and deep branches supplying the lateral and anterior leg compartments respectively. Damage causes loss of foot dorsiflexors. To compensate, the patient develops a high-stepping gait to prevent the foot hitting the floor while the foot swings forward during walking.

4. A Axillary nerve. It has a branch (upper lateral cutaneous branch) that supplies the skin of the lateral aspect of arm over the deltoid.

5. E Median nerve. This supplies the skin over the thenar eminence and the palmar surface of the lateral three and a half digits. Damage causes loss of sensation in this area as well as loss of abduction and opposition of thumb due to thenar eminence paralysis. Flexor pollicis longus still allows flexion.

3.

1. I Scaphoid. This carpal bone is situated at the base of the anatomical snuffbox. Its blood supply enters distally; thus, a fracture in its middle (waist of scaphoid) can disrupt its blood supply causing necrosis of its proximal part.

2. F Medial femoral condyle. (See Chapter 6)

3. H Neck of femur. The axis of rotation runs through the femoral head and medial condyle. A fracture of this structure causes the axis to lie in along the shaft of femur and the pull of iliopsoas becomes a lateral rotator.

4. A Adductor tubercle. (See Chapter 6)

5. G Medial epicondyle. The ulnar nerve supplies the structures mentioned in the paragraph. It winds around the posterior aspect of the medial epicondyle to enter the forearm between the two heads of flexor carpi ulnaris.

4.

1. H Superior vena cava. See Chapter 3 for explanation.

2. A Angle of Louis. See Chapter 3 for explanation.

3. B Azygos vein. See Chapter 3 for explanation.

4. J Ventricular apex (Apex of heart). See Chapter 3 for explanation.

5. C Brachiocephalic trunk. See Chapter 3 for explanation.

5.

1. H Right atrium. Blurring or loss of the right atrium border on X-ray suggests middle lobe pathology in the right lung, e.g. pneumonia.

2. A Atrioventricular (coronary) groove. It is a superficial feature demarcating atria from ventricles.

3. J Sinoatrial node. Its inherent rhythmicity causes the heart to beat 70 times a minute.

4. F Left atrioventricular bundle branch. It conducts electrical impulses to the left side of the heart via an anterior and a posterior branch.

5. C Chordae tendineae. They are composed of collagen and hold the atrioventricular valves closed during ventricular contraction.

6.

1. A   The middle meningeal artery lies just behind this region of the skull and may be damaged in a fracture.

2. C   As the name implies, via bleeding into the subarachnoid space.

3. G   Blood fills the potential space between the two.

4. J   Subdural haemorrhage may be caused by vessels involved with dural venous sinuses.

5. H   This gives rise to a 'danger area of the face' centred on the nose.

7.

1. B   Arises from the dorsal surface of the midbrain.

2. A   Sympathetic fibres carried by this nerve innervate levator palpebrae superioris.

3. G   Sympathetic control causes pupil dilation (imagine a wide-eyed shocked person).

4. J   Due to paralysis of lateral rectus muscle.

5. C   Tested in a corneal blink test, along with the facial nerve.

8.

1. B   Indirect hernias are common in young children.

2. G   Or inside the inguinal triangle.

3. F   Sometimes within a persistent processus vaginalis.

4. J   An indirect inguinal hernia enters via the deep inguinal ring.

5. I   It may lie within a persistent processus vaginalis.

9.

1. A   They pierce the diaphragm to synapse in the coeliac ganglion.

2. G   The sympathetic trunks do not give branches to abdominal viscera.

3. D   If these nerves are impaired, continence problems and impotence can result.

4. F   Distally the hindgut is supplied by pelvic splanchnic nerves.

5. J   This then gives origin to several subsidiary plexuses, innervating pelvic viscera.

10.

1. A   It commences at the level of L4 in children.

2. C   Level with the highest points of the iliac crests.

3. J   Composed of lumbar and sacral nerve roots.

4. H   It contains fat, connective tissue and the internal vertebral venous plexus.

5. E   CSF is taken from the subarachnoid space.

Index